The Obesity Epidemic

What caused it?

How can we stop it?

First published in Hardback by Columbus Publishing Ltd 2010
Paperback Published by Columbus Publishing Ltd 2015

ISBN 978-1-907797-47-7
Rev:20150615

www.zoeharcombe.com
www.theobesityepidemic.org

Cover design by Lewis Kokoc

A catalogue record for this book is available from the British Library.

Brand and product names are trademarks or registered trademarks of their respective owners.

Disclaimer:
The content of this book is intended to inform, entertain and provoke your thinking. This is not intended as medical advice. It may, however, make you question current medical and nutritional advice. That's your choice. It's your life and health in your hands. Neither the author nor the publisher can be held responsible or liable for any loss or claim arising from the use, or misuse, of the content of this book.

COLUMBUS PUBLISHING

The Obesity Epidemic

"If we have been eating real food for 24 hours, agriculture gave us large scale access to carbohydrates four minutes ago and sugar consumption has increased twenty fold in the past five seconds. I wonder which food is more likely to be responsible for the obesity epidemic or any modern disease..."

Zoë Harcombe

The Obesity Epidemic

Review comments

"The Obesity Epidemic is an absolutely brilliant masterpiece in the art of demolition of myth and wishful thinking-based dietary dogma. I have never seen a better dissection of the unmitigated disaster that is called 'healthy eating'. It should be required reading not only in schools and universities that purport to teach nutrition and dietetics, but also in law libraries for the convenience of those victims of the system who will wish to sue the authorities who have caused them so much ill-health and misery by promoting such unhealthy practices because of their ignorance and arrogance."

Barry Groves, Author "Trick and Treat: how 'healthy eating' is making us ill."

"In The Obesity Epidemic Zoë Harcombe blows the lid off much of our current thinking about food, and uses her knowledge and commitment to pack a mighty punch in her analysis of standard food beliefs. For those of us bombarded by the weight loss message of 'eat less - do more' this book is an opportunity to espouse a different mantra: read more – learn more. Then do it all differently."

Julie Hurst, Director of the Work Life Balance Centre.

"This is not an easy read but its message is simple and terrifying – that everything we think we know about eating right and how to control our weight is, in fact, wrong. Clearly, patiently and with detailed references to support her every argument, Zoë Harcombe explains how today's obesity epidemic has come about – and the colossal shift in our thinking that will have to take place before we can beat it."

Alice Hart-Davis, Award-winning beauty and health writer.

"The truth and nothing but the truth! Zoë is a voice of well-researched reason amongst the sea of nonsense that is regularly spouted about why so many people are overweight or obese. It's obvious that current tactics are not working and that dramatic changes need to be made. This book should be mandatory reading for all health professionals and for anyone who needs to lose weight!"

Julia Smurthwaite, Freelance health writer.

"In her new and controversial book, Zoë Harcombe moves her Holmesian lens to an examination of the underlying causes of the current obesity epidemic. Clue by clue, and drawing on a breath-taking range of scientific disciplines including biochemistry, physiology, archaeology, statistics, nutrition and physics, she carefully deconstructs the misleading 'expert' opinions that have guided our eating habits since the late seventies and early eighties. This rigorous analysis is leavened with a fresh and accessible prose style and a crusading passion for her subject.

"The book describes her odyssey to track down and confront researchers, agency officials, food company representatives, (and even the first lady of the USA), in an effort to investigate the scientific basis behind those opinions and the programs formulated around them. That basis is found to be woefully lacking in almost all cases, and compromised by clear conflicts of interest in others. (The bumbling and inadequate responses of various officials to her letters of inquiry was one of the shocks of the book.) By the time she is done it is clear: citizens, patients, and consumers, have been systematically misled by governments, medical researchers, and corporations. The vast majority of nutritional advice offered to us is not substantiated or sound, and far from being the cure for the current obesity epidemic, it is actually the major cause."

Phil Read, M.A. (Cantab), M.Sc., Author "Games at Work."

"In a series of rigorously sourced chapters Harcombe pulls apart many of the key tenets in the diet and nutrition industry. The science behind them is found to be contradictory and often based on repeated mantras with little idea about where they originated.

"Harcombe painstakingly dissects obvious statements such as people are fat because they eat too much and exercise too little and demonstrates they are based on a mixture of prejudice, myth and bad science.

"There have been a number of books in recent years looking at the politics of food production and consumption. Harcombe's is a welcome addition which adds new insight and evidence."

Phil Chamberlain, Freelance journalist.

"Zoë Harcombe belongs to that growing band of writers who succeed in making science interesting as well as relevant. Zoë uses pertinent data and insightful analysis along with humour to show that we have cast aside the most nutritious and natural foods to replace them with the less nutritious. Most importantly, she shows how our need for nutrition has been exploited by food manufacturers with official complaisance. The book's message is to urge a return to the natural and normal: the consumption of real food as provided by nature and not the processed products of the food industry. It is a message that we would be wise to heed and act upon."

Dr Trefor Lewis, Designer and author "Intentional Neuroplasticity: the Brain Changing Programme."

"Zoë Harcombe unravels one of the biggest paradoxes of today: why levels of obesity are rising despite the fact our supermarkets are producing more products designed to help people lose weight and boost their health. Harcombe overturns long held myths about weight gain – and shows how processed foods are at the heart of the problem. Unless the food industry takes responsibility for this, the future health costs will become unsustainable; no matter how efficient our system."

Lucy Johnston, Health Editor, Sunday Express.

"Zoë Harcombe understands that the promotion of a natural diet, which works with the body rather than against it, is essential but not sufficient to beat today's obesity epidemic: it is also necessary to destroy the calorie and exercise theory which, backed by governments and the food industry, created the epidemic in the first place. The Obesity Epidemic does that, comprehensively and definitively."

David Lewis, Editor of Diaeta.

"Zoë Harcombe has taken a surgeon's scalpel to the Alice In Wonderland World of obesity. For years we have been told that the answer to obesity is to eat less and exercise more. Advice that is based on no evidence whatsoever. This advice works on the strange assumption that the body is like some man-made machine. You eat more, and the body then stores it as excess weight. You exercise more, and this energy is lost, along with the weight.

"Whilst this is, partly true, it represents what I call concrete thinking, or maybe idiot thinking. The possibility that the body is capable of adapting, reacting, hoarding energy stores when starved, and shedding excess weight, is dismissed by people who honestly believe that they are using science to support their simplistic energy in − energy out argument. Zoë exposes this argument as the facile and ridiculous nonsense that it truly is. She also supports what she has to say with clear and inarguable evidence.

"By the end of this book I had been convinced, where I have never been before, that switching from a high fat to a high carbohydrate diet is the single greatest cause of the recent obesity epidemic. Ironically, carbs are the very foodstuffs that we have been instructed to eat by the new army of obesity 'experts.'

"This book is not a simple, quick, easy read. However, if by the end of it, you have not changed the way you think about food and obesity - forever - you have clearly not understood what you have just read."

Dr Malcolm Kendrick, Author "The Great Cholesterol Con."

The Obesity Epidemic

What caused it?

How can we stop it?

Thank You...

To all the pioneers who are leading the way in this vitally important field of diet and nutrition (alphabetically): Natasha Campbell-McBride; Sean Croxton (a.k.a. Underground Wellness); Sally Fallon Morell; Barry Groves; Malcolm Kendrick; Uffe Ravnskov; Gary Taubes and many more. Who would have thought "eat real food" to be such a controversial message? Your determination to find and communicate the truth is an inspiration to others. I am particularly indebted to Gary Taubes. I would not have found the Tanner or Taggart quotations without your brilliant *The Diet Delusion*. I am immensely grateful for your ground breaking research.

To all the academics who so generously and helpfully make their work available to researchers. Especially to Colleen Rand who helped me locate the original work for the opening to this book.

To all the fans and followers of The Harcombe Diet – one of the biggest *eat real food* studies taking place in the UK and spreading.

To Justin Stoneman, for believing in the cause and for using his journalistic skills to challenge the thinking of the media.

To Simon Mansfield, Sarah Broughton and Sarah Howells at Modern TV for realising what is at stake so quickly and so well. We are ready to present all the themes in this book with any channel.

To Matthew Gough and James Shawe from Eversheds for publishing and copyright advice.

To Pan Macmillan, London, for permission to use the quotation from one of my favourite books – Helen Fielding's *The Diary of Bridget Jones* (1996) – for the opening to Part Two of this book.[i]

To Elsevier, for permission to use the illustration in Chapter Seven, from the *Journal of the American Dietetic Association* (October 2007).

To Dr. Roger and Dr. Lorna Finlay at Barlow Moor Books, for helping me find the books and journals that no one else can.

Last and always most, to Andy and Roxy – many of the ideas in this book were seeded on our numerous dog walks. Thank you Andy especially, for being my partner in every sense of the word and for being an unquestionable example that man descended from the ape!

---

[i] Other quotations are deemed to be covered by Section 30 of the Copyright Designs and Patents Act 1988, as they are for the purpose of criticism or review, are publicly available and have been fully referenced.

Contents

The Obesity Epidemic

What caused it?

How can we stop it?

"The previous nutritional advice in the UK to limit the intake of all carbohydrates as a means of weight control now runs counter to current thinking and contrary to the present proposals for a nutrition education policy for the population as a whole... The problem then becomes one of achieving both a reduction in fat intake to 30% of total energy and a fall in saturated fatty acid intake to 10%."

Proposals for nutritional guidelines for Health Education in Britain (1983)

And so started the obesity epidemic...

Introduction

The Obesity Epidemic

In a study of formerly obese people, researchers at the University of Florida found that virtually all said that they would rather be blind, deaf or have a leg amputated than be obese again.[1] That is the extent of our desire to be slim and yet two thirds of people in the UK, USA and Australia are overweight and one quarter obese.[ii] Why?

To be slim, to achieve the thing we want more than our sight, hearing, or mobility, we are told that we just need to "eat less and/or do more." Quite specifically, the advice is "One pound of fat contains 3,500 calories, so to lose 1lb a week you need a deficit of 500 calories a day."[2]

So, why don't we just follow the advice? Why on earth do we have an obesity problem, let alone an epidemic, when we so desperately want to be slim?

I set out to answer that question in the late 1980's and this book is the culmination of that quest. At the time of starting my research, obesity levels for men and women in the UK had reached double figures. The World Health Organisation published BMI statistics for the UK for five comparator years: 1966; 1972; 1982; 1989 and 1999 (presented in the tables below).[3] The UK health service was devolved in 1999, with England, Scotland, Wales and Northern Ireland managed separately from this point forth, thus losing the opportunity for UK data beyond the turn of the Millennium.

Table 1: Percentage of men in each BMI category (UK):

Men (%) [iii]	1966	1972	1982	1989	1999
BMI < 18.5	2.3	1.9	1.3	0.6	0.3
BMI 18.5-24.9	83.7	72.6	54.7	44.0	27.9
BMI 25.0-29.9	12.8	23.0	37.8	44.7	49.2
BMI > 30	1.2	2.7	6.2	10.6	22.6

[ii] Overweight is defined by a body mass Index (BMI) of over 25 and obese as a BMI of over 30.
[iii] Totals for men in 1972 and 1989, and for women in 1966 and 1989, deviate slightly from 100% due to rounding.

2

Table 2: Percentage of women in each BMI category (UK):

Women (%)	1966	1972	1982	1989	1999
BMI < 18.5	7.8	5.4	3.7	1.6	0.3
BMI 18.5-24.9	81.1	78.0	70.4	58.5	37.6
BMI 25.0-29.9	9.2	13.9	19.0	25.8	36.3
BMI > 30	1.8	2.7	6.9	14.0	25.8

We can make a number of observations about this data, but there is only one key point to note. UK obesity levels were remarkably constant and small for decades. Indeed, throughout the tens of thousands of years before the 1966 data, there is no record of an obesity problem, let alone an epidemic. Suddenly, in evolutionary terms, and dramatically, in amounts, obesity levels increased from 2-3% in the 1970's to 25% today. Two thirds of UK citizens are now overweight or obese.

The USA started from a slightly higher base and displayed a virtually identical trend, with 70% of Americans currently overweight or obese:

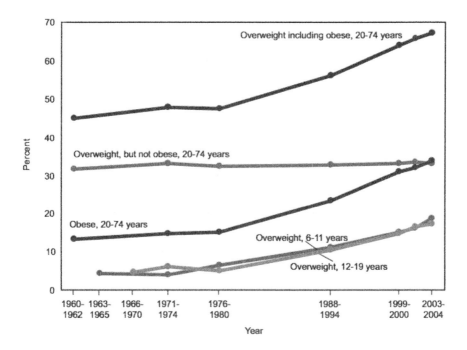

Figure 1: Overweight and obesity, by age: United States, 1960-2004.[4]

It seems so obvious that the starting point for understanding the obesity epidemic should be – what changed in the late 1970's/early 1980's? Was there one thing that happened that could explain the sudden and dramatic increase in obesity?

Yes there was. In 1977 the USA changed its public health diet advice. In 1983 the UK followed suit. A more accurate description would be that we did a complete U-turn in our diet advice from "Farinaceous and vegetable foods are fattening, and saccharine matters are especially so"[5] to "base your meals on starchy foods". Obesity has increased up to ten fold since – coincidence or cause?

There are so many more questions that we need to ask (and answer) to understand the worst health crisis that we have ever faced:

1) Have you heard the sayings "energy in equals energy out" and "you can't change the laws of physics"? What precisely do the laws of thermodynamics say? Which law have we oversimplified and which law have we neglected to consider?

2) Are you familiar with the formula "one pound equals 3,500 calories, so to lose one pound of fat, you need to create a deficit of 3,500 calories"? When and where did this originate? Would you be able to prove that the formula holds true? Would you be interested to know the responses given by seven UK government and obesity organisations when asked those same questions?

3) Is a calorie a calorie? Is one sugar the same as any other?

4) What happens if we manage to get humans to eat less and/or do more over a period of six months? What happens afterwards? What is the scientific evidence for sustained weight loss in the seminal obesity studies from the past 100 years?

5) Are obese people greedy, or lazy, or both, or none of these? Can obesity be caused by anything other than greed or sloth?

6) Where does five-a-day come from? What are the five most nutritious foods on the planet?

7) Why is fructose being called the lipogenic (fattening) carbohydrate?

8) Would you be able to prove that saturated fat consumption causes heart disease? If I told you that the study to consider this has not even been done, would you believe me? If the UK Food Standards Agency said this, would you believe them?

9) What remains if you take the public health list of 'saturated fat' and cross out processed food (primarily carbohydrates)? Would you be open to the idea that we could have a heated agreement with a clarification of terminology?

10) Where does cholesterol fit in to the obesity debate?

11) What is human fat tissue? How do we (biochemically) store fat? How do we burn fat? Which macronutrient[iv] determines fat storage and fat utilisation?
12) Does sedentary behaviour explain the timing and the increase in obesity? Can exercise be a cure for the obesity epidemic?
13) How embedded are the food and drink industry in our dietary advice and agencies? Would you be concerned if the likes of Coca-Cola, Kellogg's and the sugar industry were working in partnership with our national dietary associations?

This epidemic has become far too serious for us to continue with tautologies (a calorie is a calorie), or platitudes (eat less/do more), or marketing slogans (five-a-day). It is time for some facts.

I will keep everything as simple as possible, but, as Albert Einstein so rightly advised "It can scarcely be denied that the supreme goal of all theory is to make the irreducible basic elements as simple and as few as possible without having to surrender the adequate representation of a single datum of experience."[6] I.e. make things as simple as possible, but not simpler. We have made some serious simplifications thus far and we must make no more.

This book will examine some of the classic literature in some detail: The Seven Countries Study; the Minnesota Starvation experiment; Newburgh and Johnston; Kekwick and Pawan; Stunkard and McLaren-Hume; systematic reviews of the efficacy of different weight loss methods and other evidence relied upon by our public health advisors today. Some studies have shaped our current advice and shouldn't have and some have been overlooked and shouldn't have been. We need to know what stands up to scrutiny, what can explain the obesity epidemic and what, therefore, can stop it. This book is fully referenced and evidence based. If I proffer an opinion, I make it clear that I am doing so by saying "I believe" or "I think". I invite you to come to your own conclusions along the way.

This book will take you on the journey that I have been through, as an obesity researcher, from thermodynamics and peanuts under Bunsen burners to obesity organisations sponsored by food manufacturers and carbohydrates being confused with fats. Out of an illogical assumption that people have made themselves obese (when this is the last thing that they want to be), through being greedy and lazy, may come a different logical conclusion that our current diet advice a) doesn't work and b) worse – that it is actually the cause of the obesity epidemic that it is supposed to cure.

The final part of this book looks at what needs to happen to reverse the obesity epidemic. This can be achieved, but crises require major interventions, not the same things done in different ways. One definition of madness is doing the same thing again and again and expecting a different result. Revolutionary change will not be achieved with the UK Change4Life campaign, for example, advising people to have a banana instead of a bag of crisps. Swapping one starch

---

[iv] Macronutrient(s) is the collective term for carbohydrate, fat and protein.

for another is going to make no difference to the obesity epidemic. Some of the proposals may appear extreme, but, if they do, how does "90% of today's children being overweight or obese by 2050" sound?[7]

There is so much conflicting information about diet and nutrition, and the public is rightly confused and mistrustful of current advice. The same conflict can arise for a researcher, so I have established two fundamental principles, to which I return for grounding every time I find myself questioning issues.

1) I believe that nature knows how to feed humans better than food manufacturers. Nature has no vested interest, no profit to be made from us and no reason to provide us with anything other than nutritious food. I therefore believe that the human race must return to eating food in the form closest to that provided by nature: meat, eggs and dairy from naturally reared animals; fish; vegetables and salads; nuts and seeds; fruits and whole grains. I call this *real food*.

2) I believe that the job description of the human body is to keep itself alive. I therefore believe that, in normal circumstances, the human body will *not* do anything that is intended to kill us.

I have a one in four chance that you, the reader, are obese. I have a two in three chance that you are overweight. Given your interest in the subject matter, I have a virtual certainty that you know and/or work with overweight people. If I can prove to you that eat less/do more has never worked and will never work – are you prepared to consider an alternative that will? For yourself or for your patients or for our children facing a fat future?

All I ask is that you read this book with the most open mind possible. My experience of calories started at the age of 15 and I believe nothing now that I believed then. When I started studying nutrition professionally, I was a vegetarian. Within weeks of learning about food and nutrients, I started eating fish. When I started the manuscript for this book I was still a non-meat eater, believing that I could be optimally healthy without meat and that animals could concomitantly be better for this. After 20 years of abstinence, I now eat red meat until, or should I say when, the cows come home. That is how much my own thinking has changed as a result of the research I have undertaken. Please be open minded to your own views changing even a fraction of this, rather than have the following apply to you:

"My mind is made up; don't confuse me with the facts." (Anon)

Thank you

Zoë Harcombe

Part One

The General Principle

Part One

The General Principle

Eat less, do more

In 2002, the British politician, Ann Widdecombe, took part in a television show called *Celebrity Fit Club*. It was a follow up programme to *Fat Club*, which featured ordinary people, weighing up to 30 stone, prepared to be photographed in swimsuits in a desperate bid to have access to people who, they believed, could help them to lose weight. At the end of her experience, Widdecombe said that if she ever wrote a diet book it would be just two pages long. Page one would say "eat less" and page two would say "do more."

It is an almost universally held belief that the only way to lose weight is to eat less and/or do more. Check any newspaper diet article posted on line and look at the comments on the message boards at the end of the article. Here are some of my favourites from just one site following the Dr. Geoffrey Livesey article (21 July 2009) about the calorie content of fat and carbohydrate being wrong:

- "Eat less, move more. The four word diet that can't fail." Youpushedtoohard, USA;
- "Its (sic) not hard really is it. Eat less, move more." Sue, London;
- "If you eat and drink too much and do no exercise you will put on weight. If you eat and drink less and exercise you will lose weight and then stay slim. End of Story." Carol, Germany.[8]

I saw a categorical comment at the end of an article on the role played by genetics in weight. Surely any sensible person would agree that genetics play a part in weight – the only debate can be how big a part. There would be no animal husbandry if genetics were not passed on. Two 'column-like' parents are highly unlikely to have short, stocky, off-spring. We can inherit: skin, hair, eye colour; intelligence and psychological characteristics; health and serious illnesses; height, hand and foot size. It would be absurd to suggest that there is no way whatsoever that shape or frame size can be passed on. And, yet, Ellen in Dorset wrote at the end of "Size 8 jeans; size 12 genes: are some people naturally disposed to be bigger?" (*Mail on Sunday*, 14 February 2010):

- "It's about how much you put in your mouth and how much you move around and that's it... nothing more, nothing less – no excuses!!"

The UK *Daily Mail* ran yet another new diet on 6 April 2010 eliciting the following responses:

- "Less calories (sic) + More exercise = Lean body". Paul Swan, Manchester;
- "Just eat less and move more, that is the way to loose (sic) weight but it would be a very short book !!" Heardit Allnow, Somewhere Insane;
- "Two ways to lose the tyre that work and costs nothing. Eat less and exercise more ...simples (sic)." Rodney, swiss cottage.[9]

Pick any diet story, in any country, on any day of the week and the comments will be dominated by people arrogantly asserting "which bit of 'eat less/do more' do fat people not understand?" Why have these confident 'experts' never thought to question the basis of the belief that we need to eat less/do more?

I got quite excited when I started reading Anne Diamond's *Winning the Fat War* and, on p13, she said "I am so fed up with self-righteous men and women telling me that 'losing weight isn't rocket science, you know. All you have to do is eat less and exercise more.' Because that sort of advice has landed us with an obesity epidemic."[10]

At last, I thought, we have an intelligent, high profile person challenging 'energy in equals energy out'. My excitement was premature as, just two sentences later, Diamond continued, "It's not that it's incorrect advice. Of course it's right. We all know that energy in must equal energy out, but that is not helpful enough." She then went on to talk about sedentary lifestyles, the widespread availability of branded food, heavily advertised to make it seem desirable and, what looked like original thought, returned to the traditional view.

The laws of the universe

Columbia University physiologist John Taggart said in his opening remarks at an obesity conference in the 1950's, "We have implicit faith in the validity of the first law of thermodynamics. A calorie is a calorie. Calories in equal calories out and that's that."[11] Applied to humans, all three of Taggart's statements are incorrect.

The laws of the universe, also called the laws of physics, are collectively captured under the term thermodynamics. It is worth noting at the outset that the term thermodynamics derives from the Greek language and it literally means 'heat power' (thermo for heat and dynamic for power). It is the study of heat and the work needed in the conversion of heat to other forms of energy. This is worth remembering every time you see the laws of thermodynamics applied (incorrectly) to humans. The laws are about the transference of heat. At the most simplistic level, the laws say that, if we drop a hot stone into cold water, the stone will cool and the water will warm to achieve equilibrium in temperature.

There are four Laws of thermodynamics – the zeroth, first, second and third. The two we need to be aware of, in the obesity debate, are the first and second. Let us include the others for completeness:

The zeroth law was added after the other three. This states that "If object A is in thermal equilibrium with object B, and object B is in thermal equilibrium with object C, then object C is also in thermal equilibrium with object A."

The third law is "As a system approaches absolute zero, all processes cease and the entropy of the system approaches a minimum value."

To the best of my knowledge, the zeroth and third laws of the universe are not considered to have relevance to the weight loss debate. Interestingly, the zeroth law, combined with the second law, may suggest that we should eat cold food, so that the body expends energy warming the food to body temperature. However, we will not risk misapplying any more laws of the universe to the human body, so I will not go any further with that thought.

The two laws that we need to take into account when researching obesity are the first and the second. The belief that humans need to eat less and/or do more to lose weight is based on a fundamental misapplication of the laws of thermodynamics to the human body and to the world of dieting. There are three crucial errors that have been made:

1) The first law has been oversimplified: The concept of eat less/do more comes from a mistaken belief that energy in equals energy out. It follows that people are overweight because they have put too much energy in and/or expended too little energy out. (We will come back to how less energy in is supposed to lead to weight loss, rather than less energy out). However, there is no law of the universe that says energy in equals energy out. The first law, known as the conservation of energy law, states that in a closed system, in thermal equilibrium, "Energy can be neither created nor destroyed". (Robert Mayer 1841)[12] (Please note the implicit assumption that energy can be changed from one form to another). The implications of this over simplification are significant.

2) The second law has largely been ignored: The first law of thermodynamics, even when correctly interpreted, only applies to a closed system in thermal equilibrium. The first law, therefore, cannot be applied in isolation to the human body. In an open system, not in thermal equilibrium (i.e. a human), the second law must therefore also be applied. The second law, known as the law of entropy (from the Greek word "entrope", meaning change) states that "The increase in the energy of a closed system is equal to the amount of energy added to the system by heating, minus the amount lost in the form of work done by the system on its surroundings." Entropy takes into account *insensible* energy, as it is often referred to in early obesity journals – energy used up in making energy and energy unavailable or lost to the system in any way. The implications of ignoring energy lost and energy used in making available energy are also significant.

3) Our third error has been to assume a direction of causation. We have assumed that energy in ('too much') and/or energy out ('too little') causes overweight. Why don't we assume the converse? Why don't we assume overweight determines energy in (heavier people need more fuel) and energy out (heavier people find it more difficult to move). Thermodynamics does not say anything about causation. The laws of the universe do not say "we put a gallon of petrol in a car and caused it to move (say) 30 miles".

Thermodynamics is more likely to say the car was *able* to move 30 miles because we put in a gallon of petrol. The energy didn't cause the movement – it enabled it. We have assumed that energy in and/or out determine weight and have neglected to consider how weight may determine energy in and/or out. We actually position the direction of causation more plausibly when we insult people – we say "fat people are lazy", we don't say "lazy people are fat". The significance of this will also be explored.

All of the above three points are about pure thermodynamics and how we have misapplied the laws of the universe as they stand, to the human body. There is potentially an even greater error that we have made. With the first calorimeters, Max Rubner and Wilbur Atwater did rightly consider the first and second laws of thermodynamics together and they demonstrated that they held for a dog and a human respectively.[13] They demonstrated that energy was conserved, correctly accounting for energy lost and energy used up in making available energy.

However, these early studies were done on the basis that the required amount of energy (calories) was given to the dog and human. Rubner and Atwater did not study what happens if *insufficient* energy is given to a living creature. Francis Benedict is often credited as being the first person to do such an experiment, in 1917.[14] In this study and every subsequent study that has been performed, where an energy deficit has been created in a human, less energy in is more likely to result in less energy out than in the system using itself up (losing weight). This is not surprising. Notwithstanding the fact that the first law is about energy conservation, the logical corollary of energy in and energy out is that less energy in will equate to less energy out.

Although Benedict's study may have been the first proof of this, the Ancel Keys' 1945 Minnesota starvation experiment is the definitive study.[15] Albert Stunkard and Mavis McLaren-Hume summarised the consistent findings from the first half of the twentieth century, in their 1959 paper.[16] The Marion Franz et al study from 2007 confirms the Stunkard and McLaren-Hume, results.[17] All such studies prove that there is no direct relationship between calorie deficit and weight loss. This will be covered in detail.

When we no longer view excess weight as a simplistic outcome of energy in (overweight people eat too much) and/or energy out (overweight people are too sedentary), we can more usefully focus on what enables fat to be stored and what facilitates fat being utilised. We can then see that the very macronutrient, which we eat more of when we try to eat less (carbohydrate), is the macronutrient that enables fat to be stored and disables fat from being utilised, through the concomitant role of insulin. We come to see carbohydrates and not calories as the key determinant of weight gain and weight loss.

In my more challenging moments I do question the merits of applying the laws of the universe to the human body *per se*. They are not called the laws of the universe for nothing. The first law is invaluable in helping us understand things like the finite supply of energy in the world and the peak oil schedule. The second law ended the quest for perpetual motion and gave practical applications for the first law, not least the principle of the irreversibility of our energy consumption. Laws, as absolute principles, should help, not hinder, scientific research. At best I think that our obsession with calories (in and out) has constrained our approach to the obesity epidemic. At worst I think that it has made us miss the real issues (how we store vs. un-store human fat tissue). Either way, a century of calorie obsession later and we are in the midst of a crisis.

Let us proceed with the notion that the laws of thermodynamics have some use when applied to human beings, but with the strong caveat that although putting sufficient energy in to a system is one thing, putting *insufficient* energy in to a system is quite another. We must also proceed with extreme caution for every occasion when we observe a seamless interchange between energy and weight. The dieting world currently flits between energy and weight, but thermodynamics says nothing about *weight* being conserved. We will see that the assumed energy to weight conversion is incorrect at every level, starting with a taste of this in Chapter One. In this context, looking purely at the application of the laws of thermodynamics to the world of dieting, I can see three fundamental errors that we have made.

Chapter One

Energy balance vs. fat storage

The first law of thermodynamics

The first law of thermodynamics has been oversimplified to the slogan "energy in equals energy out". However, the first law does not say that energy in equals energy out. (And, if it did, surely the corollary would be less energy in equals less energy out?) The first law says that, in a closed system, in thermal equilibrium, the form of energy may change, but the total is always conserved.

Let us take a simple example – we can put a gallon of petrol into a petrol car and it will go, say, 30 miles. At this point we may be confident that energy in equals energy out. However, we can then put a gallon of diesel into the same car and it will go nowhere. Immediately we can no longer argue that energy in equals energy out. We can see that energy has been conserved – which is what the first law of thermodynamics says. We have not created or lost energy, but energy in does not equal energy out. Energy in equals energy out (none in this case), plus energy stored – this is crucial.

What if, for example, the vast numbers of empty calories, such as sugar, which we consume today in unprecedented quantities, are the nutritional equivalent of putting diesel into a petrol car? Citizens of the UK consume 1.6 pounds of sugar per week,[18] which translates into approximately 400 empty calories, per person, per day. Citizens of Australia consume an average 600 empty sugar calories per person per day.[19] Are we absolutely sure that the human body is designed to run on sugar, emulsifiers, yeast autolysate, high fructose corn syrup (also known as glucose-fructose syrup amongst other names), maltodextrin, hydrogenated fat, butylated hydroxyanisole (BHA), butylated hydrozyttoluene (BHT), dextrose, Acesulfame-K and many other common ingredients that we will find in processed foods consumed daily? I doubt that we will get any better performance out of a human, by putting the wrong fuel into the body, than we will by putting diesel into a petrol car. This is just a question to pose to you – my arguments to follow do not rely upon it.

Energy in and out is often simplified further to energy balance. I have used this term for the chapter title, to capture the extreme of one simplification on top of another, but I won't use it again. I apologise in advance if energy in and out become a bit repetitive, but we need to be precise in our language, to correct errors constantly being made. The term energy balance has many underlying assumptions at best and can be a tautology at worst.

Angela Tella, a spokesperson for the British Dietetic Association, was quoted in *The Sunday Times* as saying "... there are a few constants, such as the 'energy balance' equation, which means if you burn off more calories than you eat, you will lose weight. That will never change."[20] At one level this can be restated as if you burn fat, you lose fat, making it a tautology. At any other level, it can be shown to be wrong.

The first and second laws of thermodynamics together tell us that, in a closed system in thermal equilibrium, *energy* will be conserved, but that the human being is not a closed system in thermal equilibrium, so energy will be lost and energy will be used up in making available energy. Even if we ignore for now energy lost and energy used up in making available energy we are making sweeping assumptions about energy and weight which do not hold. The diet world currently assumes that the form in which energy goes in to the human body (calories) translates directly into weight at the conversion of four calories for a gram of carbohydrate or protein and nine calories for a gram of fat and that the conversion holds for weight out as well as weight in. It simply does not hold in this way, as we will prove for both a calorie deficit and a calorie surplus repeatedly throughout this book.

So that you can start to see this for yourself, let's have a bit of fun with numbers – the very numbers used by the calorie theorists. If you eat 1,000 calories of carbohydrate, at an approximate four calories per gram, you have eaten 250 grams in weight. If you burn more calories than this – let us say 1,008 calories of fat, at an approximate nine calories per gram, you have lost 112 grams in weight. Holding everything else equal, for the time it would take to measure this, you will have gained weight – 138 grams to be precise. Furthermore, (not least because Tella was not precise about weight vs. fat, or the order of events), if you burn off the 1,008 calories of fat first and then eat 1,000 calories of carbohydrate and don't burn this off, this can be stored as glycogen.[v] There is some debate as to how much water is stored with glycogen, but four parts water to one part glycogen is a common and long-standing conversion.[21] Our person who has just lost the 112 grams of fat is now holding 250 grams of glycogen and one kilogram of water. They have therefore gained over 11 times in weight, what they have just burned off in fat.

You would need to eat all 1,000 calories in the form of fat (111 grams) to register an immediate weight loss of one gram having burned 1,008 calories (112 grams) of fat. Even if you ate 1,000 calories in the form of 110 grams of fat (990 calories) and 2.5 grams of carbohydrate (10 calories), you would register an immediate gain of half a gram vs. 112 grams of fat lost. You can eat 444 carbohydrate calories *or* 1,000 fat calories for the same *weight* of food intake (111 grams). You can have a lot of fun with maths and "the energy balance equation", as defined above, will still not be "a constant".

I hope that this example alone illustrates how specific we need to be about energy in and out and not energy balance and, far more importantly, the precise form in which the energy goes in, because it makes a significant difference. As for weight, that's another factor entirely.

---

[v] Glycogen is the form in which the body stores glucose.

Correcting the oversimplification of energy balance to the correct principle of the conservation of energy has the following significant implication. Energy stored, not just energy in and energy out, becomes of critical importance. It seems so obvious that gaining weight is about fat stored and losing weight is about fat 'un-stored'. The simplification of energy in and energy out would be understandable if it had a perfect correlation with fat stored and un-stored, but it doesn't. Obesity then becomes a far more considered study of what facilitates fat (adipose tissue) storage and what debilitates fat utilisation. Similarly, losing weight then becomes the challenge of preventing fat storage and enabling fat utilisation.

Fat storage

There are two forms of fat in the human body: triglycerides and fatty acids.[vi] Human fat (adipose tissue) is stored as triglycerides. Fatty acids are burned for fuel. Triglycerides are three fatty acids bound together on a backbone of glycerol.[vii] Fat enters and exits fat cells as fatty acids (triglycerides are too big to move across the cell membrane).

When we talk about fat stored in human fat tissue, we are talking about triglycerides. Inside the fat cell, fatty acids continually 'cycle' across the cell membrane and back out again. Fatty acids can be used as fuel during this process (or recycled/stored if they are not used). If three fatty acids are bonded by glycerol to form a triglyceride, they can't get back out of the fat cell until the triglyceride is broken back down into glycerol and fatty acids (we will see how this happens under fat utilisation in the next section).

The critical role in this triglyceride, fatty acid, and fat storage process is, therefore, played by glycerol. Glycerol provides the backbone needed to bind three fatty acids into a triglyceride. It therefore determines the rate at which fatty acids become triglycerides within fat cells i.e. the rate at which humans store fat. If we make more glucose available to fat cells, more glycerol can be made. If more glycerol can be made, more fat is stored in the fat cells. Anything that works to transport more glucose into fat cells will lead to the conversion of more fatty acids into triglycerides and more storage of fat. The easiest and most effective way of achieving this fat storage environment is to eat carbohydrates. Carbohydrates are broken down into glucose by the body, causing blood glucose levels to rise and making glucose widely available to the body.

Essentially the body is in a carbohydrate/glucose/fat-storing environment or a carbohydrate-free/fatty acid/fat-burning environment. This is not new. In the 1920's we knew that fat was metabolically active and not an inert 'receptor'. In

---

[vi] Fatty acids are a somewhat 'sexed-up' term for fats, but they provide a useful distinction between fat generally and a single fat, so I use the term.

[vii] Glycerol is a sugar alcohol and it has many other names – glycerine, 1,2,3-trihydroxypropane etc. The 1,2,3 reference indicates that glycerol has three hydrogen/oxygen groups that can bond with the COOH group at the end of fats (we will learn more about fats in Chapter Twelve).

the 1930's, Rudolph Schoenheimer and David Rittenberg[22] demonstrated that fatty acids constantly 'cycle' in and out of fat cells, being bonded together as triglyceride and then broken back down into glycerol and fatty acid component parts with lipolysis.[viii] In 1948, Ernst Wertheimer and Benson Shapiro stated the following in their article "The physiology of adipose tissue": "Mobilisation and deposition of fat go on continuously, without regard to the nutritional state of the animal."[23] Declaring that "The 'classical theory' that fat is deposited in the adipose tissue only when given an excess of the caloric requirement has finally been disproved", they might be shocked to know that we still hold the 'disproved' belief 60 years later.

The rightful focus on energy storage and utilisation shifts the study of obesity internally into everything that happens in between energy in and energy out – most usefully towards the endocrine (hormone) system. Most routes then lead to the hormone insulin and consequently to carbohydrates, since only carbohydrate calories stimulate the production of insulin.[ix]

The primary role of insulin is to return the blood glucose level to within the normal range. In performing this role, insulin converts glucose from the carbohydrate eaten into glycogen, a starch stored in the muscles and liver for energy use. If all the glycogen storage areas are full, insulin will convert the excess to fatty tissue, which, at a simplistic level, is why insulin has been called the fattening hormone. Insulin is the primary facilitator of fat storage.

We need a quick review of diabetes to develop this concept. Rosalyn Yalow and Solomon Berson are credited with having taken Sir Harold Himsworth's distinction between what we now know as type 1 and type 2 diabetes,[24] and demonstrating that type 1 diabetes was an insulin-deficient state, whereas patients with type 2 diabetes had substantial amounts of insulin in the blood and could be classified as insulin resistant.[25] Type 1 diabetes can therefore be simplistically described as the type where the pancreas does not release insulin at all. In type 2 diabetes the pancreas is effectively releasing too much insulin and yet this still fails to regulate blood glucose levels normally, as cells have become resistant to insulin. This is a critical distinction and helps to explain why this Yalow and Berson study remains one of the most cited articles from the *Journal of Clinical Investigation*.

It follows that type 1 diabetes requires the administration of insulin and type 2 diabetes can be managed through medication to help optimise the insulin available and to help overcome insulin resistance. Both types of diabetes, I would argue, could be far better managed through diet, and I actually fail to see how type 2 diabetes can manifest itself in the absence of carbohydrate. Obesity in diabetics would be far less common if we adopted the low-carbohydrate

---

[viii] Lipolysis is the breaking down of triglycerides into fatty acids.

[ix] Of further interest is the fact that a number of things with zero calories can stimulate the production of insulin. The 'S's: sweeteners, stimulants (caffeine) and/or stress have a similar effect, thereby creating a 'fattening environment' in the body, with no calories consumed.

principles from the nineteenth century, before the discovery of insulin in 1921, openly shared by William Banting in 1869.[26]

In their 1965 article, Yalow and Berson teamed up with Seymour Glick and Jesse Roth to review the relationship between insulin, obesity and diabetes.[27] They opened with "Here we summarize several well established observations: A relatively high percentage of adult-onset diabetics[x] are obese and were so long before the onset of clinical diabetes. Diabetes occurs far more frequently in obese than in nonobese subjects. Obese patients without diabetes exhibit impaired glucose tolerance with abnormally high frequency." With no claims of causation in any direction, the authors are merely observing associations between diabetes, obesity and insulin resistance. At the end of a rigorous study of blood glucose levels and insulin responsiveness in all permutations of lean and obese, diabetic and non diabetic people, their conclusion was as follows: "Thus, there is some degree of insulin insensitivity in obesity without diabetes and a greater degree of insensitivity in diabetes without obesity. When the two conditions coexist, insensitivity is greatest and results in the highest insulin concentrations if pancreatic reserve is adequate."

This confirms that obese people are more likely to have type 2 diabetes and, even if not diabetic, they are more likely to display insulin sensitivity. Those who are both diabetic and obese are likely to be the most insulin resistant of all. The causation is likely circular, as obesity increases the person's chance of developing type 2 diabetes and the accompanying insulin resistance makes obesity more likely. The subject of fat storage is very interesting to compare in type 1 and type 2 diabetes.

The first life event to trigger my interest in the subject of weight, insulin and carbohydrates was my brother developing type 1 diabetes when he was aged 15 and I was 13. As is classic in the onset of the condition, he lost approximately 20 pounds in a similar number of days (the condition took an inexplicably long time to diagnose, given the classic nature of the symptoms). His 'energy in' had undoubtedly increased – as he was sending me to the corner shop to buy litre after litre of sugary fizzy drinks. His 'energy out' undoubtedly decreased, as he seemed unable to move from his armchair. Having shared this story a number of times – the most common response is curiosity about any possible violation of the laws of thermodynamics – how could energy in go up and energy out go down and a human lose so much weight?

When type 1 diabetes occurs, sugar is lost in the urine. Indeed, diabetes means 'sweet urine' in Greek and diabetes is diagnosed by testing for sugar in the urine. At the 2010 Wales obesity conference Dr. Jeffrey Stephens a diabetologist, estimated that glycosuria (literally weeing out sugar in the urine)

---

[x] "Adult onset" was the common terminology used for type 2 diabetes at the time of the 1965 article. Type 1 diabetes similarly used to be called juvenile diabetes, as it manifested itself in children, adolescents or young adults. Type 1 and 2 are the favoured terms nowadays, not least because we are observing new cases of type 1 diabetes in middle aged people and, extremely worryingly, type 2 diabetes in children. The vast majority, 90-95%, of diabetics have type 2 diabetes.

may account for 500 calories a day. That still doesn't allow the first law of thermodynamics alone to explain the notorious weight loss in the sudden onset of type 1 diabetes. We seem more interested in calorie reconciliation than thinking about possible implications for obesity. I was always more interested in what this told us about the role of insulin in weight and weight loss.

What we observe, at the onset of type 1 diabetes, is, essentially, a human body incapable of storing fat in the absence of insulin.[xi] As soon as the condition is diagnosed we (unforgivably in my view) advise the person to eat carbohydrate at every meal and administer insulin regularly and the ability to store fat resumes. Invariably the person then struggles to avoid obesity for the rest of their life.

Conversely, just as onset type 1 diabetics, before diagnosis, are unable to store fat, type 2 diabetics are masters at this. Pre-diabetic individuals are often efficient 'fat storing machines' while insulin resistance is developing and before they are officially diagnosed with type 2 diabetes. Whereas the onset of type 1 is sudden and dramatic, type 2 diabetes can emerge over time and remain undiagnosed for months, even years. Any insulin resistant type 2, diagnosed or otherwise, would be well advised to avoid carbohydrates, as this is the one macronutrient that they cannot handle. Instead, we advise all citizens, diabetic or non-diabetic, to base their meals on starchy foods and to eat little and often and we maintain an excellent fat storage environment in so doing.

Edgar Gordon wrote in the *Journal of the American Medical Association* (JAMA) 1963 "It may be stated categorically that the storage of fat and therefore the production and maintenance of obesity cannot take place unless glucose is being metabolized. Since glucose cannot be used by most tissues without the presence of insulin, it also may be stated categorically that obesity is impossible in the absence of adequate tissue concentrations of insulin. Thus an abundant supply of carbohydrate food exerts a powerful influence in directing the stream of glucose metabolism into lipogenesis, whereas a relatively low carbohydrate intake tends to minimize the storage of fat. "[28]

There are enough journal articles and medical references connecting insulin and weight to keep an obesity researcher engaged for years on this subject alone. The conclusion of all references, however, is that insulin leads to weight gain (and, therefore, by inference, that carbohydrate leads to weight gain). Nothing illustrates this better than medical journal forums seeking ways to encourage diabetics (especially young females) to take their insulin, because the doctors know that the diabetics know that insulin makes them fat.

[xi] There is a debate about the role of acylation stimulation protein (ASP) in fat storage. I have ignored this for now on the basis that there is no consensus on whether it can play a role and there is some consensus that any role it might play is negligible compared with the fat storing role played by insulin.

Fat utilisation

Just as fat storage requires insulin, fat utilisation requires the opposite environment to this. Fat utilisation can *only* occur when there is no carbohydrate and glucose available. When a non diabetic person consumes carbohydrate, insulin is released by the functioning pancreas. This has the role of: converting glucose to glycogen; facilitating the cellular uptake of glucose and converting excess glucose to fat.

The lesser known hormone secreted by the pancreas is glucagon, which converts glycogen to glucose. Insulin and glucagon are working almost in equal and opposite ways to regulate blood glucose levels. When blood glucose levels rise, insulin is released to return blood glucose levels to normal. Insulin does this by turning the glucose in the blood stream into glycogen. The pancreas releases glucagon when blood glucose levels fall too low. Glucagon causes the liver to convert stored glycogen into glucose, which is released into the bloodstream. Glucagon also stimulates the release of insulin, so that glucose can be taken up and used by insulin-dependent tissues. Thus, glucagon and insulin are part of a feedback system constantly working to keep blood glucose levels stable.

The hormone glucagon also plays a key role in fat utilisation (i.e. weight loss). When there is no more glycogen available and the body requires fatty acids as an energy source, glucagon stimulates the breakdown of the triglycerides (via lipase[xii]) to release free fatty acids. An alternative driver to demand fat breakdown can be the brain. As the brain cannot use fatty acids as an energy source (unless converted to a ketone), the glycerol part of triglycerides can be converted into glucose, (via gluconeogenesis[xiii]), for brain fuel. Either the body needing fatty acids or the brain needing glucose from glycerol can encourage the breakdown of triglyceride (human fat tissue) into those component parts. Please note that it is the pancreas, the absence of insulin and the presence of glucagon that breaks down fat – not a simple energy imbalance.

The misapplication of the first law

I cannot stress enough how critical this misapplication of the first law of thermodynamics has been for the obesity epidemic. If you believe energy in equals energy out, it is 'somewhat' logical to think that we need to put less energy in and/or get more energy out. I say 'somewhat' logical, as this belief still fails two logical tests:

[xii] Lipase is a fat-digesting enzyme produced by the stomach, small intestine and pancreas. (An enzyme is a protein (or protein based molecule) that speeds up a chemical reaction in a living organism. It acts as a catalyst).

[xiii] Gluconeogenesis is the process by which glucose is formed from non carbohydrate sources.

1) Even if energy in equalled energy out, surely less energy in would equal less energy out?
2) Even if energy in equalled energy out, we would still need to apply the second law of thermodynamics and consider whether different types of energy (different macronutrients) use up different amounts of energy in making available energy and/or if some energy can be 'lost' by the body.

It would be more logical to believe:

1) 'Eat less' will lead the body to try to restore energy intake to the level needed a) through hunger driving the person to eat more and b) through energy conservation driving the person to do less. Similarly,
2) 'Do more' will lead the body to try to restore energy intake to the level needed a) through hunger driving the person to eat more (to meet the extra fuel requirement) and b) through energy conservation driving the person to do less (to resist the demand for fuel that has not been supplied).

So, 'eat less' leads to eat more/do less and 'do more' leads to eat more/do less. The counter productive response is exacerbated as follows. By 'eat less' we specifically mean eat fewer calories and this has an immediate and direct impact on food choices. The person who tries to restrict calories eats a greater proportion (if not greater absolute amount) of their diet in the form of carbohydrate. As carbohydrate approximates to four calories per gram and fat approximates to nine, calorie counters choose carbohydrate over fat to get the most food for their limited intake.[xiv] In case they don't work this out for themselves, the government advice is there to tell them "eat less fat", "base your meals on starchy foods" and so on.

As we have already noted, weight gain and weight loss is not a simplistic matter of energy in and energy out, but a matter of fat storage and fat utilisation. As carbohydrate facilitates fat storage and debilitates fat utilisation, dietary advice that leads someone to eat more carbohydrate is, therefore, fundamentally flawed.

A common theme of this book will be that all routes lead to carbohydrate and that the single most damaging part of our diet advice has been the drive to get humans to eat more carbohydrate. I stand to be corrected, but, as Edgar Gordon concluded, I cannot conceive of how the body can store fat in the absence of insulin. As insulin is only present when the body has consumed carbohydrate, it follows that I cannot conceive of the circumstances in which the body can store fat in the absence of carbohydrate. Insulin will, of course, automatically be released by the pancreas, in response to carbohydrate consumption in a non-diabetic. In a type 1 diabetic, insulin only needs to be administered when a carbohydrate is consumed. In a type 2 diabetic, the body only tries to release insulin when carbohydrate is eaten. The absence of

---

[xiv] Some people opt for high protein diets on the basis that protein also approximates to four calories per gram. Eating protein, without the fat that nature delivers purposefully with it, is not natural or healthy.

carbohydrate is accompanied by the absence of insulin (including the need for insulin) and therefore the absence of the ability to store fat.

Tragically, if you believe that energy in equals energy out and you, therefore, want a person to put less energy in, you will tell them to eat more carbohydrate (because of the comparative calorie content). If you correctly apply the first law of thermodynamics and you understand that energy is conserved (in a closed system in equilibrium) and that energy in does *not* equal energy out, you will tell an overweight person to eat less carbohydrate because they will be less able to store fat. This misapplication of the first law of thermodynamics has led to completely the wrong advice being given to overweight people.

Chapter Two

Is a calorie a calorie?

The second law of thermodynamics

We cannot place any faith in the first law of thermodynamics alone. The first law can only be applied in isolation to closed systems, in thermal equilibrium. Living organisms (human beings) are open systems, far from equilibrium (although continuously trying to achieve this state); carrying out continual metabolic reactions and so we must also take into account the second law of thermodynamics.

The second law of thermodynamics is effectively the law of common sense. This second law of thermodynamics came about while looking into optimal efficiency of machines during the Industrial Revolution. The first law alone implies that perpetual motion could be possible (if energy is neither created, nor destroyed, could a system go on for ever?) The second law introduces the pragmatic fact that energy will be lost to its surroundings and energy will be used to convert energy and the quest for perpetual motion was thus ended.

To give an everyday example, when we put the kettle on, electricity or gas energy is converted into heat energy to heat the water. Some energy is used up heating the filament to then heat the water (that's energy used in making available energy) and some energy is lost out of the spout and some more is 'wasted' as the sides of the kettle inevitably heat (that's energy lost because the system is not closed).

The second law also introduces the irreversibility concept. We can turn coal into heat, but we can't turn the heat back into coal. Where we can turn something back into the form it once was, we can't turn it back into the same amount. E.g. electricity can produce steam and steam can produce electricity, but the energy lost throughout the process is such that the electricity at the end would be a fraction of the electricity with which we began.

In every human being, energy will be lost and so the second law, entropy, must be applied. This is almost universally ignored by the 'calorie is a calorie' proponents and yet, from a weight loss perspective, entropy is the Holy Grail. Dieters should want as much energy to be lost from the body as possible and they should want as much energy as possible to be used up in making energy available to the body. Indeed, the weight loss pill orlistat (branded as Xenical/Alli) works on the basis that fat is not digested by the body until it reaches the small intestine, so this drug tries to ensure that some fat rushes from the small intestine into the colon and then the toilet, before it can be digested. In this way energy is lost from the body. The F-Plan diet had similar (if gentler) aims – to try to have energy pass through the body and to be lost to the body and therefore unavailable as fuel.

As regards the second aspect of entropy in a human – energy used up in making useable energy – Eric Jequier, who works in the Institute of Physiology, University of Lausanne, Switzerland found that the thermic effect of nutrients (thermogenesis) is approximately 6-8% for carbohydrate, 2-3% for fat and 25-30% for protein.[29] I.e. approximately 6-8% of the calories consumed in the form of carbohydrate are used up in digesting the carbohydrate and turning it into fuel available to be used by the body. In contrast, 25-30% of the calories consumed in the form of protein are used up in digesting the protein and turning it into fuel available to be used by the body. This also makes intuitive sense; carbohydrates are relatively easy for the body to turn into energy (indeed they start being digested, and turned into glucose, with salivary enzymes, as soon as we start chewing). Protein needs to be broken down into amino acids, which is a far more complex process.

Richard Feinman and Eugene Fine, a biochemist and a nuclear physicist respectively, have done some outstanding research in the area of thermodynamics and metabolic advantage of different diet compositions. In their 2004 paper,[30] they took Jequier's mid points (7% for carbohydrate, 2.5% for fat and 27.5% for protein) and applied these to a 2,000 calorie diet comprising 55:30:15 proportions of carbohydrate:fat:protein. This demonstrated that 2,000 calories yielded 1,848 calories available for energy. I repeated the calculation for a 10:30:60 high protein diet, as another example, and the yield drops to 1,641 calories.[xv]

With this Jequier, Feinman and Fine research the first law of thermodynamics is satisfied – the books balance – we can account for all 2,000 calories in and out. And the second law holds – we have 'useful' energy (1,848 calories in Feinman and Fine's example) and 'useless' energy (152 calories), the energy used in conversion. I don't understand why this alone has not ended the debate and proven, once and for all, when it comes to eating and weight, a calorie is *not* a calorie.

As Feinman and Fine so beautifully put it, if a calorie were a calorie, the second law of thermodynamics would be violated. That is to say – if all calories gave the same energy available to the body then there would be no difference in energy used up in making energy available and the law of entropy would be invalid in the human body. Pure carbohydrate calories are very different to pure protein calories once ingested.

The notion that a calorie is a calorie is also naive in terms of nutrition. 100 calories of tuna or pork have excellent nutritional value and complete amino acid protein representation vs. 100 calories of sugar, which have no nutritional

---

[xv] I first repeated the Feinman and Fine (F&F) experiment and my calculation for a 55:30:15 carbohydrate:fat:protein diet gave a yield of 1,825 calories, not the 1,848 recorded by F&F. I contacted Dr. Feinman who confirmed that there had been an arithmetical error in their calculations, but the difference is small and would have only served to make their point more profound.

value and no protein, let alone amino acid provision. If we could only replace the 400 sugar calories per average (UK) person per day for the same calories of brown rice and stir-fry vegetables (still essentially carbohydrate) we could make a significant difference to the obesity epidemic with one change.

Macronutrients – because a calorie is not a calorie

One of the most brilliant obesity experiments ever done was by Professor Alan Kekwick and Dr. Gaston Pawan, published in *The Lancet* (1956).[31] They worked in the Middlesex hospital, so they could control the food given to their patients (where they observed "inadequate personalities", they would isolate patients, or discard those results):

- In experiment one, they gave their patients the 'normal' (in 1956) UK daily food intake of 47:33:20, carbohydrate:fat:protein. They kept these proportions the same as they put the patients on 2,000 calories a day, then 1,500 a day, then 1,000 a day and finally 500 a day. They found that there was a relationship between lower calories and weight lost, when the diet composition was maintained, in the 7-9 days they looked at for each calorie level. However, they found no straight line relationship, let alone the loss of one pound of fat for each and every deficit of 3,500 calories.

- In experiment two, they gave 14 patients 1,000 calories each, but split the patients into three groups and varied the types of food that they were given. Group A had 90% fat, Group B had 90% protein and Group C had 90% carbohydrate. Their findings were revolutionary. The 90% fat group lost the most, the 90% protein group was just a fraction behind this and the 90% carbohydrate group were way behind. Their conclusion was "So different were the rates of weight-loss on these isocaloric[xvi] diets that the composition of the diet appeared to outweigh in importance the intake of calories."

- In experiment three, they took five people who, they observed, maintained weight at 2,000 calories a day (in the normal 47:33:20, carbohydrate:fat:protein, ratio of the time) and they put them on 2,000 calories of carbohydrate a day and they all gained weight. They then put the five people on 2,600 calories (yes – more) of fat/protein and all but one lost weight (they noted in the paper that one woman was impacting the results, as she seemed able to retain more than three litres of water at her time of menstruation). They alternated members of the group between 2,000 calories of carbohydrate (which resulted in weight gain) and 2,600 calories of fat/protein (which resulted in weight loss).

Kekwick and Pawan ruled out glycogen and concomitant water retention playing a part in experiments two and three. Their conclusion on glycogen was "it is unlikely that the patients became depleted of carbohydrate reserves. These reserves are small and could not account for the amount of weight lost (Soskin

---

[xvi] Isocaloric = same calories/different composition of carbohydrate, fat and protein.

24

and Levine 1950)." Body water content and nitrogen balance were studied throughout the experiments enabling Kekwick and Pawan to say "in all the patients, the available water initially represented 50-52.5% of the body-weight. By the end of about four weeks on the diets the proportion of body-water to weight remained the same (50-52%)."

Many studies, including and since Kekwick and Pawan's 1956 paper, show that low carbohydrate diets are more effective than low calorie diets and isocaloric studies also show that low carbohydrate diets have a distinct advantage. As Feinman and Fine observe "These reports have not been refuted, but rather largely ignored."[32]

Marjorie R. Freedman, Janet King, and Eileen Kennedy wrote an article called "Popular Diets: A Scientific Review", where 17 studies of weight loss with different macronutrient (carbohydrate, fat and protein) composition, are reported with the concomitant results.[33] The authors state that "no published studies are excluded", so I have assumed that these are the only studies between 1956 and 2001. The three authors concluded "Caloric balance (calories in vs. calories out), rather than macronutrient composition is the major determinant of weight loss." Yet I analysed all the data for these 17 studies and found *no* relationship between low calorie intake and high weight loss (0.009 correlation coefficient), but a significant relationship between low carbohydrate intake and high weight loss (0.79 correlation coefficient) (Appendix 1). How can the authors have concluded as they did, unless they set out to prove an already held point of view?

Chapter Three

Greed and sloth, or something else?

The laws of thermodynamics do not imply causation

There is no direction of causation in the principle of energy conservation. This brilliant idea dates back to Hugo Rony's *Obesity and Leanness* (1940) and it has been resurrected by Gary Taubes in *The Diet Delusion* (2007). Taubes uses the example that a teenage boy gains weight not because he is overeating and sedentary. He eats and sleeps all the time because he is growing and the growth hormone is driving his energy intake and expenditure and weight gain is but a result of this.

The implications of this concept for the treatment of obesity are significant. To solve something, you need to know what has caused it. It is universally assumed, in the world of dieting, that overweight people have eaten too much and/or not done enough activity. Hence the prescribed solution is to eat less/do more. Notwithstanding the fact that weight gain is about fat stored, and not just energy in and out, if there is a separate factor, which has caused the person to eat in a way such that fat can be stored, this separate factor is a cause and needs to be addressed.

Over 25 years ago, we had already questioned even an association between overweight people, food consumption and exercise. The 1983 Royal College of Physicians report on Obesity states: "The traditional view that the majority of overweight subjects are eating more or exercising less than those of a normal weight is now recognised as not being uniformly true."[34] We missed an opportunity to build on this observation and look at what was going on within the body, rather than spending another quarter of a century obsessing with calories in and calories out.

Even if we did observe an association between, let's say, being overweight and doing less, we must be open to the idea that (quite logically) people are not, for example, overweight because they are sedentary, but they are sedentary because they are overweight (a larger frame is quite simply more difficult to move around). This then leads the researcher to look at sedentary behaviour as an effect and not a cause. (There is likely an element of both, of course, but I am making the point that we have assumed only one direction of causation. Rare and useful are the studies that assert "Fatness leads to inactivity, but inactivity does not lead to fatness."[35]

The observation that the law of conservation of energy describes an association, rather than any direction of causation, raises another interesting point. Surely a key determinant of activity has to be fuel consumed – both quantity and quality. If we don't put enough fuel in a car, it won't get as far as we want it to go. If we put the wrong fuel in the car, it will go nowhere. I fail to see how you can give an overweight person 1,000 fewer calories a day than they actually need and for those meagre calories to come from sugary cereals, white bread, calorie counted processed products, starchy foods (not necessarily wholemeal) and then expect the overweight person to have the energy to do anything other than watch TV. The precursor to doing more is surely eating better.

Despite the fact that there is no direction of causation in the first law of thermodynamics, we have assumed that there are only two causes of obesity – gluttony and sloth. When we move away from this erroneous and patronising simplicity, we can see both an endogenous system and exogenous medication as clear causes of obesity.

The endocrine (hormone) system – an endogenous theory

The Taubes /Rony example above of the teenage boy is not unique in being a hormone driven weight change. The endocrine system is the most likely source of other 'separate factors', so let us look at this in some detail. (Please don't be put off by the medical terms that follow and read at the level that works for you. You don't need to understand the detail, just enough to appreciate the role that hormones can play in weight gain).

The endocrine system is made up of the endocrine glands that secrete hormones. The endocrine glands are:

1) Pineal;
2) Pituitary;
3) Thyroid (and parathyroid);
4) Thymus (not strictly part of the endocrine system);
5) Adrenals;
6) Pancreas;
7) Ovaries in females; and
8) Testes in males.

Just as the central nervous system sends motion and sensory messages to control and co-ordinate the body, so the endocrine system has a similar job, but using hormones to communicate. The endocrine glands are ductless, which means that their secretions (hormones) are released directly into the bloodstream and travel to elsewhere in the body to target the organs upon which they act. Although there are eight major endocrine glands scattered throughout the body, they are still considered to be one system because they have similar functions, similar mechanisms of influence, and many important interrelationships.

Let us go through the functions of the endocrine system and draw attention to the roles that can clearly have an impact on weight:

1) The pineal functions as a gland, secreting the hormone melatonin during the hours of darkness, which regulates the pituitary gland and is associated with the biological clock. Melatonin is derived from serotonin, with which it

27

works to regulate the sleep cycle. There have been some important studies on weight and sleep patterns and we know that shift work is conducive to weight gain. We also know that hours of sunlight per day and the mood aspect of serotonin play an important part in weight, but I do not intend to go further into the pineal gland, as there are bigger hormonal targets to catch.

2) The hypothalamus, which is part of the brain, links the nervous system to the endocrine system via the pituitary gland. The pituitary is thus known as the master gland and this part of the brain consists of two lobes called the anterior and the posterior. The anterior releases the following hormones: human growth hormone (HGH); thyroid stimulating hormone (TSH) (to release thyroxin); adreno cortico trophic hormone (ACTH), which stimulates the adrenal cortex to produce cortisol and androgens, amongst other corticosteroids; luteinizing hormone (LH), which brings about ovulation; follicle stimulating hormone (FSH) – another key hormone in the menstrual cycle; and the interstitial cell stimulating hormone (ICSH) to produce sperm. The main secretion from the posterior lobe is the anti-diuretic hormone (ADH).

Every one of the above can have a significant impact on size and weight. To share just a few examples:

- Too much (hyper) HGH can lead to the condition crudely known as gigantism and too little (hypo) HGH can lead to the condition equally crudely known as dwarfism.
- Cortisol is deemed to play a role in hormone related weight gain from literally stressing the body with intense exercise. This would benefit from further investigation, as we observe abdominal fat in a number of otherwise very fit people.
- Androgens play a crucial role in poly cystic ovary syndrome (PCOS). Dr. Nuha Haboubi, a chemical pathologist, has been instrumental in reviewing the contribution of PCOS to the obesity epidemic. Speaking at the Wales National Obesity Forum conference in May 2010 she noted that PCOS affects approximately 10% of women and that in some countries one fifth of PCOS sufferers are obese and in other countries it is as high as three quarters. Haboubi presented evidence that 69% of PCOS sufferers in the USA are obese. This concurred with a UK 2009 health sciences research audit where dietitians were surveyed to request information about how many of their patients with PCOS were obese. The result was that 24% of PCOS sufferers remained lean while 76% were found to be obese. It is uniformly noted that the fat storage, in PCOS patients, is more commonly observed around the abdominal area. Excess production of androgens is noted with PCOS sufferers and obese women produce more androgens. So we have a vicious circle of raised androgen production and PCOS and obesity and I have made no assertions about causation thus far. If, however, you are a pure calorie theorist, you will believe that putting too many calories in (or not expending enough calories) is the cause of obesity and this in turn

(somehow) causes PCOS and the pituitary master gland is telling the adrenal cortex to produce too many androgens, all because the woman ate too much.

The Rotterdam Consensus workshop (2003) on PCOS defined the condition as "PCOS is a syndrome of ovarian dysfunction along with the cardinal features hyperandrogenism and poly cystic ovary morphology."[36] The diagnosis of PCOS can be made on the basis of two out of three of the following:

- Oligoovulation (infrequent, irregular ovulation) – or anovulation (absence of ovulation);
- Clinical or biochemical signs of hyperandrogenism;
- Polycystic ovaries on ultrasound or direct inspection.

The third point brings in the influence of another part of the endocrine system – the ovaries. PCOS is also characterised by excess production of oestrogens and fertility problems (this is often the route through which PCOS is diagnosed). So we have an enormously complex, multi faceted, medical condition, integrally linked with at least three parts of the endocrine system. Surely it is *not* reasonable to claim that any obesity observed with this condition is driven purely by energy in and energy out. We must start looking more at the body itself – not just the simple measures of what goes in to the body and what goes out.

Finally, in this brief review of the pituitary gland, we have the known impact of hormones on weight even during the menstrual cycle, let alone from puberty to menopause. During a typical 28 day menstrual cycle, luteinizing hormone (LH) is fairly constant other than the significant rise a couple of days before ovulation and the rapid fall away at day 14. Follicle stimulating hormone (FSH) has a smaller peak also at the middle of the month and rises slightly at the end of the cycle to start the next cycle at one of its higher levels. Most women report small to considerable weight gain during days 21-28 of this cycle.

3) The thyroid gland secretes thyroxin, which is critical to metabolism and basal metabolic rate (BMR). We know that the thyroid gland is a clear and definite factor in weight. With no change in calories consumed, we could remove the thyroid gland in a thin person and make them fat. This is an extreme scenario, but an underactive thyroid, also known as hypo-thyroidism, will lead to a decrease in BMR, weight gain, lethargy and other unpleasant symptoms. Conversely, an overactive thyroid, hyper-thyroidism will lead to an increase in BMR, weight loss, hyper-activity and equally unwelcome symptoms. Indeed a blood test for thyroid functioning is one of the first tests done to investigate seemingly inexplicable weight loss or gain.

The parathyroid is primarily concerned with the growth of muscle and bone and the distribution of calcium and phosphate in the body and needs no further mention in this brief review of hormones and weight.

4) The thymus is strictly an immune system gland, but it is invariably included in reviews of the endocrine system. It activates the immune system and regulates lymphocytes (white blood cells associated with antibody production). It plays a critical role in transplant situations, but we need not devote more time to it here.

5) Adrenalin is the most common hormone secreted by the adrenal glands. This prepares the body for the fright, fight or flight mechanism and, in so doing, the action of the heart is increased, the rate and depth of breathing is increased, the metabolic rate is increased and muscular contraction improves – all excellent responses by the body, for the need to act.[xvii]

Noradrenalin is also released by the adrenal gland (also called adrenal medulla) and this has similar effects to adrenalin.

The adrenal cortex produces corticosteroids such as cortisol, cortisone, corticosterone and aldosterone. The first three of these are collectively known as glucocorticoids. The most interesting function amongst these, from a weight perspective, is the role of glucocorticoids on the utilisation of carbohydrate, fat and protein by the body. With the name derived from a combination of abbreviations of *gluco*se, adrenal *cort*ex and ster*oids*, glucocorticoids play a key role in glucose metabolism and thus fat storage and utilisation. Aldosterone has a key role to play in the regulation of salt and water balance, which can impact weight to a more transitory extent.

6) The pancreas is the single most important part of the endocrine system for our review of hormones and weight. It is actually both exocrine (ducted) and endocrine (ductless). As an exocrine gland it secretes the following enzymes into the small intestine:

- Pancreatic amylase (which breaks down polysaccharides into simple sugars – more on this in Chapter Thirteen);
- Lipase (which breaks down triglycerides into fatty acids and glycerol);
- Protease (which breaks down protein into amino acids).

We covered the critical role of insulin in fat storage and fat utilisation in Chapter One. The weight gain resulting from insulin is so well known that, as far back as 1925, Wilhelm Falta began using insulin to treat underweight adults and anorexia.[37] The weight loss at the onset of type 1 diabetes is equally long known and remarkable. The non diabetic person can produce the same fattening effect of administering insulin by eating carbohydrates frequently and causing the pancreas to release insulin. The impact of insulin on weight is irrefutable and substantial, as we will also see in the next section on medication.

[xvii] For those interested in why such stress makes you want to go to the toilet, the blood supply to the bladder and intestines is reduced – as it is needed elsewhere – and the muscular walls in these regions relax.

7) Experiments with rats have shown that the removal of ovaries (and therefore the hormone oestrogen) can lead to excessive hunger and inactivity (and weight gain).[38] This can be observed in females following the removal of ovaries, as may happen with certain types of hysterectomy or treatment for ovarian cancer. The ovaries effectively cease to function with any hysterectomy or during the menopause, when the ovaries cease production of eggs and the levels of oestrogen fall measurably. The Wade and Gray study (referenced in this paragraph) of the gonad hormones (oestrogen, progesterone and testosterone) in 1978 noted four interesting things:

- "Estradiol (i.e. oestrogen) and testosterone decrease adiposity, while progesterone increases carcass fat content." It is interesting to note that progesterone is the hormone that rises from day 14 of the menstrual cycle, coinciding with noticeable weight gain for many women. Additionally, the most common hormone taken by females, "The Pill", typically contains 150 milligrams of progesterone and 30 milligrams of oestrogen for the combined pill and 350 milligrams of progesterone (usually norethisterone) for the progesterone only pill (POP). Women taking the pill commonly report weight gain.
- "These hormone-induced changes in body weight and composition are accompanied by changes in food intake and voluntary exercise, suggesting that the hormones induce behavioral changes which alter body weight and adiposity.
- "However, several lines of evidence indicate that these behavioral changes are neither necessary nor sufficient to produce the hormone-induced body weight shifts.
- "From this perspective, estradiol and progesterone-induced changes in food intake are viewed as consequences, rather than causes, of changes in fat metabolism."

Taking the final three points together, the argument is that hormone changes *do* drive weight changes both directly, with a metabolic impact, and indirectly, with an effect on appetite and activity levels, and that the metabolic impact is likely the greater.

There are many examples of the impact of hormones on weight, which get completely disregarded if you are stuck in the narrow view that all that matters are calories consumed and calories expended in activity.

Medication – an exogenous theory

We move on now from the natural endocrine system, which can impact weight in numerous different ways, to prescribed medication and the impact that this can have on weight. Such medication is called 'obesogenic' – meaning tending to favour weight gain.

The UK *Independent on Sunday* ran a sensational story on 24 June 2007 "Huge weight gains reported by patients on prescription drugs". "Researchers, who found that some patients were putting on up to 22lbs in a year, say that the drugs may even be contributing to the nation's rocketing obesity epidemic... All of the patients they studied, on medication for conditions as diverse as diabetes, epilepsy, depression, high blood pressure and schizophrenia, showed evidence of weight increase."

The newspaper article was based on research conducted by Wilma Leslie, Catherine Hankey and Mike Lean, presented in the *QJM*, June 2007, called "Weight gain as an adverse effect of some commonly prescribed drugs: a systematic review."[39] This is an extremely useful study, undertaken in Glasgow, Scotland, where the research team systematically reviewed papers from Medline 1966-2004, Embase 1980-2004, PsycINFO 1967-2004, and the Cochrane Register of Controlled Trials, to establish the effect on body weight of some drugs that are believed to favour weight gain. They included studies where drugs considered obesogenic were compared with placebos, with an alternative drug or with other treatment; and where the trial was for a duration of at least three months. 43 studies involving 25,663 people met these criteria. Interestingly, weight gain was a primary outcome measure in only six of the studies (i.e. weight was not a key area of interest in the majority of the studies). The conclusion was "There was evidence of weight gain for all drugs included, up to 10kg at 52 weeks."

The study needed to start from a list of drugs known to favour weight gain, so that the medical journal databases could be searched for evidence of studies involving these drugs. (Again, please don't be put off by the drug names – you will be more familiar with the conditions than the drugs associated with them. It is important to list the drug types in case you, the reader, are taking or prescribing any of these). The drugs chosen were:

1) Insulin, sulphonylureas and thiazolinidiones for the treatment of diabetes;
2) Betablockers for hypertension;
3) Corticosteroids for inflammatory disease;
4) Cyproheptadine for allergy and hay fever;
5) Antipsychotics for psychosis;
6) Sodium valproate for epilepsy;
7) Tricyclic antidepressants for depression; and
8) Lithium for bipolar disorder.

The results were as follows:

1) The large-scale studies, such as the diabetes control and complications trial (DCCT) in patients with type 1 diabetes and the United Kingdom prospective diabetes study (UKPDS) in patients with type 2 diabetes, have quantified the weight gain resulting from the administration of insulin. The DCCT was a prospective trial involving 1,441 patients with type 1 diabetes randomised to either an intensive (three to four insulin injections/day or insulin pump) or conventional (one to two insulin injections/day) treatment protocol.[40] At the nine year follow up, approximately 30% of men and 35% of women, receiving the intensive insulin dosage, were five points higher on their BMI scale. Men and women on the more conventional dose still gained

weight, but far less. The study quantified the average (mean) weight gain as 4.75 kilograms greater for the three to four injections a day group.

The UKPDS study had 3,867 participants, newly diagnosed with type 2 diabetes.[41] They were randomly assigned to either an 'intervention' group, with insulin or alternate drug treatment, or to a 'managed through diet' group. Weight gain over the 10 year study was a mean of 6.5 kilograms. Weight gain was significantly higher in the insulin/drug group (mean 2.9 kilograms) than in the diet group. Furthermore, of the drug treatment options, patients assigned insulin had a greater gain in weight (4.0 kilograms) than those given chlorpropamide (2.6 kilograms) or glibenclamide (1.7 kilograms). (The latter two named drugs are from the family of medication called sulphonylurea. They act to stimulate the release of insulin from the beta cells in the pancreas, thus trying to optimise any insulin that can be 'squeezed out' from the body more naturally than insulin administration).

The Glasgow report presented numerous other studies confirming the same observed weight gain with the administration of either insulin or sulphonylureas. The latter produced lower weight gain than insulin, but gain none the less.

The weight gain with insulin is immediate and sustained, as the Yki-Jarvinen 1992 study showed, with a mean gain of 1.8 kilograms to 2.9 kilograms in 12 weeks with two injections and multiple injections respectively. Similarly the Yki-Jarvinen 1997 study, carried out over a one year period, showed a mean weight gain of 5.1 kilograms with 2-4 injections per day. All of these studies were done for management of type 2 diabetes, not type 1.

The people taking sulphonylureas fared better than those taking insulin, but still recorded notable weight gain. The largest weight gain, over a one year period, for a sulphonylurea, was a mean of 3.6 kilograms recorded by Marbury (1999) for glipizide.[42]

2) Three different drugs for hypertension were reviewed (atenolol, metoprolol and propranolol) across five different studies and weight gain was negligible. One study (Berglund 1986) recorded a 0.6 kilograms mean weight *loss* and the largest recorded gain was 1.5 kilograms.

3) Only one randomised controlled trial was found comparing prednisone with radiotherapy in the treatment of inflammatory disease. The weight change was recorded as a side effect and was noted to be a mean of two kilograms after 24 weeks.

4) Although cyproheptadine, for the treatment of allergy and hay fever, was deemed to be an obesogenic drug worthy of review, no studies were found in the wide and systematic search undertaken.

5) 6) and 8) are worth reviewing together, as many drugs are used for a number of different conditions – psychosis, epilepsy, schizophrenia and bipolar disorder. The drug valproate, for example, is used for epilepsy and bipolar

disorder and the lowest mean weight gain recorded in the four studies reviewed was 1.2 kilograms and the highest was 5.8 kilograms. One study of lithium for bipolar disorder recorded a mean weight gain of four kilograms. The headline for the *Independent on Sunday* article came from clozapine, for schizophrenia, with a mean weight gain of 9.9 kilograms over a one year study. Perhaps even more shocking was the mean recorded gain of 7.1 kilograms, in just 12 weeks, for olanzapine for the treatment of psychosis.

7) The Tricyclic drugs for depression include: doxepin (brand name Adapin or Sinequan); amitriptyline (Elavil); nortryptyline (Pamelor); clomipramine (Anafranil); amitriptyline (Endep); maprotiline (Ludiomil); desipramine (Norpramin); desipramine (Pertofrane); trimipramine (Surmontil); imipramine (Tofranil); protriptyline (Vivactil). The three drugs reviewed in the Glasgow study were the first three: doxepin; amitriptyline and nortryptyline. The latter recorded a mean weight gain of 3.7 kilograms at 12 weeks.

I am surprised that the study did not look at one of the most widely prescribed drugs – The Pill. This is the most common of all hormones taken regularly by women. Add to this hormone replacement therapy (HRT) and hormone treatment for males, for example with prostate cancer, and we have examples of how regularly we administer hormones, alongside the body producing them continually with the functions of the endocrine system.

Dr. Stephens, the diabetologist mentioned in Chapter One, gave a presentation on obesogenic drugs at the Wales obesity conference in May 2010. The opening slide said "It is estimated that 9% of adult weight gain can be attributable to prescribed medication". Dr. Stephens is working in the ideal field to become familiar with obesity because the incidence of type 2 diabetes is strongly and positively correlated to weight. The *JAMA* (1999) article "The Disease Burden Associated with Obesity and Overweight" estimated that a male under 55 and with a BMI of over 40 has 90 times the chance of developing type 2 diabetes than a normal weight male of the same age.[43] Although this study found the risk for women slightly lower, other studies have corroborated this multiple for women. Colditz et al (1995) found that women with a BMI of more than 35 had 93 times the risk of developing type 2 diabetes than women whose BMI was less than 22.[44] A BMI of 35 is also not breathtakingly high – 1.2 million people in the UK currently have a BMI of over 40. An average height woman (5'4") who is 14 stone seven pounds has a BMI of 35 and an average man (5'9") who weighs 17 stone has a BMI of 35.

Dr. Stephens' patients, therefore, are almost all obese. He has seen a clear connection between people gaining weight and the prescribed medicines they are taking. When he questioned colleagues about drugs that they were prescribing he was invariably told "we prescribe a particular drug because we find it works best for the condition". Faced with an obesity epidemic, we need doctors to consider prescribing an alterative that is sufficiently efficacious but that doesn't, or is less likely to, cause weight gain.

Drug treatment for a relatively common condition can spiral into a scenario of 'thick note patient syndrome'. An individual could be prescribed an antidepressant and gain some weight. A female, particularly, would likely take steps to correct this. If they follow the current advice of basing their meals on starchy foods, they will create the perfect biochemical environment for storing, rather than burning, fat. As the weight condition worsens, and as carbohydrate consumption has likely increased, the chance of type 2 diabetes increases. If picked up as pre-diabetes, because the patient is seeing their doctor regularly for depression, they can be put on metformin or a sulphonylurea. This may cause further weight gain. With additional weight and with the concomitant water retention from a high-carbohydrate diet, the person can develop blood pressure problems and be prescribed a hypertensive drug, which can cause further weight gain. A small problem can escalate into a patient horror story.

If you think that this story would be an unlikely exception, the closing passage of the journal article was perhaps the most sobering part. In Scotland alone, a country with a population of five million people, during the year April 2004 to March 2005, there were 2,936,456 prescriptions issued for beta blockers, 81,252 for lithium and a further 275,114 for other psychotic drugs, 1,134,611 for tricyclic antidepressants and 1,003,028 prescriptions in total for insulin and other diabetes medication. The Association of the British Pharmaceutical Industry reports that a total of 912 million prescriptions were dispensed in 2007.[45] That's an average of 15 prescriptions per British citizen.

Patients should be far more vociferous and challenging before starting any medication. If the average patient knew the findings of the Glasgow review, no doubt they would think twice, even three times, before taking any medication. Doctors also need to be given more time in consultations to consider the side effects of prescription medicines. The patient leaflet for clozapine (Clozaril) says "may cause weight gain."[46] It does not say that you may gain an average of 9.9 kilograms in one year. On-line chat rooms are useful places for both patients and doctors to read about first hand experience of people gaining weight on different medications. People are listing drug and brand names and dosage in such a comprehensive way that this would be valid as an obesity study of medication if collated.

One of the best tests of causation is the 'had not' test, holding other things equal. Had not the teenager been growing, all other things being equal, he would not have gained weight, (and been observed to eat more and sleep more). Had not the teenage girl gone through puberty, she would not have gained weight. Had not the teenager developed type 1 diabetes, s/he would not have initially lost weight dramatically and then struggled to maintain their weight for life. Had not the schizophrenic taken clozapine, s/he would not have gained several kilograms. I hope that there are enough examples to show even the most ardent calorie theorist that there can be many more *causes* of obesity than energy in and out.

Chapter Four

What happens if we try to eat less/do more?

The Minnesota 'Starvation Experiment'

The bombing of Pearl Harbour brought the Americans into World War II on 8 December 1941. Europe had already been at war since September 1939. Fuel rationing started in the UK later that year and food rationing started in January 1940. The first food product to be rationed in American history was sugar (from May 1942 until 1947).

As Europe continued to be decimated and the future impact on America remained unknown, an American doctor, Ancel Keys, realised that it would be crucial to know what would happen if the war did not end soon and rationing turned to starvation. He set about one of the most ambitious health experiments ever undertaken – to provide the definitive study of hunger and re-feeding. Keys achieved this goal and also, unintentionally, he provided one of the most crucial insights into dieting and weight loss to this day. Many, if not most, current diet advisors have never heard of this experiment, let alone studied it.

The Minnesota Starvation Experiment started with an advert, posted across America in May 1944. "Will you starve that they be better fed?" Two hundred conscientious objectors volunteered, as an alternative to war, and Keys and his team of researchers whittled these down to 36 men. The men (all aged 20-33) were chosen for their physical and mental resilience. The results, 1,385 pages in total, were published in *The Biology of Human Starvation* (1950).[47] Todd Tucker's *The Great Starvation Experiment* (2006) is useful as a reflective accompaniment to the Keys' report of 1950.[48]

The year long experiment was split into four phases:

- The Control Period (12 weeks): The key goal of this period was to determine the calorie requirement for the men. It was established that the men maintained their weight at approximately 3,210 calories a day while walking 22 miles each week – an average of three miles a day (45-60 minutes walking).
- The Starvation Period (24 weeks): The fact that the study was referred to as a "starvation experiment" is interesting, because the six-month 'starvation' was actually a calorie controlled diet of approximately 1,570 calories per day (more calories than many modern diets allow) with 45-60 minutes walking per day. The meals were made up of foods typically available in Europe during the latter stages of the war: potatoes, turnips, bread and macaroni – i.e. starchy carbohydrates. Keys set out to try to induce a 25% weight loss in each man in 24 weeks.

- Restricted Rehabilitation Period (12 weeks): The men were divided into four groups of eight (four had been dismissed for stealing food and binging) and given different calorie, protein and vitamin levels to see what would best re-nourish them back to health.
- Unrestricted Rehabilitation Period (8 weeks): For the final period, the men could eat as much as they wanted and the research team carefully recorded what they did in fact eat.

This invaluable study tells us the following about dieting and weight loss:

1) Hunger is comparable with war in terms of the devastating effect it has on humans. Many of the volunteers came to believe that military service would have been an easier option than their chosen path.

The men were required to keep diaries and Sam Legg noted "I have been more depressed than ever in my life… I thought that there was only one thing that would pull me out of the doldrums, that is release from C.P.S. (the experiment) I decided to get rid of some fingers. Ten days ago, I jacked up my car and let the car fall on these fingers. It was premeditated."[49] A few days later Legg cut three fingers off his left hand while chopping wood. Legg was subsequently unable to explain whether this was deliberate self harm, possibly in an attempt to overcome the pain of starvation, or whether it was the result of an inability to perform normal tasks with insufficient food.

Keys put 36 physically and mentally healthy men on a calorie controlled diet, with a moderate amount of exercise, and, in a matter of weeks, he turned them into physical and emotional shadows of their former selves.

Physically, the men reported incessant hunger, weakness, exhaustion and they lost 21% of their strength in the first 12 weeks alone. They experienced dizziness, muscle wasting, hair loss and reduced coordination. Several withdrew from their university classes, because they simply didn't have the energy or motivation to attend.

Psychologically, the men became obsessed with food, meal times and everything to do with eating. The study documented "For some, the fascination was so great that they actually changed occupations after the experiment; three became chefs, and one went into agriculture."[50] They had to 'buddy up' to avoid breaking their diets, as their drive to binge was so enormous. Before the buddy system was put in place, a couple did get hold of some forbidden food and binge and suffered extreme guilt and self-loathing as a result. (It is fair to assume, therefore, that, had this not been a confined experiment, all men would have given up on their diet). The men reported extreme depression, irritability, a sense of deprivation and they lost all interest in sex. (They actually lost all interest in anything other than food – such is the human drive to overcome hunger).

2) Part Two of this book dissects and destroys the claim "To lose one pound of fat you need to create a deficit of 3,500 calories." However, the Minnesota experiment alone rendered this statement invalid over 60 years ago.

Tucker's book noted that the men lost, on average, 1.76 pounds in the control period. Hence the deficit in the Keys' study was at least 1,640 calories a day from the outset.[xviii] The calorie deficit (at least in theory) was further increased during the experiment, as Keys needed to continually reduce the calorie allowance to try to induce further weight loss. Assuming that the deficit remained at 1,640 for the 24 week 'starvation' period, if the 3,500 formula were correct, during the 24 weeks, every man should have lost at least 78 pounds in fat alone and more on top of this in water and lean tissue. The average *weight* loss of the men was less than half of this – 37 pounds – 1.5 pounds per week. If the 3,500 formula were correct, the lightest man in the study, Bob Villwock from Ohio, should have finished the study below three stone (he would, of course, have died long before this).

3) The less you eat, the less you must continue to eat to have any chance of losing more weight and weight loss will stop, at some point, whether you like it or not.

Interestingly, Keys rejected the 3,500 formula from the outset and relied instead on adjusting the calorie intake every week to try to induce his desired weight loss of 25%. Keys found he needed to limit some men to 1,000 calories a day to try to induce further weight loss (the men should have been losing over five pounds per week, at this calorie intake, having created a deficit of almost 2,500 calories a day from their original calorie need. In reality the body had adjusted energy need to resist any further weight loss).

I said 'in theory' above as we cannot ignore the fact that a circular reference exists. The original deficit, in Keys' study, was 1,640 calories a day. The deficit is a function of energy need. The energy need is a function of weight and weight is a function of the deficit. As Keys showed, the men needed 3,210 calories, on average, to maintain their weight. When the men were given 1,570 calories a day in the 'starvation period', they lost weight and their energy need fell and therefore the calorie level needed to fall to maintain the deficit. All reached a plateau around week 20 and further weight loss could not be induced. At least one diary recorded weight *gain* in the final month of the 'starvation' period.

4) The body will do whatever it takes to reverse the effects of starvation/dieting.

During the restricted rehabilitation period, the four different groups of men were given 400, 800, 1,200 or 1,600 additional calories per day. Within each group of eight men, some were also given additional vitamin and protein supplements. Keys concluded that the only thing that determined the speed at which the men recovered was the calorie intake. The body didn't respond to vitamins or protein – it just wanted the energy (calorie) deficit to be reversed.

[xviii] 3,210 calories needed minus 1,570 allowed gives a deficit of 1,640 calories a day.

It can be no surprise, therefore, that when given free access to food, in the final two months, the men overate and binged to correct the calorie deficit they had suffered. One man managed to eat 11,500 calories in one day and men still felt hungry consuming twice the number of calories that had maintained their weight in the control period. The researchers noted in the study: "Subject No. 20 stuffs himself until he is bursting at the seams, to the point of being nearly sick and still feels hungry"; "No. 1 ate until he was uncomfortably full"; and subject "No. 30 had so little control over the mechanics of 'piling it in' that he simply had to stay away from food because he could not find a point of satiation even when he was 'full to the gills'."[51]

They all gained all their weight back and approximately 10% more than they weighed before the experiment. Men who had previously shown no awareness of body size and image reported 'feeling fat'.

Surely we have just observed the pre-requisite for an obesity epidemic? Eat less, get hungry, slow the metabolism, increase the desire to consume energy, reduce the desire to expend energy, gain weight, try to eat less and so on. We have certainly just described the western world, since we started our obsession with calorie counting.

Why doesn't eat less mean weigh less?

This raises the obvious question – if we eat less than we 'need' (leaving aside 'do more' for now) – why don't we lose weight? The more obvious question for me is – why would we? The ultimate naivety in the world of dieting is that the body is a 'cash machine' for fat. The energy in and out assumption about dieting is that, if you don't put enough calories in and then try to force a requirement for energy, the body will just say "there's 100 calories – off you go". The body will use energy that is easily available, but relinquishing potentially life saving fat deposits is its last resort.

The body's first option, when faced with a calorie deficit, is to look for glucose in the blood stream. If we have recently eaten a carbohydrate, which has been converted into glucose, this will be used first. The body can also look for fatty acids available in the blood stream. If no energy is readily available, the body then has glucose stored, as glycogen, for this purpose. If we follow the current dietary advice to "base our meals on starchy foods", we will eat carbohydrates in quantity and with regularity and this should optimise our glycogen storage performance within the body. This constant intake of carbohydrate should enable us to store approximately 100 grams of glycogen in the liver and 250-400 grams in the muscles. (The glycogen in the muscles can only be used by the muscles, but the glycogen in the liver can be used wherever energy is needed by the body). Even if the regular carbohydrate eater has the lower end of 350 grams of glycogen in the body – that represents 1,400 calories available for energy. At the higher end, it represents 2,000 calories available.[xix]

[xix] Glycogen is a carbohydrate and therefore approximates to four calories per gram.

I'm curious to know at what point people who base their meals on starchy foods ever get the chance to dip into fat reserves.

In parallel with this search for energy, the body will simultaneously produce hunger signals to try to get the person to eat to recover the deficit. This alone ruins most diets. The body has many such signals to try to make us eat – shaky hands, rumbly tummy, irritability, inability to concentrate, indecisiveness and an unusually high preoccupation with food. Many people experience these symptoms at approximately 11am and 4pm on a daily basis, when their blood glucose level drops. These are the times when we most want food; our body is literally commanding us to eat.

If the body fails to find fuel to meet a calorie deficit, it will likely use lean tissue before fat (particularly if the calorie deficit becomes more prolonged). Lean tissue requires three times more calories than fat just to maintain itself, ("resting metabolic rates of skeletal muscle 13 kcal/kg per day and adipose tissue 4.5 kcal/kg per day")[52] so the body needs to 'dump' the part of it that needs the most energy. This has a direct impact on our basal metabolic rate (need for fuel), which is counterproductive for weight loss.

The final key point, which we seem to have overlooked, is that the body has the option of shutting down internal operations. It is important to note how much our daily energy requirement is determined by our basal metabolic rate (BMR). The Harris Benedict Equation can be used to estimate metabolic rate and additional energy required beyond this for differently active people.[53] An inactive person (little or no exercise) is estimated to need their BMR plus 20%; a light activity individual (exercise 1-3 days per week) is estimated to need their BMR plus 37.5%; the individual doing moderate exercise (3-5 days a week) is estimated to need their BMR plus 55% and very heavy exercise (twice a day, intense workouts) is estimated to need BMR plus 90% – even this level of activity does not double daily calorie requirement. As an example, the BMR for a 160 pound female, 5'4", aged 40 is 1,464 calories.[xx] If our average woman exercises 1-3 days per week, her overall calorie requirement is 2,013 – close to the 2,000 calories we often hear are needed by the average woman. This means that 73% of her energy requirement is determined by basal metabolic needs.

Let's keep the numbers simple and assume that this woman needs 2,000 calories per day and that 1,500 of these are for basal metabolic requirements. The energy in and out belief is that, if she consumes only 1,500 calories and then uses up 200 calories exercising, she will lose one fifth of a pound (700/3,500). This makes far too many assumptions, which are not legitimate to make. First it assumes that no compensation is made in the basal metabolic rate. Secondly it assumes that no adjustment is made to the 500 calories needed above BMR. It assumes that the calories consumed *can* be used for BMR needs – a huge and erroneous assumption if the woman is eating the per capita average for processed food. We cannot 'ring fence', 'red circle', 'protect' – whatever

---

[xx] This is the imperial version of the formula. Our same woman has a metric BMR of 1,456 calories. This is a significant difference if you believe the 3,500 formula.

terminology is meaningful for you – calories in this way. We cannot force the body to do its basic maintenance – we can only create the right environment for the body to have *no* reason *not* to do this. Given that we cannot guarantee that the body can or will use 1,500 calories for basal metabolic needs, less energy in will lead the body to cut back on these activities. The body can save cell repair, building bone density and fighting infection for another day. Exercising serves to further reduce the planned maintenance list for the body that day. Both reduced energy in, and any attempts to increase energy out, can also reduce the normal energy requirement beyond BMR (the 500 calories in this case). As we see in Chapter Fourteen, those who exercise may be tired and therefore less likely to do, say, household activities, which they otherwise would have done. The 'cash machine for fat' view also assumes that the body is able to 'un-store' fat on demand and that the biochemical environment does not matter.

Here's a simple analogy – if we lose our job and less income is coming in to the household, we don't automatically raid savings, we cut back on spending. If you go on a diet and less energy is coming in, the body doesn't automatically raid fat reserves, it cuts back on the energy it expends. The body can turn off its heating system, for example, in the same easy way that we turn off the home heating system to try to save money. I use the expression eat less and/or do more as "The General Principle", but, the advice is more typically to eat less *and* do more. The analogy works well – where is the sense in going out partying when you've lost your job. You don't even feel like partying when you've lost your job and you don't feel like going to the gym when you've had 1,000 calories of processed food. Think also of the damage done to the household if you try to do more with less coming in. We can see what happens to the human body when people try to eat less *and* do more. Just watch *The Biggest Loser* – the modern day equivalent of Gladiators.

I unwittingly did the Minnesota Starvation Experiment aged 15-16. I did not know this to be anorexia at the time, not least as this condition had only recently been defined so perfectly by Gerald Russell.[54] This gave me first hand experience of what the body will do to reduce its need for food. With reference to the nine systems of the human body, this is what happened to me within a few weeks of being on a 1,000 calorie a day diet:

1) The nervous system, my control room, slowed dramatically and it is astonishing that I managed to study for and take O-Level exams;
2) The skeletal system would have been damaged and I may suffer osteoporosis in later life from the detriment caused to my bone density at this time;
3) The endocrine system would have gone into minimal operation mode and hormone requirements would have been eased by the shutting down of ...
4) ...the reproductive system. At the age of 15 my periods stopped for two years, as my body stopped putting energy into any non-essential bodily operations. It was only after I started to gain weight (involuntarily) and my body detected that I was no longer starving that my menstrual cycle made an irregular return;

5) The digestive system also started a 'work to rule' and I recall very infrequent bowel movements, as there was so little waste to evacuate – my body needed every morsel that it could get;
6) One of the most pronounced changes that I noticed was with my circulatory system. My extremities were particularly cold and I never felt warm – even in the height of summer;
7) The dual roles of the lymphatic system, drainage of fluids and protection against infection, were obviously compromised as I was puffy, despite being skeletal and I frequently succumbed to colds and flu viruses;
8) I severely tested my urinary system and contracted regular and painful bladder and kidney infections through abuse of diuretics and mistakenly thinking that drinking less would make me weigh less;
9) My respiratory system slowed – a friend at a sleepover said that she thought I had died in the night as I just didn't seem to breathe. My pulse was rarely over 50 despite (or because of?) the fact that I was playing hockey, tennis, rounders and badminton for the school; throwing the discus for the county and swimming to lifeguard standard throughout my teens.

All the bodily systems working together ensured that I fainted regularly. This is the ultimate action that the body can take to try to shock its host into taking corrective action. I cursed these warning signs at the time, in case adults might spot them and force corrective action upon me.

1,000 calories a day is the approximate intake for more than a million people worldwide (mostly women) on 18-20 Weight Watchers points each day. That we allow this to happen is bad enough. That we are contemplating prescribing slimming clubs as a public health weight loss method, when the above describes the impact on the human body, is scandalous.

I mirrored the Minnesota experiment perfectly. I did lose weight in the short term, but in no way did this weight loss follow any mathematical formula. I lost approximately 25% of my starting weight, as the Minnesota men did, not my entire body weight twice over, as the 3,500 formula would have guaranteed. I regained it all, plus a further 20% (more than the Minnesota men, but then I did try to starve for longer). Just as happened with Keys' men, I turned from a physically and psychologically healthy person into a shell of my former self – obsessed with calories, hungry, cold, unable to concentrate or think about anything other than food. It will be invaluable for your understanding of weight loss if you have done the same, or a similar, experiment yourself.

There is a wonderful anecdote, sometimes attributed to George Bernard Shaw (GBS) and sometimes to Winston Churchill, which goes along the lines of:

GBS: "Madam, would you sleep with me for a million pounds?"
Actress: "My goodness, Well, I suppose… we would have to discuss terms, of course…"
GBS: "Would you sleep with me for a pound?"
Actress: "Certainly not! What kind of woman do you think I am?!"

GBS: "Madam, we've already established that. Now we are haggling about the price."

I share this because it has much relevance for those who believe that weight is determined by calories in and calories out. Those who believe that we need to create a calorie deficit to lose weight differ only in their view on the level of deficit. The UK National Institute for Clinical Excellence (NICE) defines very low calorie diets (VLCD) as those delivering fewer than 1,000 calories a day (some definitions of VLCD's set the bar at 800 calories a day).[55] The NICE definition for low calorie diets (LCD) is 1,000-1,600 calories a day (other sources define a LCD as 1,200 calories a day or fewer). The UK National Health Service booklet *Your weight your health* advises "eating 500 to 600 fewer calories each day than your body needs is a realistic way to lose weight. That means around 1,500 calories a day for adult women and 2,000 calories a day for adult men." So, the principle is the same – we're just haggling over the deficit.

A significant calorie deficit will likely result in short term weight loss, particularly the first time a person attempts to 'starve'. Weight loss becomes increasingly less successful with further attempts to restrict calorie intake, as the body has no intention of letting the same devastation happen twice. After any initial weight loss, calorie intake will need to be continually reduced to try to achieve further weight loss. The dieter is more likely to have to maintain a debilitating low calorie intake, not to lose more, but to avoid the seemingly unavoidable regain. If they manage this, they will be fighting hunger on a daily basis.

The anthropologist Melvin Konner acknowledged this: "There is only one way to lose weight, and that is to grow accustomed to feeling hungry."[56] Konner makes an interesting point here and one relevant to calorie restricted diets. However, it is completely unacceptable to condemn human beings to a lifetime of overweight or hunger. Both options are equally intolerable and, I believe, unnecessary.

Part Two

The Calorie Formula

Part Two

The Calorie Formula

Introduction

"How many calories are you supposed to eat if you're on a diet?" Tom said.

"About a thousand. Well I usually aim for a thousand and come in at about fifteen hundred", I said, realizing as I said it that the last bit wasn't strictly true."

"A thousand?" said Tom incredulously. "But I thought you needed two thousand just to survive."

"How many calories in a boiled egg?" Said Tom.

"Seventy- five."

"Banana?"

"Large or small?"

"Small."

"Peeled?"

"Yes."

"Eighty", I said, confidently.

"Olive?"

"Black or green?"

"Black."

"Nine."

"Hobnob?"

"Eighty-one."

"Box of Milk Tray?"

"Ten thousand, eight hundred and ninety-six."

"How do you know all this?" said Tom.

Bridget thought about it "I just do."[57] (*Bridget Jones's Diary*)

The underlying principle of eat less/do more goes hand-in-hand with a mathematical formula, which every Bridget Jones can recite on demand: "One pound of fat contains 3,500 calories, so to lose 1lb a week you need a deficit of 500 calories a day." This particular quotation comes from the British Dietetic Association's (BDA) leaflet *Want to lose weight & keep it off...?*[58]

Sometimes the concept of 'deficit' gets forgotten. The joint BBC/Welsh Assembly Government campaign *The Big Fat Problem* (2004) said: "To lose 1lb of fat per week, you need to either reduce your calorie intake by 3500 a week, or increase your exercise, or do a combination of both."[59] This then gives us the conundrum I call 'Dave': Dave needs 3,000 calories a day, but is currently eating 5,000. First, is he putting on weight at the rate of four pounds a week every week, week in week out (i.e. 208 pounds every year)? Secondly, if he reduces his intake by 1,000 calories a day – will he *lose* two pounds a week or *gain* two pounds a week?

Most surprisingly, the 'bible' of nutrition makes the same mistake. Gordon Wardlaw and Anne Smith's "Contemporary Nutrition", now on its seventh edition, states "Adipose tissue, mostly fat, contains about 3500 kcal per pound... to lose 1 pound of adipose tissue per week, calorie intake must be decreased by approximately 500 kcal per day, or physical activity must be increased by 500 kcal per day."[60]

The BUPA, *Healthy Living*, booklet does the same: "For steady, safe weight loss of around half to 1kg (1 to 2lbs) a week, aim to reduce your calorie balance by 500 to 1000 calories a day, either by eating less or burning more or, ideally, both."[61]

Sometimes the whole formula is wrong. I found the following on the UK National Health Service Weight Loss pages "To shift 900g (2lbs) a week, you need to reduce your calorie intake by around 500 calories a day." This diet must be very popular – you lose two pounds, not the usual one pound, with a 500 calorie-a-day deficit. This has since been corrected, but not before there was quite a debate in the comments below the advice with as many people thinking you would lose two pounds as those thinking you would only lose one pound with your 500 calorie a day deficit.[62]

As mentioned in Chapter Four, the National Health Service booklet *Your weight, your health* advises "eating 500 to 600 fewer calories each day than your body needs..."[63] The National Institute for Clinical Excellence (NICE) advice is to eat "about 600 calories less (sic) than your body needs to stay the same weight."[64]

The advice from the American Department of Health and Human Services is (specifically from the National Heart, Lung and Blood Institute: obesity education initiative) "A diet that is individually planned to help create a deficit of 500 to 1,000 kcal/day should be an integral part of any program aimed at achieving a weight loss of 1 to 2 pounds per week."[65]

The American Academy of Family Physicians states "A pound of fat is about 3,500 calories. To lose 1 pound of fat in a week, you have to eat 3,500 fewer calories (that is 500 fewer calories a day), or you have to 'burn off' an extra 3,500 calories."[66]

The American weight loss programme, Anne Collins, states "About 3,500 calories adds up to about 1 pound. If you eat 3,500 more calories more than your body needs, you will put on about 1 pound. If you use up 3,500 calories more than you eat, you will lose about 1 pound in weight."[67]

Even Wikipedia tells us "There are 3500 calories in 1lb (0.45kg) of body fat... if someone has a daily allowance of 2500 calories, but they reduce their intake to 2000, then the calculations show a 1 pound loss every 7 days."[68]

The absolute belief in this formula is fundamental to all official (and almost all unofficial) weight loss advice. You will struggle to find a diet book on the shelves that doesn't state this formula as fact. As often as not, the 'fact' is presented incorrectly, so, even a fact that is incorrect to start with becomes even more incorrect. Here are some examples from just a few of the diet books on my shelves:

Flat Belly Diet (p69): "It takes an excess of 3,500 calories to create 1lb of body fat. If you ate 700 more calories than your body could burn in 1 day, you'd put on 1/5th of a pound. Do that for 5 days in a row starting on a Monday, and by the end of the working week, you've accumulated 1lb of fat."[69] (You will find that you haven't).

Bikini Fit: The 4-week plan (p14): "Since 500g (1lb) of body fat is equivalent to 3,500 calories, you need to burn calories through physical activity and/or reduce the number of calories you eat for a total of 3,500 calories in order to lose 500g (1lb) of fat." (The incorrect gram to pound conversion here makes this an example of an incorrect version of an incorrect formula. One pound equals 454 grams, so 500 grams would equal 3,855 calories according to the 3,500 formula itself. The implications of this are that readers of the Bikini Fit diet book can eat 10% more than everyone else without gaining weight, but, sadly, they will need to cut back by 10% more than everyone else to lose that magical one pound).[70]

A-Z of calories (p4): "Eat 3,500 calories fewer than normal and you will lose 1lb of weight." This one is also wrong. This is the 'Dave' problem above – you can eat 3,500 calories fewer than 'normal' and still create no deficit. You can start to see very quickly that a) no one knows where this formula comes from and b) it is wrongly quoted almost as often as it is quoted.[71]

Lorraine Kelly's *Nutrition Made Easy* (p98): "If you eat 3,500 calories more than you need, they will be stored and add half a kilo (1lb) to your weight. On the other hand, burn 3,500 more calories than you eat and you'll lose half a kilo (1lb)." (Here we have the pound to kilo error again, which, according to the formula itself, would make the average woman, needing an average 2,000 calories, either 20 pounds lighter or heavier at the end of one year, depending on whether this 10% error were in her favour or against).[72]

The Little Book of Calorie Burning (p28): "...a pound is roughly 3,500 calories. So, for every kilo you want to lose, you must: eat 7,700 kcal fewer or burn 7,700 kcal by taking extra exercise or try a combination of both." (This one gets the pound to kilo conversion right, but misses the concept of deficit, so we are back to the 'Dave' conundrum).[73]

Fat Bloke Slims (p121): "It takes a deficit of 500 calories per day to burn off one pound of fat."[74] This neglects to define the time period during which this deficit needs to be maintained; it assumes that people 'know' that they need to do this every day for one week. Notwithstanding the fact that it takes a great deal more biochemistry than a simple deficit before the body will relinquish that much treasured pound of fat.

Newspapers quote the formula as complete fact in almost every calorie/weight loss article they print – and they print several. On 14 March 2010, *The Times* (UK) article "Chew on this – calorie counts on foods are too high" claimed "An extra 20 calories a day can lead to an annual weight gain of 2lb." Just four days later, the UK *Daily Mail* ran an article "The tweaks to your diet that could transform your life". The article stated "Halving the quantity of rice can cut calorie intake by 200 calories (400 calories for a generous 250g portion of rice compared with 200 for a more modest portion). Do this once a day and within two weeks you should have cut out enough calories (nearly 3,000) to lose a pound of hard-to shift body fat. "

Television, also, uses the formula as a fact. The Endemol programme *Larger than Life: 33,000 calories a day*, first aired on 13 December 2009, was a documentary about four morbidly obese people – Paul, Larry, Lisa and Jacqui. Larry was eating 14,349 calories a day (such a precise number). The narrator (Samantha Bond) quoted the usual statement that the average man needs 2,500 calories a day. Dr. Ian Campbell, former head of the UK National Obesity Forum, estimated that Larry needed about 4-4,500 calories a day "and so that extra 10,000 calories a day would equate to three pounds of weight gain on a daily basis." The unproven calorie formula was applied directly as if fact without even being quoted. Dr. Campbell has divided 10,000 by 3,500 to get (approximately) three pounds and has assumed that every excess of 3,500 will gain one pound (in fat alone – we are forgetting water and lean tissue for now).

"We eat too many calories. Each day an average man should eat 2500 calories. A woman should eat no more than 2000. But just 500 calories a day over that limit can increase our weight by a pound a week." This was one of the opening statements in the ITV A Tonight Special programme *The World's Best Diet.*[75] The programme, in turn, quoted their source as NHS Direct. I have been involved in the research for a Channel 4 (UK) programme and the rigour with which facts are checked is impressive. However, if a government source provides a piece of information it is taken as fact. The problem is that, as we will see in Chapter Seven, our governments use this formula without knowing from whence it came or being able to prove its validity.

The chair of the National Obesity Forum, Dr. David Haslam has written a book with Terry Maguire called *The Obesity Epidemic and its management.*[76] The following quotation can be found on p149: "From national surveys, it has been shown that English activity patterns have fallen in recent decades and, even though overall dietary calories have also fallen, there is an average net gain of 15 kcals per day. Over a week this is over 100 kcal; in a month is it 400 kcal; in a year 4800 kcal; in 10 years 48,000 kcal, all of which can translate into an increase in weight of approximately 1 stone". This is quite possibly the most ludicrous literal application of the formula that I have seen. This relies absolutely on energy in exactly equalling energy out. No entropy, no energy used by the body in making available energy or energy lost in the open system. No difference in protein calories vs. carbohydrate calories. It also relies on a human body being able to discern calorie intake to a fraction of one percent accuracy every day for 10 years (from both energy in and out). Woe betide the person who slips pouring the porridge oats each morning and adds 15 calories to the daily intake, or the person who makes one fewer trip upstairs, thereby missing out on the opportunity to burn a handful of calories. Even if you believe such nonsense, you would have to allow for the person needing more energy as they gained weight and therefore the 15 'extra' calories becoming 14, 13, 12 etc over time and then see where the circular reference calculation takes you. If this weren't so serious, it would actually be quite funny.

If you do an internet search on "how to lose weight" or "3,500 calories", you will be overwhelmed with results. Find your own 'expert comment', boldly asserted with no backup whatsoever. My personal favourite is *Binch – Cool Cruiser's* message board comment (Aug 2008): "Why is 3,500 calories = 1lb of fat so hard for many to understand? This is really basic math…"[77] OK Binch, let's see how the 'math' holds up over the following pages…

What is a calorie?

The definition of a calorie is "The amount of energy required to raise the temperature of 1 gram of water from 14.5°C to 15.5°C, at standard atmospheric pressure." For the famous Bunsen burner experiment, in school science lessons, we were able to measure the rise in water temperature and determine that a standard peanut contains approximately two calories.

The Système international, developed in 1960, should have rendered the use of the term calorie redundant. However, worldwide adoption of the standard metric system of measurement has two important exceptions – the United States and the United Kingdom. The USA, Burma and Liberia have not adopted the metric measurement system at all. The UK has officially adopted the metric system, but imperial measurements, such as pound, pint, gallon and mile, for example, are still very commonly used.

The definition of the calorie above is, strictly speaking, the definition for the "gram calorie". The definition for the "kilogram calorie" is the amount of energy required to raise the temperature of one kilogram of water by one degree Celsius. The Kilogram calorie is also known as: the large calorie; a food calorie and/or Calorie with a capital C.

When calories are used in nutrition, and especially in food labelling, they are, strictly speaking, 'large calories', i.e. kilo calories, denoted by kcal as an abbreviation. However, the word kilo is invariably dropped to avoid confusion with kiloJoules and that just returns us to the word calorie.

The definition of a kiloJoule (kJ), as used in the context of food energy, is the amount of solar radiation received by one square meter of the earth in one second. One kiloJoule is 1,000 Joules. The kiloJoule is the unit officially recommended by the World Health Organisation and other international organisations. In some countries only the kiloJoule is found on food packaging, but the calorie is still the most common unit in many countries and in almost every diet book.

One kilocalorie (kcal) is approximately equal to 4.1868 kiloJoules (kJ). The example I have readily to hand is a 100 gram bar of 90% cocoa dark chocolate. The label says that this has 580kcal and 2,400kJ, which gives a conversion of 4.1379 – close enough considering likely rounding to both 580kcal and 2,400kJ.

The notes above give the text book position on calories, kilocalorie, joules and kiloJoules. Throughout this book I will simply use the word "calorie", which should strictly be 'large calorie', but Bridget Jones and I know what we mean. The simple word calorie is also the term used in "The Calorie Formula", which we have got so badly wrong.

The Calorie Formula" (also known as the calorie theory) states "One pound of fat contains 3,500 calories, so to lose 1lb a week you need a deficit of 500 calories a day." (British Dietetic Association).

There are three errors with this:

1) One pound of fat does not equal 3,500 calories;
2) The body is not a Bunsen burner;
3) There is no evidence that a repeated deficit of 3,500 calories will lead to a loss of one pound of fat. Equally there is no evidence that a repeated excess of 3,500 calories will lead to a gain of one pound of fat.

Let us look at each of these in turn.

Chapter Five

What is one pound of fat?

Introduction

The first part of the calorie formula is the assertion that one pound of fat contains 3,500 calories. You will struggle to find anyone who can demonstrate the precise calculation behind this, so I have sourced the following to get as close as possible to 3,500 calories:

1) One pound equals 454 grams (decimal places aside, this is a fact);
2) Fat has nine calories per gram (this is the universally accepted conversion, but it is an estimate and materially rounded down from even the original estimate);
3) Human fat tissue is approximately 87% lipid (this is a widely accepted conversion, but it is also an estimate).

Putting these together, we can derive the sum that 454 grams of body fat tissue has *approximately* the calorific energy of 395 grams of pure fat (454 grams x 87%), that is 3,555 calories (395 grams x 9).

3,555 is close enough to 3,500 you may think, until you see the absurdity of how precisely the formula is applied. According to those who believe this formula, this difference of 55 calories (in this case from the calculation being approximate) would make five to six pounds difference a year. The National Obesity Forum web site states "one less (sic) 50 calorie plain biscuit per day could help you lose 5lbs (2.3kg) in a year – and one extra biscuit means you could gain that in a year!"[78] No it won't. I can't even get an estimate of the formula to closer than 55 calories 'out'. Even if the 3,555 were correct (and it isn't), this would mean we all need a 55 calorie biscuit, no fewer, every day or we will be five pounds lighter in a year anyway. Every person who *didn't* have that biscuit every day should have lost 141 pounds over the past 25 years.

The only part of the calculation, which is not subject to question, is one pound equals 454 grams. The decimal places on the pound to gram conversion would make a difference over time, if the rest had any validity. The other two components, being estimates within wide ranges, negate the entire calculation. This variability has also been known all along – it is not something that has been discovered since, or questioned since (with the Livesey exception noted below).

The original calorie estimates for different macronutrients are generally credited to the American chemist, Wilbur Olin Atwater and the German physiologist, Max Rubner. (It is interesting to make connections with other great scientists, as both were also working with Francis Benedict and Carl Voit at this time). In 1901, carbohydrate, protein and fat were estimated to have 4.1, 4.1 and 9.3 calories per gram respectively[79]. (Rubner recorded the calorific value for olive oil as 9.4, so even his 9.3 was an average of four fats reviewed). This has never been a precise science.

The 1911 article by Bozenraad[80] is the seminal work for the estimation of the lipid content of human fat tissue. This German article registered the fat content of adipose tissue as being anywhere from 72% to 87%, so the widely used number is the top point of the original range.

Dr. Geoffrey Livesey has estimated that fat has 8.7 calories per gram.[81] Back in 2002, the United Nations Food and Agriculture Organization (FAO) assembled an international group of nutritionists, including Livesey, to investigate the possibility of recommending a change to food labelling standards to update the four, four and nine calories attributed to carbohydrate, protein and fat respectively. The group, with the exception of Livesey, decided to stick with the long-standing values because, the report concluded, "the problems and burdens ensuing from such a change would appear to outweigh by far the benefits".[82] I would have supported Livesey, but with the recommendation that he go way further and challenge the entire application of these estimates.

(Please note that, if we do adopt Livesey's work, we would need to take care with double counting if we separately allow for entropy. In large part, Livesey's work is an attempt to adjust the approximate calorie estimates, for different macronutrients, by accounting for energy used up by the body in making available energy. I welcome the day we may have the dilemma of having considered entropy twice, rather than not at all).

Max Wishnofsky (1958) set out to understand how many excess calories would produce a gain of one pound of weight and, conversely, what caloric deficit would determine a loss of one pound of body fat.[83] There is some interesting information in this brief article on the role of nitrogen equilibrium, as a guide for whether lean tissue or fat is being lost. However, the relevant content of this obesity journal, for our current discussion, is Wishnofsky's estimate that fat has 9.5 calories per gram. Indeed, his second paragraph states "It was shown by Bozenraad that the average fat content of human adipose tissue taken from various parts of the bodies of well nourished subjects is 87 per cent. One pound (454 grams) of human adipose tissue, therefore, contains 395 grams of fat. The caloric value of one gram of animal fat is 9.5; consequently, the caloric equivalent of one pound of human adipose tissue may be considered to be about 3,750 cal."

I have calculated the range of options, from the values I have seen in journals, using both the variation in calories for fat and lipid content of adipose tissue. It is important to note that there could be even wider variations in other journals, but the ones that I have found (with moderate effort) will suffice to make my point.

Taking one extreme, the lower (Livesey) estimate of the calories in a gram of fat and the lower (Bozenraad) estimate of the lipid content of fat tissue; one pound of human fat would then equal 454 grams, at 8.7 calories, multiplied by 72% i.e. 2,843 calories.

At the other extreme, the higher (Wishnofsky) estimate of the calories in a gram of fat and the higher estimate of the lipid content of fat tissue is calculated exactly as shown by Wishnofsky, giving a precise number of 3,752 calories. The latter is more likely the number to which we should have been referring for the past century. The Rubner estimates were much closer to 9.5 than 9.0 and, for some reason I know not, the top end of the Bozenraad range has been the accepted number for adipose tissue.

So, using just a couple of the alternatives for each of the two variables underpinning the 3,500 number, we have established a range whereby one pound of fat could contain anywhere between 2,843 and 3,752 calories. Given that it is currently held that one pound is 3,500 calories we could (according to this formula) inadvertently gain six stone every year at the low end of the calculation and lose almost two stone in the same year if one pound is 3,752 calories.[xxi]

You will find numerous examples in government literature, books and media articles where people try to apply this mathematical formula to the letter. Brian Wansink's book *Mindless eating: why we eat more than we think* was featured in a National newspaper article in the UK in September 2009. Brian was quoted as saying "Just ten extra calories a day – one stick of gum or three jelly beans – will make you a pound heavier in a year. And 140 calories a day – or one can of soft drink - will make you put on a stone. And you won't even notice." No it won't. The formula would have to be perfectly accurate for even the first part of the calorie theory to hold true. (We've got two more errors to review).

Please take a moment just to reflect on how completely and utterly nonsensical this formula is and to ask yourself if you have ever challenged its validity or accepted it as fact, as it has been so widely quoted. (No criticism or blame is intended here – I kick myself for not blowing this formula apart over 20 years ago, when I should have realised, as an anorexic teenager, that I would be dead if it did work). The key thing is what we do now that we know it is untrue. We need to stop quoting it anywhere, let alone widely. It does not even hold at the first hurdle.

Let us move on to the second error.

[xxi] This calculation is done as follows: It assumes that a person can maintain weight at a daily intake of the calories assumed to equal one pound of fat. If we think one pound equals 3,500 calories and in fact one pound equals 2,843 calories, over a year, 657 'extra' calories a day, simply from the formula 'being wrong', would add up to 239,805 extra calories and this, divided by 2,843 gives 84 pounds, or six stone. Adjust the calculations for women more typically maintaining at 2,000 calories a day and men more typically at 2,600 calories a day and the inaccuracy of the formula still creates wide disparity.

Chapter Six

Where does the calorie formula come from?

Introduction

I am still trying to find the earliest reference to the 3,500 formula and then to trace it through to when it became 'folklore'. To date, I have found a book called *Diet and Health* by Lulu Hunt Peters (1918).[84] Hunt Peters states "Five hundred Calories equal approximately 2 ounces of fat. Two ounces per day would be about 4 pounds per month, or 48 pounds per year. Cutting out 1000 Calories per day would equal a reduction of approximately 8 pounds per month, or 96 pounds per year."

An article from the *Chicago Daily Tribune* (Sept 15, 1959) asserts "a pound of fat is lost whenever the body burns up 3,500 calories by diet or exercise".[85] The way that this is asserted, suggests that it is already a well known 'fact' by this date, but did Hunt Peters start it or perpetuate it?

A couple of extracts in *Diet and Health* make me think that it is entirely plausible that Hunt Peters did effectively originate "The Calorie Formula":

1) On the opening page, Hunt Peters says: "I am sorry I cannot devise a key by which to read this book, as well as a Key to the Calories, for sometimes you are to read the title headings and side explanations before the text. Other times you are supposed to read the text and then the headings. It really does not matter much as long as you read them both. Be sure to do that. They are clever. *I wrote them myself.*" (Hunt Peters own emphasis in italics).

2) Chapter 2 "Key to the calories" has the following: [Sidenote: *Pronounced Kal'-o-ri*]. So calories were so little known at the time, that Hunt Peters needed to tell people how to pronounce them. If only we had stayed so blissfully ignorant about calories, or at least had come to see them as fuel for the body – which is all that they are.

If Hunt Peters had the right to be proud of her 'cleverness' and if she really did break something revolutionary to the women of Los Angeles in 1918, we may indeed have one woman to 'thank' for "The Calorie Formula", which is the foundation of weight loss advice to date. If anyone else knows of a reference earlier than 1918, I would be most interested for research sake, but it actually matters less from where this originated and more that it has held as 'fact' for at least 90 years and yet it cannot be proven to hold true.

There are a couple of obesity journal articles that have been cited as proof of the 3,500 calorie formula. The earliest and probably most well known is the Newburgh and Johnston article *The Nature of Obesity* (1930).[86] Newburgh and

Johnston sum up by saying "In conclusion we wish to commit ourselves to the statement that obesity is *never* directly caused by abnormal metabolism but that it is *always* due to food habits not adjusted to the metabolic requirement – either the ingestion of more food than is normally needed or the failure to reduce the intake in response to a lowered requirement." I have italicised the words 'never' and 'always', as they are strong words. I am trying to conceive of the circumstances in which I would use such strong words. What led Newburgh and Johnston to be so convinced that they had found the complete answer to the problem of obesity?

The article is not long – approximately 3,000 words (p197-212 of an A5 size journal). It is quite difficult to read, not least because the language of 80 years ago differs to terminology used today. For example, "undernutrition" is taken to mean giving someone fewer calories than they need and "insensible loss" is a crude measure of entropy (the difference between the weight of the subject at the start of a 24 hour period and their weight at the end, allowing for the weight of food and water in and out).

The opening statement in the article is "The medical profession in general, believes that there are two kinds of obese persons – those who have become fat because they overeat or under-exercise; and those composing a second group whose adiposity is not closely related to diet, but is caused by an endocrine or constitutional abnormality." Newburgh and Johnston refer to the arguments in the second 'camp' as "endogenous obesity" – obesity caused by something within the body – rather than anything to do with energy going in and out.

The article then proceeds with two approaches – on the one hand it tries to dismiss any evidence for "endogenous obesity" and, on the other hand, it tries to present evidence that energy in and energy out can exactly be reconciled.

The dismissal of "endogenous obesity" is superficial and illogical. In just three pages of A5, Newburgh and Johnston present and claim to have knocked down the following three theories for "endogenous obesity":

1) Theory 1: Some obese persons have an abnormally low basal metabolic rate. The dismissal here was the illogical claim that "many persons of normal stature show abnormally low metabolic rates". Many people of normal weight may indeed have low metabolic rates, but that doesn't mean that an overweight person can't have a low metabolic rate.

2) Theory 2: Some obese people metabolise food less efficiently. The dismissal was as follows: "Our prolonged study of this question has convinced us that the inherent error in the method to date, when it is applied to the human subject, is such that it precludes the possibility of making quantitative statements regarding the specific dynamic response to food in man." This can be interpreted as – we can't study this to reach an accurate conclusion, so we will dismiss it as an argument anyway.

3) Theory 3: Some writers think that the body cells don't allow fat to be broken down in a way that helps the obese person lose weight. The dismissal for this third and final case for "endogenous obesity" was:

a) "...the well known fall in basal metabolic rate caused by undernutrition in the normal subject often fails to occur in the type of obesity under consideration" and
b) "the obese subject uses more energy to perform a given piece of work than does the normal person."

In (a) Newburgh and Johnston seem to be saying that reducing calories leads to a fall in the metabolic rate of 'a normal' person, but that this often fails to occur in an overweight person. Benedict had already refuted this by 1917, but this is still illogical as an argument. (b) has never been in dispute to the best of my knowledge – larger people need more energy to perform the same task as smaller people. I find the logic most strange – whether or not (a) or (b) are valid, they both seem irrelevant in the context of the body breaking down adipose tissue. Newburgh and Johnston seem to be saying that larger people need more energy and this energy requirement doesn't seem to lessen if they eat less and therefore there is no reason why they should not use up fat reserves, but this is completely missing the point. Fat requires certain biochemical circumstances for its breakdown and any person, overweight or 'normal', who has carbohydrate/glucose/insulin present in the body will not be in a fat break down environment. Newburgh and Johnston are to be forgiven for this not being fully known at the time, but we should not take this article as presenting any evidence that the 3,500 calorie formula holds.

The conclusion of this part of the article is worth quoting, not least because it will jar in our politically correct world: "These considerations lead to the conclusion that the fundamental cause of endogenous obesity is not to be found in some type of metabolic aberration; but rather, that these individuals, in common with all obese persons, are the victims of a perverted appetite. In normal people there is a mechanism that maintains an accurate balance between the outgo and the income of energy. All obese persons are, alike in one fundamental respect, – they literally overeat." i.e. fatties are abnormal, perverted and greedy.

The next bit is the key part of the article – having 'dismissed' the only three cases for "endogenous obesity", which Newburgh and Johnston proposed in the first place, they go on to look at energy in and energy out. Two pages are devoted to working out the basal metabolic rate in their subject – something we take for granted in being able to calculate nowadays.

For their first experiment, Newburgh and Johnston used one of their lab staff as a guinea pig and the experiment was conducted over five days. They recorded the man's weight in grams (56,815) at the start of the experiment (125 pounds). He stayed in bed during the experiment – except to urinate and defecate – both of which he did into containers, so that bodily outputs could be weighed and analysed. Body inputs were 1,078 calories – made up of 63 grams of protein, 26 grams of fat and 148 grams of carbohydrate (this assumes, not unreasonably at the time, that carbohydrate and protein were four calories per gram and fat nine). The diet consisted solely of milk, sugar and water. Newburgh and Johnston calculated that the total calories used by the man averaged 1,688 for each day. They analysed, to the gram, food and water in, urine and excretions out, and calculated what the basal metabolic energy expenditure should have been, with the conclusion that the man should have lost 95 grams daily. Can you believe that they go on to report "He gained 115 grams in 5 days instead of losing 475 grams"?

Undeterred by this, Newburgh and Johnston went on to examine a handful of other subjects for no more than 27 days (most for just nine days) and concluded that "We found that departures from the predicted weight were always accounted for by storage or loss of water." So, work out what a person should lose on the basis of the calorie formula and then any deviations from this should be explained by water retention and/or water loss. This begs the question – are we trying to see if a formula is valid or assume that it is and then find reasons to explain when it isn't.

The critical bits of the article are the following two quotations:

- "It is a relatively simple matter to cause either variety of weight curve. If it is desired to have the subject, whether normal or obese, lose weight regularly day after day, he is fed a diet whose calorific value is less than the energy used by him, but containing an abundance of carbohydrate. When the intention is to obtain a plateau in the weight curve, a diet is fed that not only yields less than the maintenance calories but is also poor in carbohydrate. (NB – for 'poor' read 'low') This restriction of the dietary carbohydrate will cause the organism to deplete its store of liver glycogen and will inevitably cause a rapid loss of weight." (This is surely an error – in successive sentences a low carbohydrate diet is assumed to produce both a plateau and rapid weight loss).
- Newburgh and Johnston go on to say "When an individual is undernourished, the shape of the weight curve is determined by the quality of the diet, and is in no sense dependent upon the constitutional or endocrinal state of the individual."

They have categorically stated that *what* a person eats is of critical importance to weight loss and not how much a person eats. However, Newburgh and Johnston don't present this as their conclusion. They conclude instead "Our evidence leads to the generalization that obesity is always caused by an inflow of energy that is greater than the outflow".

I spent quite a bit of time on this article, as it is seen as the first proof of the 3,500 calorie formula and hopefully I have shared enough (I could share more) to illustrate that it did far from prove this. There is anecdotal evidence (not least in Montignac[87]) that Newburgh and Johnston were quite concerned at how literally their article was taken as proof of a mathematical formula for weight loss. They should not have used such strident language as *always* and *never* had they not wanted this article to be taken so literally.

Proof of the assertion "if you create a deficit of 3,500 calories you *will* lose one pound of fat" requires a seriously high level of evidence. It needs to happen each and every time a deficit of 3,500 calories is created – no matter the gender, the weight of the person to start with, what calories are eaten and it needs to hold time after time after time. This is a straight line formula, which needs to hold for me going from 110 pounds to just six pounds by cutting 1,000 calories a day for precisely one year. We will see just how much evidence there is for this formula in the next chapter.

Let us return to Hunt Peters now, as the earliest proponent of the 3,500 formula that I have found. Reading the simplicity of her assertion, one can surmise that it has been assumed that, if a pound of human fat placed under a Bunsen burner did yield 3,500 calories (notwithstanding the fact that it doesn't) then, if a human needs 3,500 calories (because a deficit has been created) it will burn one pound of fat, just as if the fat were placed under the Bunsen burner. The mantra 'energy in equals energy out' (the misapplication of thermodynamics to the human body) would suggest that the whole theory may indeed be based on the idea that a body will behave exactly like a Bunsen burner. Forget the nine systems of the human body, not least the digestive system and the endocrine system, just pop to the shops and 100 calories come off your love handles. Please someone tell me that there is more evidence than this? Could any assertion possibly be more naïve?

If we burn a peanut under a Bunsen burner, the only available energy comes from the peanut. If we deprive the body of energy, we don't have a packet of peanuts sat inside us to release two calories every time we need two calories. The body has a choice from where to get energy and, possibly even more critically, as we saw in Chapter Four, the body also has the option of reducing the need for energy – neither of these options are replicated with the Bunsen burner experiment.

In Chapter Two, we noted the work of Richard Feinman and Eugene Fine, our Biochemist and Nuclear Physicist respectively. They took their analysis of thermogenesis further, and analysed each amino acid, within the highly thermogenic category of protein, and the various pathways of macronutrient conversion into the body's energy currency, Adenosine TriPhosphate (ATP).[88] Feinman and Fine demonstrated that there was up to 27% energy loss in converting, as an example, amino acids to protein and back. (They note that higher inefficiencies have been found in other studies). They don't mention Bunsen burners, but they go to the heart of this issue when they say "1g carbohydrate =4 kcal; 1g fat = 9kcal, these relations only apply to the reaction with oxygen...if an ingested macronutrient undergoes some other reaction in vivo, e.g. conversion from amino acid to carbohydrate, or multiple metabolic cycles before oxidation, then calories cannot be directly substituted for mass."

To put this into terms that we can all understand: I can eat a banana and use the glucose available for energy immediately. I can eat a banana and not need the energy immediately; I can eat a banana and need some of it immediately and use up some energy converting the rest for storage for later on. The banana may be turned into glycogen and I may need this later on. Or the banana may be turned into glycogen and I don't need it, so it can be turned into triglyceride. This may get stored as fat, or I may need fat for energy (if I have no glucose or glycogen available at some stage) and then the fat cycling in and out of fat cells can become available and I can burn this for fuel. There are virtually infinite combinations of pathways that a simple banana can take within the human body. At every stage, energy is being used up in storing or making available energy and the body has different needs and energy options continuously.

Then imagine what would happen if I ate the following: Water, sugar, glucose fructose syrup, skimmed milk powder, wheat flour, glucose powder, cocoa powder (2%), fructose syrup, milk chocolate (1.5%, sugar, cocoa butter, whole milk powder, cocoa mass, emulsifier – soya lecithin, natural flavouring), whey powder, inulin, chocolate (1%, cocoa mass, sugar, cocoa butter, emulsifier – soya lecithin, natural flavouring), vegetable oil, white chocolate (1%, sugar, cocoa butter, whole milk powder, whey powder, milk sugar, emulsifier – soya lecithin, natural flavouring), chocolate (1%, cocoa mass, sugar, cocoa butter, butter oil, emulsifier – soya lecithin, natural flavouring), dextrose, chocolate (1%, cocoa mass, sugar, cocoa butter, fat reduced cocoa powder, emulsifier – soya lecithin), stabilisers – pork gelatine, locust bean gum, guar gum, sodium alginate, carrageenan, xanthan gum, sorbitol syrup, egg powder, modified potato starch, barley starch, egg albumen, gelling agent pectin, natural flavourings.

There is no accidental repetition here. This really is the full list of ingredients for Weight Watchers Double Chocolate Brownies.[89] Only 163 calories and three points; with all three macronutrients, and one of the worst ingredient lists I have come across. Would a biochemist like to work out how many different pathways could be set in motion with this "Rich chocolate brownie with an indulgent Belgian chocolate & vanilla mousse, oozing chocolate sauce?"

And we think that energy in equals energy out.

Chapter Seven

Is the calorie formula true?

Evidence on weight loss from obesity journals

Benedict (1917) is believed to be the first to look at weight lost under calorie restriction.[90] He put 12 young men on diets of approximately 1,400-2,100 calories a day with the goal of lowering their body weight by 10% in one month. Their diets were then adjusted to maintain the lower weight for another two months. The men reported hunger, extreme cold and their energy expenditure dropped so dramatically that, if they consumed more than 2,100 calories a day (a third less than they had been eating) they put on weight. The men then overate and regained all the weight lost in less than two weeks. Within another three weeks they had gained, on average, eight pounds more.

James Strang and Frank Evans (1928) observed that obese patients get hungry on calorie restriction diets and their energy expenditure "diminishes proportionately much more than the weight".[91]

As we saw in Chapter Four, the Keys' (1944) Minnesota Starvation experiment is the most comprehensive study ever undertaken and the best documented evidence for the futility of calorie controlled diets.[92] Even after the definitive Keys' study, researchers continued to study the effect of low calorie diets on obesity.

Having reviewed the literature from the first half of the twentieth century and having done their own study Stunkard and McLaren-Hume (1959) concluded "Most obese persons will not stay in treatment for obesity. Of those who stay in treatment, most will not lose weight, and of those who do lose weight, most will regain it."[93] Stunkard and McLaren-Hume's own statistical study showed that only 12% of obese patients lost 20 pounds, despite having stones to lose, only one person in 100 lost 40 pounds and, two years later, only 2% of patients had maintained a 20 pound weight loss. This is where the often quoted "98% of diets fail" derives from.

By 1970, the outcomes of such experiments were so well known that George Bray entitled his journal article "The myth of diet in the management of obesity."[94] Bray referred to the Stunkard and McLaren-Hume study, amongst a number of other studies, and reached the logical conclusion: "If there was an effective diet, there would be no need for the continuous introduction of new diets: the 'Grapefruit diet,' the 'Drinking Man's diet,' 'the "Air Force diet,' the 'Mayo diet,' the 'Quick Weight Loss diet,' and so on. It seems obvious from the number of diets that have been made available and are continuing to appear, none of them provides the answer to obesity." Bray concluded, "Unfortunately, for the obese patient each new diet produces its temporary weight loss, but this is usually followed by a relapse, with weight returning to the same or higher levels."

Such insight did nothing to deter the interest in obesity. If you search pubmed.org alone, for "obesity", for the dates from the time of George Bray's article to the present day, there have been 126,982 further articles on this topic.[95] Rudolph Leibel et al opened their 1995 article with the statement "No current treatment for obesity reliably sustains weight loss."[96] Leibel et al found that restricting calories (for lean or obese people) resulted in a disproportionate reduction in energy expenditure and metabolic activity. Increasing calorie intake resulted in disproportionate increases in energy expenditure and metabolic activity.

Jules Hirsch worked on obesity for over 30 years leading him to conclude "Of all the damn unsuccessful treatments, the treatment of weight reduction by diet for obese people just doesn't seem to work."[97] For as long as we continue to think that energy in equals energy out and that we must, therefore, reduce energy in and/or increase energy out, this despair will prevail.

Why, 50 years later, are we still advocating low-calorie, low-fat diets as the solution for obesity and, worse than this, as the *only* solution for obesity? (Weight loss pills, bariatric surgery and slimming clubs all share the same aim of trying to get the person to eat fewer calories). I simply cannot understand why we are focusing all hope in resolving the obesity epidemic on the calorie theory, when we have known for so long that it won't help us. We have clever minds working on experiments such as – do people eat less at lunch if they have an apple or apple juice half an hour beforehand.[98] It doesn't matter. Even if we can get those people to eat less, we have known since 1917 how quickly and easily any calorie deficit will increase a person's desire for energy and reduce their propensity to expend energy.

The Stunkard and McLaren-Hume review was effectively updated in 2007. There is an excellent and exceptionally useful review presented in the *Journal of the American Dietetic Association* (2007).[99] Marion Franz and seven colleagues performed a systematic review of 80 weight loss studies, grouped into eight different categories, including only those trials with a one-year follow-up. The studies were all from the period January 1997 and September 2004. 26,455 participants were enrolled in the studies. At the one-year follow-up, the attrition rate was 29% across the studies. Overall attrition was 31% at study end regardless of follow-up timing.

The eight categories were (the number of studies in each category is noted in brackets): advice alone (28); exercise alone (4); diet alone (21); meal replacements (7); diet & exercise (17); very low energy diets (11); orlistat (13) and sibutramine (7). (The 28 studies for advice alone were not counted as part of the 80 studies, as they represented the baseline).

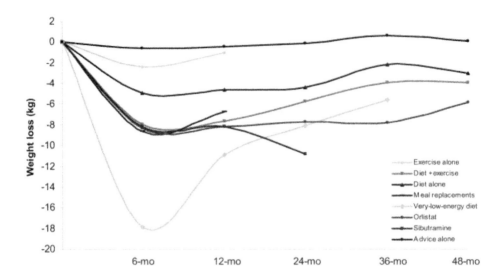

Figure 2. Average weight loss of subjects completing a minimum 1-year weight management intervention; based on review of 80 studies (n=26,455; 18,199 completers).

The original chart is in colour, making the eight interventions easier to distinguish. In Figure 2, reproduced with kind permission from Elsevier: the top line is advice alone; the second pale line, ending at 12 months, is exercise alone; the next line down is diet alone; the darker line ending at 12 months is meal replacements; the line that continues to 48 months, and is third of the four lines at 48 months, is diet & exercise; the line that dips to minus 17.9 kilograms at six months is the very low energy diets; the final line that continues to 48 months is orlistat and the only line ostensibly moving down at 24 months is sibutramine.

Before you rush out to get sibutramine, which traded as Reductil (amongst other names), please note that it was withdrawn under a European Medicines Agency directive on 21 January 2010.[100] Following concerns about the risk of cardiovascular events, such as heart attack, stroke and cardiac arrest, the SCOUT study (Sibutramine Cardiovascular Outcome Trial) was started in 2002. Approximately 9,800 patients were followed up over six years with the conclusion that the increased risk of serious cardiovascular events was not outweighed by the "modest" weight loss achieved – two to four kilograms more than with the placebo. It should also be noted in Figure 2 that only one of the seven sibutramine studies had data at 24 months, so the apparent 'bucked trend' is a data point for one study, which recorded weight loss at 6 and 12 months as 12 kilograms, so this was a regain for that study.[101]

The conclusion of the Franz review was: "A mean weight loss of 5 to 8.5kg was observed during the first 6 months from interventions involving a reduced-energy diet and/or weight loss medications with weight plateaus at approximately 6 months. In studies extending to 48 months, a mean 3 to 6kg of weight loss was maintained with none of the groups experiencing weight regain to baseline."

I first saw this graph presented by Nick Finer at the Wales National Obesity Forum conference in May 2010. The pessimistic, but realistic, conclusion was that such interventions would at best set the weight gain curve back a few years. At some point, the baseline would be 'broken through' and the dieter would merely reach a higher weight a few years later than without intervention. Finer also noted that the real baseline was not 'advice alone', but weight gain, if no weight loss interventions are made. So, you need a calorie restricted weight loss intervention not because you will lose weight, but to delay inevitable weight gain. No wonder the professional obesity world has all but given up on adults and is trying to prevent childhood obesity instead. (Any overweight readers – please do not despair at this stage – there is an alternative to starving to stand still).

USA adults alone spend more than $50 billion per year on weight loss efforts.[102] The expectations were well noted in the article: Women participating in a weight loss programme reported their goal weight as an average 32% reduction in body weight. The actual results quantified by Franz et al were closer to one tenth of this and the facts show that reduced energy diets will result in plateau and then regain at six months and therefore maintenance should be the goal at this stage. The article notes "health care professionals and participants often express frustration believing that if a reduced energy intake is maintained (or decreased even further as was done in some studies), weight loss should continue. This appears not to happen... (and) ...if weight-loss interventions are discontinued, weight regain is likely to occur."

How many dieters know that these are the facts for 'eat less/do more' weight loss interventions? To be fair, the expectations of substantially higher weight loss are not unreasonable. Dieters have been promised such weight loss by the 3,500 calorie formula.

In Figure 3, I have reproduced the Franz chart and added on the straight line weight loss promise of the calorie formula. There is a kink in the line because the horizontal axis is not uniform – with the distance between 0 and 6 months the same as that between 12 and 24 months. However, you can see quite clearly the promise that the person on a 1,000 calorie deficit will be 23.6 kilograms lower at six months, 47.2 kilograms lower at 12 months and 188.8 kilograms lower at four years. And this is all about fat alone – not weight. If the lipid content of adipose tissue is 87%, we can add approximately 13% on top of this, resulting in a loss of over 213 kilograms (470 pounds) at the four year interval.

In my experience of working with people desperate to lose weight, two pounds a week is the *minimum* they expect to lose, not about a fiftieth of what they might lose after four years. One patient said to me "With nearly half my current weight to lose, I can't cope with two pounds a week". Why was I the first person to be honest and tell this 60 year old woman that, if she lost two pounds a week, week in week out (in fat alone) until she reached target weight, she would be the first person in the world ever to do so.

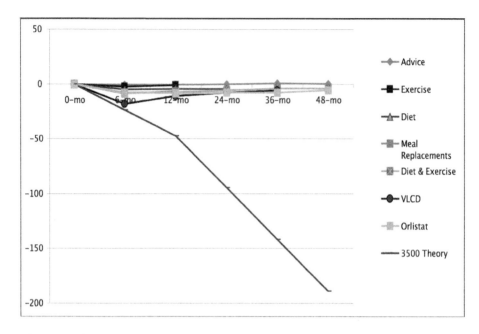

Figure 3: The 'promise' made by the calorie formula.

To see for yourself, even more dramatically, the promise made by the calorie formula, please get two sides of A4 paper and lay them below Figure 2. Please extend the Y-Axis to scale going down as far as minus 220 kilos (you will need both sheets) and then plot where the calorie formula says that the 1,000 calorie a day deficit person will be, either for fat alone and/or with some allowance for lean tissue/water. Figure 3 (for fat alone) doesn't have quite the impact that your A4 sheets of paper will have.

This Franz study should be taught in school and should be on the front page of newspapers worldwide. Would people be so blasé about weight gain if they knew how difficult it was to lose? Early in 2008 I saw a facilitator whom I had not seen for some time. He raised the subject of his noticeable weight gain by saying that he had gone to his native Australia for Christmas and New Year and had decided to 'go wild', on the basis that he would lose any weight gained when he returned to the UK. He was discovering how difficult that was to do. Sustained weight loss is probably the biggest challenge that the human body can face. The body is hard wired to both store fat and conserve energy and, ironically, our current diet advice facilitates both of these beautifully.

Evidence on weight gain

Just as every calorie reduction experiment has disproved the 3,500 formula, so calorie increase experiments have done the same. The 1967 Vermont Prison experiment showed that overfeeding sedentary prisoners up to 10,000 calories a day could not induce anywhere near 'predicted' weight increase.[103] The January 2009 BBC Horizon programme, *Why are thin people not fat?* similarly failed to validate any predictable relationship, let alone the 3,500 formula, in the presence of over feeding.

In the introduction to Part Two, we mentioned the Endemol programme *Larger than Life: 33,000 calories a day*. Let us look at two of the four morbidly obese subjects of the programme (we'll look at the other two in the chapter on exercise):

- Paul was 45 years old (at the time of the programme being made) and he weighed 48 stone (672 pounds) and consumed an estimated 36,902 calories a day. (Am I alone in wondering where the two calories came from?)
- Larry was 38 years old and he weighed 50 stone (700 pounds) and consumed an estimated 14,349 calories a day.

Dr. Ian Campbell estimated Larry's calorie requirement to be approximately 4,500 calories a day and therefore calculated that Larry would be gaining at the rate of three pounds per day (the 10,000 calorie 'difference' is approximately three lots of 3,500 calories). If we use the estimate of three pounds gain per day, Larry should be gaining at the rate of 1,095 pounds per year (i.e. 78 stone, three pounds). If we do this more accurately, (because this is a formula after all), we can calculate that Larry should be gaining at the rate of 1,027 pounds per year.[xxii] Both calculations are absurd.

If only Dr. Campbell had thought about these implications for Larry and/or done the same calculation for Paul, he would surely have discovered that the calorie formula can not hold true for weight gain (and therefore, by inference, for weight loss). Paul is actually slightly lighter and seven years older than Larry and fully bedridden (Larry managed to walk when food was being filmed in the room next to him), so he should need fewer calories. However, let's assume Paul also needs 4,500 calories per day. As Paul eats approximately 32,000 calories a day more than this, he should be gaining at the rate of nine pounds every single day. Paul is therefore supposed to be gaining weight at the rate of 3,337 pounds per year – 238 stone. According to the *Guinness Book of Records*, the World's heaviest ever man was approximately 100 stone. Paul should have reached that weight in 84 days from the time the programme was made – notwithstanding the fact that he had been bed ridden, at not far from his current weight, for six years. I personally think that Dr. Campbell did do the maths and thought "that's daft" and then moved on instead of questioning the formula. This begs the question – where do the calories go? I don't know; but I know where they *don't* go. They don't go into a gain of two stone of fat every three days.

Evidence on weight loss outside obesity journals

Not everyone reads obesity journals (including, rather worryingly, those giving out weight loss advice), but there is evidence to disprove the calorie formula

---

[xxii] 14,349 – 4,500 = 9,849. Multiplied by 365 days and divided by 3,500 = 1,027 pounds.

surrounding us at all times. If you, the reader, have ever followed a calorie restricted diet (that covers 99% of diets) and have failed to lose one pound for every single 3,500 calorie deficit created, you alone have rendered the formula invalid. If you work with patients, you must have noticed that they disprove the formula week in, week out. You may have thought that they were cheating. Hopefully, after seeing the evidence from Franz et al, you will think differently.

On July 12 2010, under the headline "Weight Watchers does work, say scientists", Sarah Boseley, health editor for *The Guardian* wrote a wonderful endorsement for Weight Watchers following a study done by the Medical Research Council (MRC), funded by Weight Watchers.[104] The original presentation of results from the MRC revealed that 772 people were studied: 395 people were simply given weight loss advice from their doctor (the GP group) and 377 were funded to attend Weight Watchers (419 of the 772 completed their respective programme).[105] The study was a year in length and the likely deficit was at least 1,000 calories per day (a typical Weight Watchers allowance is 18-20 points, which approximates to 900-1,000 calories vs. an average 2,000 calorie requirement for a woman). The article reported that the GP group lost an average of six pounds (we know from the Franz study that 'advice alone' people did well to lose anything) and the Weight Watchers group lost an average of 11 pounds. The Weight Watchers group should have lost 104 pounds in fat alone. This study provided irrefutable proof that the calorie theory is wrong, which should have been front page news in itself, but this was not the story of the article. The story was "you'll lose twice as much weight with Weight Watchers." The headline should more accurately have been "Weight Watchers works better than just going to the GP, says study funded by Weight Watchers; but you will be lucky to lose one tenth of your lowest expectation." Not as catchy, but far more honest.

Millions of people, women particularly, are living in a state of permanent calorie deprivation (i.e. hunger), which should be 'rewarding' this starvation with 50-100 pounds lost every year. The average woman, (needing 2,000 calories a day), on 1,000 calories a day, should lose 104 pounds each and every year (regardless of starting weight). Yet, instead, they lose little or nothing and put on weight when they can't stand the starvation any longer and eat close to a normal day's requirement of 2,000 calories. We cannot allow this to continue.

Television provides excellent obesity experiments on a regular basis. Watch the next series of *The Biggest Loser* and plot the weight loss on a weekly basis and see if everyone is losing in a straight line in accordance with the calorie formula. *Britain's Biggest Loser* has had no where near the success and ratings of the similar programmes in the USA or Australia, but, dedicated to obesity research, I taped 40 episodes for three months in early 2009 to record the following results. Here is the summary table for the 16 contestants:

Table 3: Results from *Britain's Biggest Loser* (2009)

Name	Start lbs	Wks on prog	lbs loss on prog	lbs loss per wk	% loss on prog	% loss per wk	lbs after 4 mths	% loss after 4 mths
Mark	363	6	-62	-10	-17%	-2.8%	-98	27%
Kevin	330	7	-60	-9	-18%	-2.6%	-132	40%
Jennifer	327	3	-8	-3	-2%	-0.8%	-34	10%
Sadie	299	7	-36	-5	-12%	-1.7%	-84	28%
Carol	221	7	-33	-5	-15%	-2.1%	-69	31%
Katey	311	7	-39	-6	-13%	-1.8%	-64	21%
Dave	325	5	-26	-5	-8%	-1.6%	-69	21%
Jamie	400	7	-52	-7	-13%	-1.9%	-83	21%
Eunice	330	2	-16	-8	-5%	-2.4%	-49	15%
Miriam	212	3	-12	-4	-6%	-1.9%	-52	25%
Rick	299	2	-15	-8	-5%	-2.5%	-29	10%
Michelle	227	2	-8	-4	-4%	-1.8%	-34	15%
Raz	211	1	-4	-4	-2%	-1.9%	-32	15%
Lisa	360	1	-6	-6	-2%	-1.7%	-58	16%
Michaela	219	7	-31	-4	-14%	-2.0%	-44	20%
Maria	221	7	-30	-4	-14%	-1.9%	-55	25%

The third column, weeks on the programme, indicates how long each person lasted before 'eviction'. Anyone with "7" in this column made it through to weigh-in seven. Michaela went home at this point and then Katey and Jamie went home in the final week leaving Kevin, Maria, Carol and Sadie going through to the final. All contestants knew they were coming back for the overall finale and so I have recorded all the weight losses at four months (final two columns) even though, arguably, the ones with the real incentive to carry on were the four in the final. Having said that, the prize for the British version of this programme is £10,000 (compared with $250,000 for the USA), so the incentive is not comparable.

Column four is pounds lost during the time each person was on the programme – in the stately home. This translates into pounds lost per week for each of the weeks they were on the programme (column five). Column six has the percentage of their original weight lost during their weeks on the programme and column seven shows this as an average percentage loss for each of the weeks they were 'contained'.

The biggest single loss was Kevin in week one with 17 pounds. Interestingly Michelle was ill in week one and stayed in bed all week and missed all the exercise and she lost 16 pounds doing nothing while Kevin exhausted himself in the gym. (She was also over 100 pounds lighter than Kevin to start with). The third biggest loss was Mark's 15 pounds in week three – this would not be the predictable week one water/glycogen loss.

There was one occurrence of weight gain – a remarkable eight pounds in week two for Michelle (she should have stayed in bed) and there were three occurrences of just a pound being lost and one person weighing the same as the previous week on one occasion. The key evidence that blows the calorie theory apart is that people should have been following a straight line formula for fat loss alone and they should have lost more on top in water and (sadly) lean tissue. Kevin and Dave were just five pounds different in starting weight, but Kevin lost 17 pounds in week one and Dave just two pounds. In week two, Dave lost 10 pounds and Jennifer (just two pounds different in starting weight) lost one pound. They were locked away in a stately home. They had no access to additional food. They had the same meals. They were put through the same exercise routine.

Jamie and Michaela needed hospital treatment during the second episode and there was plenty of vomiting in buckets kindly provided in the gym. This was evidence of the body *not* readily giving up adipose tissue for energy, but making the person collapse to a stop instead. There may have been a 10% difference in effort (when the military style trainers weren't watching), but similar sized people should have lost virtually identical amounts of weight. For a 'perfect' comparison, Carol and Maria both started at 221 pounds, Carol was 45 years old, Maria 44. They both made it to the final and Carol lost 25% more than Maria. Any deviation from a mathematical formula renders it invalid. Differences of eight to ten times make it nonsensical.

Kevin was the overall winner, by the way, losing an impressive 40% of his body weight and he did look much better during the final programme. There has been no follow up to this Britain's Biggest Loser series, but I would be astonished if the group defied Benedict, Keys, Stunkard and McLaren-Hume and Franz et al and became the first group of people to lose weight with calorie deprivation and keep it off.

Time Magazine's special supplement *The Science of Appetite* (2007) did a follow up of Ryan Benson, winner of the first series of *The Biggest Loser* in the USA.[106] Ryan lost 122 pounds (55 kilograms) to win the first series, but he confessed that he regained 32 pounds in the five days after the final just by drinking water. Apparently the contestants eat and drink nothing, and spend as much time in saunas and taking diuretics as possible, in the days before the final to win the much coveted $250,000 prize. Matt Hoover had an immediate 15 pound rebound after winning series two. Ryan Benson weighed approximately 300 pounds (136 kilograms) when the Time Magazine article was written in 2007. At the start of *The Biggest Loser* he weighed 330 pounds (150 kilograms) and he was 208 pounds (95 kilograms at the moment of winning). Chat rooms since have noted that Ryan is back at his original weight.

Evidence at a country level (The UK National Food Survey)

Let us next look at rigorous national evidence for the UK. The UK has been doing a comprehensive National Food Survey, for household food consumption, since 1940. The National Food Survey for the period 1940 to 1974 excluded alcoholic drinks, soft drinks, confectionery and eating out. To ensure a like-for-like comparison, I analysed the National Food Survey, for the period 1974 to 2000, which was consistently recorded and produced during this time by the Ministry of Agriculture, Fisheries and Food (MAFF). Soft drinks were not in the 1974 figure, but they were included for all the years from and including 1975. Alcoholic drinks and confectionery were included from 1992 onwards. I did not attempt to calculate and deduct the calorific content of these additional foods from 1999-2000 to compare exactly the same 'basket of goods' from 1974-1975. As you will see below – the point will be made, even while conceding this advantage to the calorie theorists.

The Department for Environment, Food and Rural Affairs (DEFRA) was formed in June 2001 as an amalgamation of MAFF and the Department of the Environment, Transport and the Regions (DETR). DEFRA have produced the Family Food Survey since 2000 and we will use this in Chapter Ten, for the most recent data available. For now we are able to make a consistent comparison, across a 25 year period, during which obesity increased from 2.7% for both males and females in 1972 to 22.6% for males and 25.8% for females in 1999 (World Health Organisation statistics).[107]

The MAFF National Food Survey tells us that we were eating 2,290 calories per person per day in 1975 and, by 1999, this had fallen to 1,690 calories per person per day. If we apply the 3,500 calorie formula, to the change in annual average calorie intake, all other things being equal, we should have *lost* an average of 62.6 pounds per person during this period. Instead obesity rose nearly ten fold during this time.[108]

The DEFRA report notes the continual decline in calorie intake. The Family Food Survey for 2001-02 comments on the short term: "Energy content of the household food supply has decreased considerably over the last 5 years." The Family Food Survey for 2002-03 notes the same trend over the longer term: "Average energy intake per person in the UK is unchanged in 2002-03 compared with the previous year, although it has been declining since 1964."[109]

The Food Standards Agency (FSA) web site also acknowledges the above conundrum, "Since the 60s we've been consuming fewer calories from household food (this doesn't include eating out). However, there are an increasing number of people who are overweight or obese. The reasons for this are not clear."[110]

I have a number of explanations for this, but there can only be two calorie theory reasons for this – everything in the calorie world must be explained by energy intake and/or energy expenditure. In this case, that means calories consumed outside household food (eating out), or exercise being done, or any combination of the two.

The FSA, NHS and the Office of National Statistics (ONS) were unable to provide me with weight statistics for 1975, to translate the rise in obesity into average weight per person, but the average American has gained approximately 20 pounds during this time.[111] The average UK citizen will likely have gained at least this, as we have been closing the gap on the USA obesity statistics, but let us assume that the average UK person has gained the same (we will soon see that, whether the average gain has been 15, 20 or 25 pounds, the calorie formula still produces an incredible result).

We need to make some assumptions, as the combinations of varying energy in *and* energy out *and* varying the time that any changes took place within the period are infinite. (According to the calorie formula, for example, weight could be exactly constant for 24 years and 355 days and then the person could consume a surplus of 7,000 calories a day for 10 days and gain 20 pounds). Let us take the 'extremes' for illustration and assume that the entire 20 pound gain can be explained by energy in *or* energy out. Let us also assume that the change in energy in or energy out has been constant during the period.

For energy *intake* to be the sole explanation, for an average weight gain of 20 pounds over 25 years, according to the calorie formula, the average person must have exactly maintained their calories expended per day and then consumed just 7.67 more calories, on average, each day, no more, no less.[112]

For energy *expenditure* to be the sole explanation, the average person would have had to have exactly maintained their calorie intake per day, from 1975 throughout until 1999 (whether from household food or eating out) and used up 7.67 fewer calories, on average, per day, no more, no less. This would equate to 1-2 fewer minutes walking per day.[113]

There is an implicit assumption in the above. We need to assume that calories consumed outside the home exactly accounted for the gap as calories consumed in household food fell. This would mean, as an example, if we consumed 100 calories eating out in 1975 and the known 2,290 calories from household food, we would have needed to consume 700 calories from eating out in 1999 and the known 1,690 in household food, to maintain calorie intake. *Then* we would have had to have eaten just 7.67 'surplus' calories from either eating out or eating in, each day (on average), to explain the actual weight gain. (Or walked 1-2 minutes fewer). Do we honestly believe that the worst health epidemic we have ever faced is the result of two jelly beans a day?

We can also see now that *not* having the exact average weight gain for a UK citizen matters little with the 3,500 calorie formula. Had we gained an average 15 pounds per person, that would be 1.5 jelly beans a day and 25 pounds per person would be 2.5 jelly beans a day. Indeed I debated whether or not to round the 7.67 calories a day to 8, but this would have made a one pound difference over the 25 years.

Any explanation for the current obesity epidemic must incorporate what has changed since the late 1970's/early 1980's and it must be something unique to this period. Looking at the calorie theory in another way, the weight of the average person changed remarkably little before the obesity epidemic. If you believe that energy in equals energy out, for an average person, needing 2,500 calories per day, to have maintained their weight to within three pounds, during any 25 year period (during which time they would have consumed nearly 23 million calories) would have required a 0.046% degree of accuracy of calorie management. It is absurd to think that the majority of people managed such a remarkable feat for the thousands of years up to 1975 and then two thirds of the developed world suddenly lost this ability in the 25 years that followed and that it only took two jelly beans a day to achieve this.

This *must* lead to the conclusion that we set out in Chapter Four. Energy in and out must play a minor part compared to the internal adjustment taking place endogenously, inside the human body. The vast majority of human beings stayed at a normal weight until the twentieth century. I suggest that this was the result of the satisfactory workings of the human body. We know that the human body has a unique and incredible set of internal balancing mechanisms – it can regulate temperature in a quite astonishing way. This is one of the few natural mechanisms that still seem to be intact in modern humans. We used to be able to regulate blood pressure. Now we have high blood pressure associations. We used to be able to regulate blood glucose levels. Now we have 171 million diabetics worldwide.[114] We used to have a natural appetite mechanism. Now we have human beings weighing four times as much as a baby elephant and still eating 37,000 calories a day.

What changed in the twentieth century was not how much we ate, but *what* we ate. There is something about the modern manufactured substances that we are ingesting (food, drink, drugs and pollution), which has completely changed, in many ways destroyed, our body's fundamental ability to function.

I believe that the above tells us that what we ate in 1974 vs. 2000 is of far more importance than how many calories we ate, or what we did or didn't do. The thing that has changed, and therefore the only thing that can explain the obesity epidemic, is the composition of our food consumption and we will analyse this in Chapter Ten. This was dramatically different during the last quarter of the twentieth century and I believe that this is significant. The absurdity of the above, let alone the complete absence of evidence, surely illustrates that "The Calorie Formula", upon which current diet advice is wholly and fundamentally based, must be discarded.

The search for proof of the formula

Despite all this information being equally available to any person, calorie devotees continue to state the 3,500 calorie formula as an absolute fact (e.g. "the earth is flat" – fact). So, in the face of such overwhelming contrary evidence, in June 2009, I set out to try to uncover the rationale for this continued assertion. It is the foundation of all current diet advice, so it is critical that we can source this statement and prove that this mathematical formula does indeed explain energy intake and expenditure in the human body.

My search is documented below and it stunned me. Not one of seven government and obesity organisations can provide evidence for either part of this formula. The response from five was, in essence, "We have no idea where this formula comes from or the rationale for it." The response from the other two was "If people create a deficit of 600 calories for a year they will lose approximately 5kg in weight." As opposed to the 28 kilograms of fat, let alone weight, which the formula says that people will lose.

Kevin Hall's brilliant article in the March 2008 *International Journal of Obesity*, is entitled, "What is the required energy deficit per unit weight loss?" Hall opens by noting that the 3,500 formula is "one of the most pervasive weight loss rules" and refers to it as "this rule of thumb", which he then proceeds to show is anything but. This formula, of course, cannot be a rule of thumb when its chief proponents confirm that weight loss may be approximately 17% of what the fat loss alone should be. In this article, however, Hall tries to come up with an alternative to the 3,500 'rule of thumb'. This continues to miss the point that the body does not adhere to mathematical formulae. As Hilde Bruch noted in *The Importance of Overweight*, (1957), "human beings do not function in this way."

Hall and I were quoted in the same article, *The Sunday Times*, 4 April 2010, where the reporters said of me "Her analysis of the scientific evidence is supported by other researchers. Kevin Hall, a physicist and investigator at the National Institutes of Health in Maryland, said that because the body becomes more efficient at conserving energy as calories are reduced, it would take five or even 10 years to achieve the weight loss promised in just 12 months under the formula. 'The amount of energy your body burns when you decrease the number of calories goes down,' he said."[115]

During June and July of 2009 I approached the British Dietetic Association (BDA), Dietitians in Obesity Management (DOM), the National Health Service (NHS), the National Institute for Clinical Excellence (NICE), the Department of Health (DoH), the National Obesity Forum (NOF) and the Association for the Study of Obesity (ASO) to ask all of these expert organisations for proof of the 3,500 formula (also known as the calorie theory).

On 10 June, I sent the following query to the **BDA**: "I am doing some research on obesity and I would be most grateful if you could help me. Please can you explain where the 'One pound of fat contains 3,500 calories...' comes from?"

I received a very prompt and pleasant reply, "Unfortunately we do not hold information on the topic that you have requested." It was suggested that I contact a dietitian. I happened to be with several dietitians at an obesity conference later that month, so I asked fellow delegates and no one knew where the 3,500 formula came from. No one knew where the 'eatwell' plate proportions came from.[116] One dietitian said to me "You've made us think how much we were just 'told' during our training, with no explanation. A group of us over there don't even know where the five-a-day comes from." (We will answer this in Chapter Thirteen).

So, after the conference, on 29 June, I sent the following email to the **NHS**: "I am an obesity researcher and I am trying to find out the rationale behind the statement: "One pound of fat contains 3,500 calories, so to lose 1lb a week you need a deficit of 500 calories a day". This specific reference is a verbatim quotation from the British Dietetic Association's Weight Loss Leaflet *Want to Lose Weight and keep it off?* The BDA reply was 'we do not hold information on the topic.' As this formula is the foundation of all current weight loss advice, it is critical to be able to prove it. Please can you let me know where this formula comes from and the evidence for it?"

On 30 June I received another very prompt reply: "Unfortunately our Lifestyles team do not hold this information and are unable to assist you with your enquiry. I would suggest you contact the Department of Health to see if they can help."

On 1 July I forwarded the email exchange with the NHS to the Department of Health. I had to chase on 6 July and then got a response saying they would get back to me within 20 working days. Meanwhile, I had also written to NICE (1 July) and they responded on 2 July saying they would get back to me within a maximum of 20 working days.

On 2 July I sent the same email to the **NOF** and the ASO and received a very prompt email back from the NOF (two hours later) suggesting that I contact the ASO. I thanked the NOF for this, but pointed out that their own web site quoted the 3,500 formula verbatim and also had the following classic example: "one less (sic) 50 calorie plain biscuit per day could help you lose 5lbs (2.3kg) in a year – and one extra biscuit means you could gain that in a year!" I have heard nothing back from the NOF since. I sent Dr. David Haslam, NOF chair, an email on 6 July attaching *An Essay on Obesity*, which I had written, for his interest and comment. On 10 July I also sent Dr. Haslam the exchange I had had with the ASO, so that information could be shared. I have still heard nothing since.

The **ASO** response was the most helpful by far, but it still completely failed to prove the 3,500 formula. My query was circulated to board members and two very kindly replied:

One reply was: "Basic biology tells us that 1kg pure fat, converted to energy = 9000 kcal, 1lb pure fat = 0.453 kg = 4077 kcal. The approximation to 3500 kcal is made on the basis that 'adipose tissue' is not 100% fat (some water and some lean tissue). Hence to lose 1lb pure fat = 4077 kcal deficit, or 1lb fat tissue in the body = approx 3500kcal deficit. This equates to 500kcal per day to lose 1lb in a week. This has been supported by numerous studies using whole body calorimetry." There were no sources put forward, for these "numerous studies". I asked on 21 July and again on 11 August for "even one obesity study that proves this formula" and have received nothing back.

As you will note from my mathematical exercise in Chapter Five, and I stand to be corrected, but I came up with: Fat has 9 calories per gram; one pound is 454 grams; human fat tissue contains approximately 87% lipids;[117] so 454 grams of body fat tissue has approximately the calorific energy of 395 grams of pure fat (454 grams x 87%), i.e. 3,555 calories (395 grams x 9).

The ASO member uses the word "approximation", as do many references to the calorie formula, so there may be some acknowledgement of the number of variables. However, the diet advice that follows takes no account of this word "approximation". If we take just one variation – the difference between 3,555 and 3,500 equates to five to six pounds a year. The NOF cautions that eating, or not eating, one biscuit a day could cause a person to gain, or lose, five pounds in a year. Well, the formula being inaccurate can also do this without any biscuit involvement at all. In fact, if 3,555 is correct and not 3,500 (notwithstanding the fact that there is no proof for either formula), this would have made a difference of 172 pounds over the past 30 years (the obesity epidemic period). Fortunately the error would be 'in our favour' so we should have all been able to eat nearly 11,000 biscuits and get away with it, or be over 12 stone lighter.

The second reply from the ASO was 'evidence' from NICE and a web link to the full NICE document *Management of obesity: Full Guidance*, December 2006. The specific proof offered was one study (Table 15.14) of 12 subjects, given a deficit of 600 calories a day, where the outcome was "a change of approximately -5 kg (95% CI -5.86kg to -4.75kg, range -0.40 kg to -7.80 kg) compared with usual care at 12 months. Median weight change across all studies was approximately -4.6 kg (range -0.60 kg to -7.20 kg) for a 600 kcal deficit diet or low-fat diet and +0.60 kg (range +2.40 kg to -1.30kg) for usual care".

So, let me understand this, the people on the 600 calorie-a-day deficit (the NICE recommendation) were 5 kilograms (11 pounds) lighter than those not doing this "at 12 months." Applying the basic maths formula, these 12 people should each have lost 600*365/3,500 = 62.57 pounds of fat. Not an ounce (of fat) more or less. AND, there should have been *no* range of results – everyone should have lost exactly the same (that's what happens with a mathematical formula). The least anyone lost (let's put it all into pounds) was 0.8 pounds and the most anyone lost was 17.2 pounds. Even the highest weight loss was 45 pounds lower than it should have been. This is also all about fat – we haven't even started looking at muscle or water loss. This is also a study of 12 people. There are 1.1 billion overweight people in the world and we can't prove a formula using 12 of them.

There were 15 other studies in Table 15.14, 10 of which had data for where a calorie deficit had been created over a specified period of time. This enabled me to analyse what the weight loss should have been (using the 3,500 formula) and what the average weight loss actually was (from the study data). This is detailed in Appendix 2. Again, in every single study, there was a wide range of results (which means that the formula failed *per se*). In all of the other ten studies, the actual weight loss was multiples away from what the weight loss should have been. The smallest gap between actual weight loss and 'should have happened' weight loss (according to the formula) was 28.7 pounds (we continue to ignore water to try to give the formula a chance). At the other extreme, the biggest difference between the fat that should have been lost and the fat that was lost was 143.9 pounds.

I was still digesting the immense implications of all this when the **DoH** reply arrived, on the 21 July, saying "The Department is unaware of the rationale behind the weight formula you refer to." Pause for a second – the UK government Department of Health, has no idea where their founding piece of diet advice comes from. They very kindly suggested another lead, (Dietitians in

Obesity Management UK (DOM UK) – a specialist group of the British Dietetic Association), which I followed up on 24 July.

I chased **NICE** on 27 July, as the 20 working days were 'up' in my calendar. I appeared to have been passed between NHS and NICE during July and a very helpful woman called me back to say she had found the right department to deal with the query. A couple of days later, the reply came "Whilst our guidance does contain reference to studies involving 500 calorie deficit diets we do not hold any information about the rationale behind the statement 'one pound of fat contains 3,500 calories, so to lose 1lb a week you need a deficit of 500 calories a day'." That is to say – although we are an evidence based organisation, we have no evidence.

On 10 August I received a response from **DOM** UK: "I have asked our members and this answer was returned. It's a mathematical equation, 1gram of fat is 9kcal, therefore 1kg fat equals 9000kcal. There are some losses but 1 lb of fat is approximately 4500kcal divide that by 7 days and its (sic) approximately 643kcal hence the deficit." I went back to DOM UK, on the 10 August, to request an answer to the second part of the calorie theory – if that is how 600 calories is derived (and I have never before seen the 3,500 become 4,500), how can we then say with such confidence that each and every time this deficit is created one pound *will* be lost.

On the 18 August, I received a reply from one of the DOM UK Committee members: "My understanding is that it comes from the thermodynamics of nutrition, whereby one lb of fat is equivalent to 7000kcals, so to lose 1 lb of fat weight per week you would need an energy deficit of 7000kcals per week, or 500kcals a day. In or around that, depending on whether or not you use metric system and your clinical judgement, some people use a deficit of 600kcals a day and others 500kcals a day. There is good evidence that this level of deficit produces weight differences of approx 5kg at 1 year."

This time the 3,500 deficit 'needed' has doubled to '7,000' calories. Or, to put it another way, one pound of fat has become 7,000 calories. You can start to see what I have experienced as a researcher – how widely this formula is used as fact and yet how little it is understood and how few people know how to use their own 'fact'.

So, in the example from Dietitians in Obesity Management, key proponents of the calorie formula, one year of a 600 calorie a day deficit will produce a *weight* loss of approximately 11 pounds – not the 62.5 pounds of fat alone that should be yielded.

When I pointed this out and suggested "I really think we need to fundamentally review the basis of current diet advice and stop saying 'to lose 1lb of fat you need to create a deficit of 3500 calories'", the final reply I got was "I guess a key to all of this is that weight loss doesn't appear to be linear, any more than weight gain is."

At last, an admission that the formula has no basis of fact.

The organisations approached have been very helpful and accessible, but none is able to explain where the 3,500 comes from, let alone to provide evidence of its validity.

A request

In conclusion of this section on "The Calorie Formula", I have a simple and reasonable request. I would like proof of this formula – that it holds exactly every single time – or I would like it to be banished from all dietary advice worldwide.

First of all, any proof needs to source the origin of the formula, or it needs to validate that Hunt Peters was the origin and that her 1918 assertions are correct: "Five hundred Calories equal approximately 2 ounces of fat. Two ounces per day would be about 4 pounds per month, or 48 pounds per year. Cutting out 1000 Calories per day would equal a reduction of approximately 8 pounds per month, or 96 pounds per year."

Secondly, the proof needs to hold in all cases. There needs to be overwhelming, irrefutable and consistent evidence that *each and every* time a deficit of 3,500 calories is created, one pound of fat is lost.

Since, we already have overwhelming evidence that such proof cannot be provided, it is not enough that we quietly stop using this formula – it is too widely assumed to be true for us to just sweep it under the carpet. We need to issue a public statement saying that it does not hold and should not be used again. We need to tell people that they will *not* lose one pound of fat for every deficit of 3,500 calories that they create. We need to tell people that there is no formula when it comes to weight loss and we have been wrong in giving people the hope that starvation will lead to the loss of 104 pounds each and every year, in fat alone.

Part Three

The Diet Advice

Part Three

The Diet Advice

What should we eat?

Food (noun): "Substance taken into body to maintain life and growth; nutriment."[118]

My mother told me to eat my liver, eggs and greens, to drink my milk and to take my cod liver oil. Her mother told her the same and her mother before that. Somewhere along the line we seem to have forgotten that we eat food for a reason. Food is essential for human life and health and we need to eat food because of the nutrients it provides. Let us have a quick reminder of the life sustaining roles performed by nutrients in the body, as a precursor to the argument that we need to eat the right food for the right reason.

Macronutrients are, collectively, carbohydrate, protein and fat. The Greek word macro means large and these are nutrients that we (allegedly) need in large quantities. In this Part Three of the book, we explore carbohydrate and fat in some detail and I will argue that our need for carbohydrate is not large, if there is a need at all, and that the critical macronutrients for the human body are protein and fat – but that the micronutrients provided by carbohydrate can be valuable.

Micronutrients are, as the name suggests, those needed by the body in smaller quantities. Vitamins and minerals fall into this category. (We also need water and oxygen, but I'll take those as read).

There are 13 vitamins in total: A, B1, B2, B3, B5, B6, B7, B9, B12, C, D, E and K. The fat soluble vitamins are A, D, E and K and, as their name suggests, they are found in fats and need to be consumed in/with fats for their absorption. The water soluble vitamins are vitamin C and the vitamin B group, which comprises: B1 (thiamine); B2 (riboflavin); B3 (niacin); B5 (pantothenic acid); B6 (pyridoxine); B7 (biotin); B9 (folic acid) and B12 (cobalamin).

There are two categories of minerals – macro minerals are both present in the body and needed by the body in larger amounts than the trace minerals (where only a trace is needed). The macro minerals are: calcium; chloride; magnesium; phosphorus; potassium; sodium and sulphur. The trace minerals are: chromium; copper; fluoride[xxiii]; iodine; iron; manganese; molybdenum; selenium and zinc.

[xxiii] Fluoride is one of sixteen minerals commonly listed in nutritional textbooks. It is not, however, an essential nutrient and not a substance that the body needs to (or even should) ingest. It has been added to the water supply in many developed

Eating to overcome an obesity epidemic, we have no room for empty calories. Every calorie ingested must contribute to our nutritional requirements. We cannot afford to consume manufactured foods that have been comprehensively and carefully designed to be irresistible and 'moreish'. Instead of counting calories we need to make every calorie count.

Did you know that the average UK citizen is consuming 1,150 calories a day from just two ingredients – one with no nutritional value and one with so little that it is subject to fortification legislation, with a requirement to add back in nutrients removed in processing?[119] World Health Organisation data tells us that the average UK citizen consumes 38 kilograms of sugar per year.[120] Statistics from the Flour Advisory Bureau note that UK per capita flour consumption reached 74 kilograms in 2008/9.[121] This represents a few calories short of 1,150 per person per day from those two ingredients – when did that become a healthy balanced diet?

The USA has higher corn consumption than the UK and concomitant lower wheat consumption. The corresponding figures for the USA, for 2008, were 458 calories of sugar, high-fructose-corn-syrup and other sweeteners,[122] and 618 calories of wheat flour,[123] adding up to 1,076 calories in total per day for the average American citizen.

I did an interesting experiment, using the United States Department of Agriculture (USDA) food and nutrition database and the USA per capita consumption of sugars and flour. I analysed the nutritional value for the 121 grams of sugars and 170 grams of flour consumed by the average American. I then tried to see if I could get the American Recommended Dietary Allowances (RDAs) from eating approximately the same number of calories (1,076) in *real* food.[124] The USDA database does not have information for Biotin and it only records 11 minerals. There is not even an RDA for vitamins B5, D and K or for the minerals calcium, potassium, sodium and manganese. There is an "Adequate Intake" (AI) apportioned instead. The concept of RDA is bad enough. As Sally Fallon Morell said "why am I only *allowed* a certain level of nutrition?"[125]

I compared the 12 vitamins available and eight minerals – those for which there was both information available and an RDA, plus calcium and manganese, as important macro and trace minerals respectively. The results are summarised in Appendix 3.

The outcome was that only the requirement for selenium was met by the flour and sugar intake. Every other nutritional requirement was woefully lacking. All RDA's and AI's could be achieved by eating 1,077 calories comprising the following: 35 grams of porridge oats; 125 grams of whole milk (not low fat); 75 grams of liver; 50 grams of broccoli; 200 grams of spinach; 25 grams of cocoa powder; 125 grams of sardines (oil based, bones included); 200 grams of eggs and 20 grams of sunflower seeds. The most interesting lessons were not the results, but the exercise itself. It illustrated the following:

---

countries, as it is noted to decrease dental caries. This makes it an antidote to sugar in effect. Surely humans are better off without both fluoride and sugar.

- It is difficult to get even the RDA for many nutrients and very difficult to get the RDA for some (calcium, magnesium, zinc, vitamin D and vitamin E were the most difficult) and this is with every food on the planet theoretically available.
- In our preoccupation with macronutrients, we seem to have forgotten about micronutrients. If we eat food to obtain the vital micronutrients, the macronutrients will be what they will be (take care of the pennies and the pounds/dollars look after themselves). If we eat food to try to meet some made-up macronutrient composition,[xxiv] the micronutrients are likely impossible to consume. It is an inescapable fact that processed carbohydrates have little or no natural nutrition and even nature's carbohydrates are comprehensively beaten by nature's fats and proteins. Telling people to avoid fat is the same as telling us to avoid nutrition.
- Our parents and grandparents were brought up on relatively cheap, highly nutritious, foods like liver, eggs and sardines. Cod liver oil was commonly administered by previous generations. When you see the vitamin A and D content of the latter, our elders were very sensible. We shun such foods nowadays and should not.
- This is the *most* nutrition that we can derive from even real foods. This makes no allowance for: the quality of the food; nutrients lost in harvesting or over use of the land; cooking methods; or the fact that some nutrients need others for their absorption.

What are the implications of this for the obesity epidemic? The body has a substantial and varied nutritional requirement. If we base our meals on starchy foods and consume an average 1,100 largely useless calories, we still have a nutritional requirement to be met. The body will continue to seek food in an attempt to get the nutrition it needs. We may then consume another 1,100 calories, likely as nutritionally lacking as the first batch and we arrive at a population that is both overfed and undernourished. That's another way of defining obesity.

Healthy eaters should not stop at the basket of foods mentioned above. We can have more oats and sunflower seeds, with the milk, for breakfast. The sardines and hard boiled eggs can form part of a large 'chef's salad' for lunch with lettuce, cucumber, celery, tomatoes, beetroot, celeriac, grated carrot, spring onions, coloured peppers, mixed with olive oil dressing. Dinner need not be just liver, spinach and broccoli, but any other vegetables that can be found (in butter, of course, to deliver the nutrients) and cheese or natural yoghurt for dessert – to help with calcium intake.

Eating in this way has the following advantages over calorie deprivation:

1) There is no hunger, so there is no *general* and continual drive to eat;

[xxiv] The USA recommended intake for carbohydrate is at least 130 grams per person per day; the recommended intake for protein is 46-56 grams; the recommended intake for fat is "as low as possible."

2) All nutritional needs are met, so there is no *specific* and urgent drive to eat;
3) The metabolic advantage is equivalent to having a calorie deficit, without needing to eat less.

Expanding on point (3), the real food basket comprised carbohydrate:fat:protein in the ratio 29:27:44. The flour and sugars, being consumed by the average American each day, has the macronutrients in the ratio of 93:1:6. [xxv] This gives the real food eater the benefit of energy used up in making available energy. Protein and fat calories also have vital jobs to do and can therefore be used by the body in fulfilling these roles. Up to 85% of the energy need of the body is determined by basal metabolic rate for good reason. Carbohydrate can only be used for energy. Sugar, the most nutritionally void carbohydrate, cannot do anything useful in the body. It must be used as energy or it will be stored as fat (and it can be stored as fat because it causes insulin to be released).

The obesity epidemic is being uniquely driven by processed food, primarily carbohydrates, and these are avoided in a real food diet. I work exclusively in the field of obesity and I have never heard anyone declare an addiction to, or craving for, meat, fish, eggs, salads or vegetables. We tell an alcoholic not to touch alcohol again. We tell a smoker never to touch a cigarette again and then we tell food addicts to eat everything in moderation. It is substantially easier to avoid the foods that manufacturers deliberately engineer so that we want more of them, than it is to try to eat less of them. I have not eaten a biscuit for 15 years. There were many days before that when I struggled to manage 15 minutes without one. We cannot eat foods to which we are addicted in moderation any more than we can be an alcoholic in moderation. The only real foods that I have seen over consumed are fruit and cheese. Some women particularly are eating fruit by the kilogram and would be horrified at having to moderate this. Interestingly, these are the real foods with higher carbohydrate content.

There are overall wellbeing benefits from eating only real food: people report having higher and more stable energy levels, no 11am and 4pm hypoglycaemia; bloating, bowel problems, headaches, skin complaints – diverse and seemingly unrelated conditions disappear. I firmly believe that doctors' waiting rooms would be virtually empty if people ate only real food. If you are sceptical, try eating only food in the form that nature delivers it for even a couple of weeks and the more processed your current diet, the more you will notice the difference.

The route to sustained weight loss (I believe the only way) is to return to eating food in the form that nature provides it and having carbohydrate intake driven by nutritional requirements and not by the insatiability of manufactured 'food'. Steak, rack of (Welsh) lamb, wild salmon, an omelette made from the

---

[xxv] Both calculations are based on grams (weight). The real food basket contained 62 grams of carbohydrate, 95 grams of protein and 57 grams of fat. The flour and sugars contained 250 grams of carbohydrate, 17 grams of protein and 2 grams of fat. Full details are in Appendix 3.

neighbour's chicken eggs, berries of the season and fresh cream, whole grain rice with an array of stir-fried vegetables, the finest local cheeses, English apples in August, red wine, cocoa and cocoa butter 'chocolate' – this is how nature can feed us in the modern world and it should be embraced.

There's just one small problem to overcome – we seem to have got the idea from somewhere that nature put real fat in real food to kill us. Where did that come from?

Chapter Eight

Why did we change our diet advice?

Preamble – cholesterol

There is a very important point to cover before we start the main story in this chapter. There are still many people who think that eating cholesterol in food will raise their cholesterol level. This is actually a remarkably widely held view and one without foundation.

Even the man who started the whole diet/heart hypothesis (as it has become known), Ancel Keys, accepted right at the outset that "It is concluded that in adult men the serum cholesterol level is essentially independent of the cholesterol intake over the whole range of natural human diets. It is probable that infants, children and women are similar."[126] Keys et al presented this comment as the conclusion to their article in *The Journal of Nutrition*, November 1955. This conclusion seems rather restrained when you see the full summary of the studies that were presented in this article:

"Two cross sectional surveys in Minnesota on young men and four on older men showed no relationship between dietary cholesterol and the total serum cholesterol concentration.

"Two surveys on the Island of Sardinia failed to show any difference in the serum cholesterol concentrations of men of the same age, physical activity, relative body weight and general dietary pattern but differing markedly in cholesterol intake.

"Careful study during 4 years of 33 men whose diets were consistently very low in cholesterol showed that their serum values did not differ from 35 men of the same age and economic status whose diets were very high in cholesterol.

"Comparisons made of 23 men before and after they had voluntarily doubled their cholesterol intakes and of 41 men who halved theirs failed to show any response in the serum cholesterol level in 4 to 12 months while the rest of the diet was more or less constant.

"A detailed study of the complete dietary intakes of 119 Minnesota businessmen failed to show any significant increase of serum cholesterol with increasing dietary cholesterol intake.

"In 4 completely controlled experiments on men the addition to or removal from the diet of 500 to 600 mg of cholesterol daily had no effect on the serum cholesterol fall produced by a rice-fruit diet or on the rise in changing from a rice-fruit diet to an ordinary American diet.

"In a completely controlled experiment on 5 physically healthy men the change from a rice-fruit diet containing 500 mg of cholesterol daily to the same diet devoid of cholesterol had no effect on the serum level.

"In a similar experiment with 13 men receiving 66 gm of fat daily there was no significant effect in changing from a cholesterol intake of 374 mg/day to one of 1369 mg/day. In another 12 men the reverse change was likewise without effect on the blood serum. "

That was quite a range of studies done by Keys – who clearly initially investigated whether or not eating cholesterol raised cholesterol levels. He concluded unequivocally that it did not. He never deviated from this view. He was quoted in 1997 as saying "There's no connection whatsoever between cholesterol in food and cholesterol in blood. And we've known that all along. Cholesterol in the diet doesn't matter at all unless you happen to be a chicken or a rabbit."

The reference to these animals dates back to Nikolai Anitschkow's experiment on rabbits in 1913.[127] For some reason, Anitschkow decided to feed rabbits purified cholesterol and he managed to get their blood cholesterol levels in excess of 1,000 mg/dl. He then noticed the formation of "vascular lesions closely resembling those of human atherosclerosis" in the arteries of the rabbits. The obvious flaw in the experiment should have been that rabbits are strict herbivores. They do not eat animal products, which is the only source of cholesterol. Hence rabbits are in no way designed to digest cholesterol or animal fat and no one should be surprised if cholesterol or animal fat ended up stuck in any part of the poor rabbit. The only surprise is that no one thought to ask Anitschkow why he was feeding cholesterol and animal fat to herbivores. Interestingly, far less well known is that a parallel test was done on rats and dogs (omnivores) and feeding cholesterol to these species failed to produce lesions.

Governments don't go as far as Keys (or as far as they should) and admit that eating cholesterol has no connection whatsoever with cholesterol levels. Surprisingly, the *Dietary Guidelines for Americans* don't seem to have realised what "we have known all along". American authorities apparently still think that eating cholesterol has some impact on cholesterol levels. Chapter 6 of the guidelines says:[128]

-   "To decrease their risk of elevated low density lipoprotein (LDL) cholesterol in the blood, most Americans need to decrease their intakes of saturated fat and trans fats, and many need to decrease their dietary intake of cholesterol."

Here are two examples from the UK where the government agencies do admit that dietary cholesterol has little effect on "blood cholesterol":

-   "However, dietary cholesterol has little effect on blood cholesterol. More important is the amount of saturated fat in your diet". (National Health Service).[129]

- "But the cholesterol we get from our food has much less effect on the level of cholesterol in our blood than the amount of saturated fat we eat". (Food Standards Agency).[130]

What the government advice should say is: The body makes cholesterol. The cholesterol you eat has no impact on the level of cholesterol in your blood – not "little", but "no" – (and we've known that all along). If you consume a lot of cholesterol, your body will need to make less (and this may ease the burden on your liver), but your cholesterol level will not be impacted. It would be virtually inconceivable that you could eat enough cholesterol to override what your body makes. (We will, however, look at the impact of carbohydrate on cholesterol levels later on in this chapter).

This should also have been issued as a major, stand-alone, public announcement, not a line slipped in to prose continuing to use cholesterol and fat in the same sentence. No wonder I get so many emails from people wondering how I can suggest that eggs are one of the two healthiest foods on the planet (liver being the other one), when they think that eggs equal cholesterol equals about to drop dead.

This preamble tells us two very interesting things:

1) The diet/heart hypothesis started as an attempt to show that eating cholesterol causes raised cholesterol levels causes heart disease. This is why Keys' early studies in the 1950's all focused on trying to establish a relationship between cholesterol intake and cholesterol levels. When absolutely none could be found, Keys needed to find another suspect and, for some reason, fat was the chosen one. Speaking personally, I can see some logic for trying to find a relationship between cholesterol eaten and cholesterol in the body. However, given that there isn't one, I find no logic at all in the attempt to try to establish a relationship between fat eaten and cholesterol in the body, when none has been found with cholesterol in food and cholesterol in the body – not least when point (2) has been taken into account.

2) Looking purely at real food (as provided by nature), foods that contain cholesterol also contain fat (meat, fish, eggs and dairy products). (Please note that all of these foods contain both saturated and unsaturated fat). Although there are some foods that contain fat and not cholesterol (e.g. nuts, avocados), there are *no* foods that contain cholesterol, but not fat (some seafood is high in cholesterol and low in fat, but it still contains fat).

In the eight studies summarised by Keys (some with multiple sub-studies) any dietary changes that substantially increased cholesterol intake, and therefore, by definition, substantially increased fat intake, had no impact on body cholesterol levels. So, given that animal foods contain both cholesterol and fat and a substantial increase in these foods in the diet has no impact on cholesterol levels in the body, to the extent that it is concluded that cholesterol in food has no impact on cholesterol levels in the body; why is it not also concluded that fat has no impact on cholesterol levels in the body?

In fact, having discovered that cholesterol in food has no impact on cholesterol in the body; surely the *least* logical suspect to turn to next would be fat – the macronutrient in the same foods as those supplying cholesterol? My prime suspect for any modern illness would be carbohydrates generally and processed carbohydrates particularly, which interestingly takes us to...

In Chapter Twelve we will see that we have all the makings of a heated agreement here, because our governments tend *not* to know their fat from their carbohydrate and they are, in fact, talking about processed carbohydrates most of the time that they claim to be talking about saturated fats. This will give us the opportunity to jointly condemn cakes, pastries, biscuits, pies, confectionery, ice cream, crisps, savoury snacks, and so on, but for very different reasons. Meanwhile we have an interesting story to hear and, by the end of this chapter and a couple following, I hope to convince you that the only connection between fat and cholesterol, as found in real food, is that they travel around the body in lipoproteins together. As for the role of trans fats and processed carbohydrates in heart disease, or any other modern illness, your worst suspicions can't be worse than mine.

Introduction

I think that bathing causes singing. I am so convinced (and I think that I would really make a name for myself if I could establish this) that I am going to set out to prove it. I once had a flat mate who sang in the bath and I know two other people who sing in the bath. I have also sourced four people who are not in the bath and who are not singing. So, there you go, I have a seven person study to prove that bathing causes singing.

Immediately, as a sensible person, you are spotting three fundamental errors with my argument:

1) There are people all over the world who are in a bath and not singing and people not in the bath who are singing and I have chosen to ignore these and this is biased and wrong.
2) Even if every person in the world who took a bath sang every time and no one out of the bath ever sang, this would still only establish an association, not causation. I could no more say that bathing causes singing than I could claim that singing causes bathing.
3) Even if I could establish an association, which held every single time, two things observed at the same time could be *caused* by something else. I could be taking a bath and singing because I was getting ready for an audition – the bathing and singing may have no causal relationship between each other, but both could be *caused* by something else.

Please bear in mind how ridiculous and biased the above is as we next look at exactly the same principle, but this time it was believed (and still is) by sensible people and governments worldwide.

The Seven Countries Study – background

The same Ancel Keys who did the brilliant Minnesota experiment launched the Seven Countries Study in 1956 with an annual budget of $200,000 – enormous in today's money. Having recently published his experiment in *The Biology of Human Starvation* (1950), he was the man of the moment. This was to prove important, as he was also a great orator and a very persuasive individual and he won through against much more evidence-based science and rationale. It is difficult to overstate how catastrophic the consequences of Keys' Seven Countries Study have been for the 'developed' world over the past four decades.

Critics of the Seven Countries Study position the story as – Keys set out to prove that consuming fat causes heart disease – in much the same way that I set out to prove that bathing causes singing. They assert that there can be no other rationale, as an unbiased experiment by an unbiased experimenter would undoubtedly have produced a different conclusion.

Let's get the words of Keys himself to see what his intention was. For a review of the Seven Countries Study I started with the original summary, as published in *Circulation* in April 1970. I then looked at "The 25-year follow up of the Seven Countries Study" in the *European Journal of Epidemiology*. Keys was the key author of both, so we can read and review his own words.

The original report of the Seven Countries Study was published in *Circulation* in April 1970 entitled "Coronary Heart Disease in Seven Countries". The full research was published in 20 volumes, with the final two volumes being the summary and references. Volume VII, as an example, was entitled "Coronary Heart Disease in Seven Countries: Five-Year Experience in Rural Italy" and Volume XII was entitled "Coronary Heart Disease in Seven Countries: Three Cohorts of Men Followed Five Years in Serbia", purely to illustrate that information and data is available at country and cohort (different demographic groups of people) level.

In "Volume XVII The Diet", Keys opens with the following: "From the inception of the research program reported here, an important focus was on the diet and its possible relationship to the etiology of coronary heart disease. Earlier explorations appeared to indicate that substantial differences among populations in the incidence of coronary heart disease are associated with differences in the fat content of the diets of the populations concerned, with serum cholesterol concentration being an intermediate link (Keys 1952, 1953, 1957; Keys, Kimura et al. 1958; Bronte-Stewart et al. 1955; Roine et al. 1958). It was clear that the diet probably was an important part of the reason why middle-aged men had so much higher serum cholesterol levels in Finland than their counterparts in Italy and Japan (Keys, Karvonen, and Fidanza 1958)."

This is a very illuminating opening as it tells us a) that this *is* a study of the impact of diet on heart disease, b) that Keys and a couple of others had done some studies that "appeared to indicate" that coronary heart disease and fat in the diet are associated – through cholesterol and c) that Keys had already concluded that diet explained the difference in heart disease in Finland vs. Italy/Japan – and not mass scale human displacement, as can be offered as an alternative explanation below. Interestingly, all quoted references are works of Keys himself. So, he is effectively saying I think that fat is associated (note – not causes) with heart disease (through cholesterol) and I will use the fact that I already think this as evidence for continuing to assert this. (Please also note the use of the word fat, not saturated fat, at this stage).

Keys does go on to say "Epidemiological studies alone can rarely if ever produce final proof of a causal sequence, particularly in the case of a condition such as coronary heart disease in which there is no single cause…"[131]

The trouble is, on the very same page, Keys talks about "The urgency of finding means of prevention…" If only the well phrased caution about the limitations of epidemiological studies above had been the 'press release' from the Seven Countries Study instead of what became literally a knee jerk panic of 'Oh my goodness, we must stop humans eating fat because men (and I mean men, not women) are dropping dead with every moment we delay'.

Keys opens the summary of the *Circulation* report (1970) with the words: "In an international cooperative study on the epidemiology of coronary heart disease (CHD), international teams examined 12,770 men aged 40 through 59 years in Finland, Greece, Italy, Japan, the Netherlands, the United States and Yugoslavia." So, we know the countries and number of participants and their ages from the first sentence.

We should add to this, and therefore note at the outset, that men aged 40-59 in 1956 were aged 29-48 in 1945, when World War II ended and they were between 23-42 years old when World War II started. It is important to know this context for each of the seven countries in the study, let alone particular cohort differences:

- Italy had Mussolini at the helm, a fascist like Hitler. Mussolini seemed hesitant to enter the war, but Italy eventually joined in June 1940 after Germany secured Poland. Italian men at least started off on the winning side and were not invaded by their next door but one neighbour, Germany. Italy invaded the part of France near their border, as Germany took over the rest. The Italian army was spread thin from east Africa through Greece to southern France and so World War II would have been tough for Italian men, but arguably tougher for occupied territories.
- Greece was invaded by Italy, as Italy tried to secure southern territories while Germany headed north. The Greeks initially fought well and an imminent victory for the Greeks prompted a successful German intervention. Britons, Australians and New Zealanders were despatched from Egypt to go and defend Greece, but they were beaten back to Crete. Germany then won that region in the creatively named Battle of Crete.
- Poor Yugoslavia, as it was then, signed a tripartite treaty in March 1941 to let Germany through its territory to Greece. Germany then must have ignored the 'leave us alone in return' clause and took control of Yugoslavia on the way back.

- The Netherlands was occupied from May 1940 until the end of the war. We have Anne Frank's incredible diary, not least, to understand what life must have been like in this small territory.
- Finland made Yugoslavia look like it was having a good time – the Finns fought the Winter War alone against the Soviet Union, the Continuation War *with* Germany against the Soviet Union and the Lapland War *against* Germany. Most of Finnish Karelia was lost to the Soviet Union with The Moscow Peace Treaty of 1940. Approximately 400,000 people, virtually the entire population, had to be relocated within Finland. The Winter War and Continuation War, particularly, and the resulting Soviet expansion caused considerable bitterness in Finland. The territory taken from Finland by the Soviet Union included: Viipuri, Finland's second largest city; the industrial heartland; a key canal (Saimaa) and, most critically of all, it made an eighth of Finland's citizens refugees, without chance of return. I think that I would have had a heart attack after that and I'm not being facetious.
- The American people were brought into the war with the attack on Pearl Harbour (December 1941), but were never invaded or occupied.
- Japan's most devastating involvement in World War II was the allied atomic bombing of Hiroshima and Nagasaki in August 1945.

So the men in the Seven Countries Study were war survivors. They would likely have lost loved ones, homes, structure, support and the absolute basics in the Maslow hierarchy of needs. I think that it is critical to bear this in mind as you are about to be told that cholesterol is pretty much the only relevant factor in any heart disease that these men went on to suffer in the post-war years.

Lest we move on thinking that this is a valid epidemiological study from a population perspective, even when we know it to be highly selective from a country perspective, one of the main researchers in the study, Henry Blackburn notes, "In those days, we did not consider involving women because of the great rarity of cardiac events among them, and the invasiveness of our field examinations."[132] So, it is immediately fair to say that our global dietary advice was changed for 100% of the population when no association had even been attempted for 50% of the population (women), let alone an association proven to hold every time, let alone a clear causation established.

The Seven Countries Study – the numbers

The 12,770 men came from 16 cohorts. These cohorts were located in the USA (1 cohort), Finland (2), the Netherlands (1), Italy (3), the former Yugoslavia (5), Greece (2), and Japan (2). The 12,770 men were examined to measure certain pre-determined risk factors and they were then followed-up for mortality and causes of death for 25 years. (There was a degree of presumption at the outset regarding risk factors. Smoking rates, cholesterol levels, body mass index (BMI), blood pressure, lung capacity and arm circumference were measured. Stress, divorce rates, climate, work-life balance, differential light levels in the winter, income, employment etc were not measured).

Complete re-examinations were given every five years – for those who had survived and cause of death was recorded for the others. At the first five year review, 588 of the 12,770 men had died – 158 from coronary heart disease (CHD).

Table 4 contains the original numbers from Volume I of the 1970 report. All deaths and deaths from CHD in the first five years are recorded as follows:[133]

Table 4: Deaths and CHD deaths by cohort in the Seven Countries Study:

	Men	All Deaths	CHD Deaths
USA - Railroad workers	2,571	124	62
Italy - Crevalcore	993	60	11
The Netherlands - Zutphen	878	50	16
Finland - west Finland	860	50	9
Finland - east Finland (north Karelia)	817	61	29
Italy - Rome Railroad workers	768	24	2
Italy - Montegiorgio	719	29	5
Yugoslavia - Slavonia	699	55	7
Greece - Crete	686	10	1
Yugoslavia - Dalmatia	672	24	3
Yugoslavia - Belgrade	538	5	2
Greece - Corfu	529	11	4
Yugoslavia - Zrenjanin	516	15	1
Yugoslavia - Velika Krsna	511	23	1
Japan - Tanushimaru	509	23	4
Japan - Ushibuka	504	24	1
TOTAL	12,770	588	158

The table is ordered from largest cohort to smallest, in terms of the number of participants. Given that the USA has five times the number of people in their study, as either cohort in Japan, it is important to move straight to proportions. The three things that we need to know are:

1) What percentage of people in each cohort died (in the first five years)? I.e. total mortality.
2) What percentage of people in each cohort died from coronary heart disease (CHD)? I.e. CHD mortality.
3) What proportion of deaths was accounted for by CHD in each cohort? I.e. was CHD a far more frequent cause of death in one region?

Table 5: Deaths and CHD deaths by percentage, by cohort, in the Seven Countries Study

	(1) All deaths	(2) CHD Deaths	(3) CHD/All deaths
USA - Railroad workers	4.8%	2.4%	50.0%
Italy - Crevalcore	6.0%	1.1%	18.3%
The Netherlands - Zutphen	5.7%	1.8%	32.0%
Finland - west Finland	5.8%	1.0%	18.0%
Finland - east Finland (N Karelia)	7.5%	3.5%	47.5%
Italy - Rome Railroad workers	3.1%	0.3%	8.3%
Italy - Montegiorgio	4.0%	0.7%	17.2%
Yugoslavia - Slavonia	7.9%	1.0%	12.7%
Greece - Crete	1.5%	0.1%	10.0%
Yugoslavia - Dalmatia	3.6%	0.4%	12.5%
Yugoslavia - Belgrade	0.9%	0.4%	40.0%
Greece - Corfu	2.1%	0.8%	36.4%
Yugoslavia - Zrenjanin	2.9%	0.2%	6.7%
Yugoslavia - Velika Krsna	4.5%	0.2%	4.3%
Japan - Tanushimaru	4.5%	0.8%	17.4%
Japan - Ushibuka	4.8%	0.2%	4.2%
TOTAL (Average)	4.6%	1.2%	26.9%

In the summary of the study Keys aggregated back to the country level in all the tables, only referring to different cohorts in the dialogue. At this seven country level, Keys presented several bar charts showing incidence of coronary heart disease. The summary didn't focus on death rates, but on a combined measure of deaths, non fatal myocardial infarctions (heart attacks), angina and (to quote Keys) "men given the diagnosis of CHD on the basis of less rigid and specific clinical and ECG criteria". Using this incidence approach, the countries, in order of highest to lowest incidence of CHD were Finland, USA, Netherlands, Italy, Yugoslavia, Greece and Japan.

Keys then went on to present the CHD incidence rate for each of the seven countries against the following:

- The percentage of men smoking more than 10 cigarettes a day;
- The percentage of men described as sedentary;
- The percentage of men with relative weight more than 110% (i.e. 10% heavier than the average – today we would use BMI and possibly waist measurement);
- The percentage of men with mean skin folds more than 28mm (an indicator of body fat – today we would use body fat percentage);
- The percentage of men with systolic blood pressure more than or equal to 160 (this is the first number of the two in a blood pressure test);

- The percentage of "hypertensive" men with diastolic blood pressure more than or equal to 95 (this is the second number of the two in a blood pressure test);
- The percentage of men with cholesterol greater than 250mg/dl;
- The percentage of diet calories provided by saturated fat.

This begs the question – why did Keys introduce these 'lines' and then categorise data into that above and/or below these subjective demarcations? This introduces unnecessary judgement at the outset. Why 10 cigarettes a day and not 20? Why not correlate the number of cigarettes with the incidence of heart disease – the raw data is there. More seriously on cholesterol – why 250 mg/dl? Why not 240 mg/dl or 260 mg/dl and, again, why not do a straight correlation with cholesterol and incidence of heart disease? I share this to make two points: First, this immediately makes me, as an independent researcher, suspicious that data has been manipulated to achieve desired results. Secondly, even with such manipulation, Keys still failed to prove any association, let alone causation. Hence, we can continue knowing what Keys did, but also noting that even this didn't achieve the desired outcome.

The Seven Countries Study – Keys' conclusions

At this stage, we are still reviewing the journal *Circulation* from 1970, so we are looking at data for the first five year period only. In this context, here are Keys' conclusions from the 1970 summary of the study, in his own words:

- "Cigarette smoking cannot be involved as an explanation."
  (Please note that this doesn't just say that smoking can't explain the incidence in CHD, it categorically asserts that it cannot even be involved as an explanation. We'll come back to this).
- "Differences between the cohorts in the proportion of the men who are sedentary or physically inactive do not explain the difference between the cohorts in the incidence of CHD."
- "Consideration of neither obesity nor relative weight helps to explain the population differences in CHD incidence."
- "There is some tendency for the incidence of CHD to be related to the prevalence of hypertension in the cohorts."
- "The incidence rate of CHD tends to be directly related to the distributions of serum cholesterol values."
  (Please note, for serum cholesterol, read total cholesterol).
- "The average serum cholesterol values of the cohorts tended to be directly related to the average proportion of calories provided by saturated fats in the diet."
- "The CHD incidence rates of the cohorts are just as closely related to the dietary saturated fatty acids as to the serum cholesterol level."
- "CHD incidence rates were not found to be related to the percentage of calories provided by protein or polyunsaturated fatty acids"

Although not central to the study of coronary heart disease (CHD), I can't resist sharing the following quotation from Keys:

- "Average relative body weight, as well as average body fatness, tended to be inversely related to the average dietary calories per unit of body mass." i.e. the more overweight people were, the fewer calories they were eating.

And that is it. In the summary of the whole study, those are the statements of conclusions. Interestingly there is *no* mention in this summary of monounsaturated fat. The only mention of polyunsaturated fat is that it is unrelated. Keys confidently asserts that smoking, activity levels/exercise and weight play *no* part in CHD; blood pressure has some observed pattern and CHD *tends* to be related to total cholesterol and the average proportion of calories provided by saturated fats in the diet (my emphasis).

The three assertions, made by Keys in 1970, can therefore be summarised as:

1) CHD tends to be directly related to serum cholesterol;
2) Serum cholesterol tends to be directly related to saturated fat as a proportion of the diet;
3) CHD is as closely related to saturated fat as it is cholesterol.

Please look at these assertions carefully. It should be noted at the outset that Keys did *not* say that saturated fat consumption causes anything; certainly not that it causes heart disease. The study did *not* assert that even a consistent association exists between saturated fat and heart disease and/or saturated fat and cholesterol and/or cholesterol and heart disease (although you really would not believe this when you see how entrenched diet advice has become since – and this study is the catalytic foundation of all views that saturated fat is bad for us).

In 1960, the Framingham Heart Study found that smoking increased the risk of heart disease. By 1967 the same study had found exercise had a positive impact on heart disease and weight had an adverse impact. In 1953, Morris et al demonstrated the benefit of vigorous physical activity to cardiovascular health.[134] Hence, even at the time, Keys' conclusions were implausible. Today, we are as certain as we can be that smoking, activity and weight *do* have a significant impact on heart disease. Smoking is generally recognised as the number one risk factor for heart disease. Weight and activity are also widely accepted as being significant factors. So, why do we give so much importance to a study that is so clearly wrong about smoking, activity and weight and assume it to be right about cholesterol and/or dietary fat?

Staying with the conclusions after the first five-year review for now, in Table 6 that follows, we add in the average (mean) serum (total) cholesterol level for each cohort – called the study "baseline." From Table 5, we keep coronary heart disease (CHD) deaths as a percentage of all participants (the CHD mortality rate) and we keep CHD deaths as a proportion of all deaths (to indicate how important CHD is as a cause of death in that cohort):

Table 6: Deaths, CHD deaths and mean cholesterol levels by cohort in the Seven Countries Study

	CHD Deaths	CHD/All deaths	Cholesterol mg/dl
USA - Railroad workers	2.4%	50.0%	240.3
Italy - Crevalcore	1.1%	18.3%	201.6
The Netherlands - Zutphen	1.8%	32.0%	235.6
Finland - west Finland	1.0%	18.0%	256.2
Finland - east Finland (N Karelia)	3.5%	47.5%	265.0
Italy - Rome Railroad workers	0.3%	8.3%	207.3
Italy - Montegiorgio	0.7%	17.2%	201.3
Yugoslavia - Slavonia	1.0%	12.7%	199.5
Greece - Crete	0.1%	10.0%	207.1
Yugoslavia - Dalmatia	0.4%	12.5%	189.1
Yugoslavia - Belgrade	0.4%	40.0%	211.7
Greece - Corfu	0.8%	36.4%	203.8
Yugoslavia - Zrenjanin	0.2%	6.7%	168.6
Yugoslavia - Velika Krsna	0.2%	4.3%	160.3
Japan - Tanushimaru	0.8%	17.4%	167.9
Japan - Ushibuka	0.2%	4.2%	162.2
TOTAL (Average)	1.2%	26.9%	204.8

(Please note that the USA favours mg/dl for cholesterol measurement. Europe and Australia favour mmol/L. To convert mmol/L to mg/dl, multiply by 38.67. To convert mg/dl to mmol/L, divide by 38.67. Hence, the average cholesterol number in Table 6 is 5.3mmol/L). The current UK target of 5mmol/L or lower converts to 193mg/dl and would only have been met by Japan and three of the five Yugoslavian cohorts above.

As a *prima facie* review we can simply look at where individual cohorts are relatively high (H) or low (L) i.e. above or below the cohort average. This is shown in Table 7:

Table 7: Deaths, CHD deaths and mean cholesterol levels, compared to the average, by cohort in the Seven Countries Study

	CHD Deaths	CHD/All deaths	Cholesterol mg/dl
USA - Railroad workers	H	H	H
Italy - Crevalcore	L	L	L
The Netherlands - Zutphen	H	H	H
Finland - west Finland (*)	L	L	H
Finland - east Finland (N Karelia)	H	H	H
Italy - Rome Railroad workers (*)	L	L	H
Italy - Montegiorgio	L	L	L

Yugoslavia - Slavonia	L	L	L
Greece - Crete (*)	L	L	H
Yugoslavia - Dalmatia	L	L	L
Yugoslavia - Belgrade (*)	L	H	H
Greece - Corfu (*)	L	H	L
Yugoslavia - Zrenjanin	L	L	L
Yugoslavia - Velika Krsna	L	L	L
Japan - Tanushimaru	L	L	L
Japan - Ushibuka	L	L	L
Relative to the average	1.2%	26.9%	204.8

(The five cohorts marked with an (*) are referenced in pages to follow).

Interestingly, there are only two cohorts where CHD deaths as a percentage of the number of participants and CHD deaths as a percentage of total deaths are not aligned. In Yugoslavia (Belgrade) and Greece (Corfu), CHD deaths form a higher proportion of all deaths than average while CHD deaths overall are lower than average. This is on small numbers though – five men died overall in the five year study in Belgrade and two of these deaths were from CHD. Eleven men died in Corfu in total and four of these died from CHD. What is interesting is that the higher than average cholesterol levels in Belgrade are accompanied by lower than average CHD deaths as a percentage of the population and the lower than average cholesterol levels in Corfu are accompanied by higher than average CHD deaths as a percentage of all deaths.

So, have we proven anything? Let us go back to my errors in the bathing causes singing argument and see if the Seven Countries Study can be accused of any of the same:

1) Have we ignored any people in the bath and not singing and people not in the bath who are singing?

Yes we have. Keys simply did not include, let alone prove any association for, over 95% of the countries of the world. He discounted 50% of the population in its entirety (women). Had Keys chosen France, Switzerland and Austria, to name but a few other countries, he could have demonstrated the exact opposite of what he tried to conclude. It has been suggested that Keys did not test his theory beyond seven countries, to see if it had wider validity, because he knew as soon as he brought in France et al, it would fall apart and a great deal of money and reputation was at stake.

2) If every person in a bath is always singing and no one out of the bath is ever singing, have we proven causation? Does bathing cause singing or singing cause bathing or both or neither?

Even if Keys analysed every country in the world and had proven a consistent and universal relationship between saturated fat and heart disease *and* saturated fat and cholesterol *and* cholesterol and heart disease, this would still only establish an association, not causation. He could no more say that cholesterol causes heart disease than he could say heart disease causes cholesterol or that saturated fat intake causes either. The mistaking of association for causation is one of the most fundamental errors in science and medicine (does obesity cause diabetes, or does diabetes cause obesity, or are both associated with each other and potentially caused by eating processed carbohydrates?)

3) If there is a perfect association, could both bathing and singing be caused by anything else?

Even if Keys had proven a consistent and universal relationship between saturated fat and heart disease *and* saturated fat and cholesterol *and* cholesterol and heart disease, which held every time, (which he did not), each two things observed at the same time could be *caused* by something else. A diet high in saturated fat and high heart disease could be accompanied by a high sugar/refined carbohydrate diet (we will see how this is a highly plausible suggestion, as refined carbohydrates were called saturated fats in Keys' study and have been ever since).

In conclusion, Keys' saturated fat, cholesterol, heart hypothesis failed the same three tests as did my bathing and singing. No consistent association was proven, let alone causation.

Notwithstanding the fact that the Seven Countries Study fails the same three fundamental errors as the bathing and singing argument, does it make the case for the assertions that it claims? Earlier in this chapter, we summarised the three assertions, made by Keys in 1970, as follows:

1) Coronary heart disease (CHD) tends to be directly related to serum cholesterol;
2) Serum cholesterol tends to be directly related to saturated fat as a proportion of the diet;
3) CHD is as closely related to saturated fat as it is cholesterol.

1) CHD tends to be directly related to cholesterol.

Even within Keys' own selected seven countries, there is contradictory evidence to the notion that CHD tends to be directly related to cholesterol? In Table 7, there were five cohorts, marked with (*), where CHD was not related to cholesterol:

- West Finland had higher than average cholesterol and lower than average CHD deaths in total and CHD deaths as a percentage of all deaths;
- Rome (Italy) railworkers had higher than average cholesterol and lower than average CHD deaths in total and CHD deaths as a percentage of all deaths;
- Crete (Greece) had higher than average cholesterol and lower than average CHD deaths in total and CHD deaths as a percentage of all deaths;
- Belgrade (Yugoslavia) had higher than average cholesterol, lower than average CHD deaths in total, but higher than average CHD deaths as a percentage of all deaths;

- Corfu (Greece) had lower than average cholesterol, lower than average CHD deaths in total, but higher than average CHD deaths as a percentage of all deaths.

These five cohort observations also gave rise to inconsistencies within countries, which undermine Keys' first assertion:

- Finland: north Karelia had over three times the number of CHD deaths as west Finland, at very similar cholesterol levels (which could be separately explained with the loss of 10% of Finland's territory during the war(s) and the concomitant and unprecedented stress of displacement). West Finland actually had relatively low CHD deaths (both as a percentage of all deaths and as a percentage of the participant group) and yet had the second highest average cholesterol out of sixteen cohorts.
Blackburn acknowledges 'the Finland paradox' in his account of the study:[135] "East Finland departs from the regression line on the high side, that is, it has an even higher rate of coronary heart disease than expected from the overall Seven Countries population correlation between diet, blood cholesterol level and coronary heart disease. In contrast, the West Finns have less coronary heart disease than expected from their average cholesterol level." I.e. cholesterol levels are not directly related to heart disease in both cohorts in Finland.
- Greece: Corfu inhabitants had four times as many deaths as nearby Crete inhabitants, even though mean cholesterol levels on Corfu were slightly lower (203.8mg/dl vs. 207.1mg/dl for Corfu and Crete respectively).[136]
Undermining the asserted relationship between coronary heart disease (CHD) and cholesterol, Crete had the lowest proportion of men dying from CHD and yet the seventh highest cholesterol level. Corfu had lower than average cholesterol levels and higher than average CHD deaths as a percentage of all deaths. I.e. cholesterol levels are not directly related to heart disease in both cohorts in Greece. Volume IX on the Greek Islands notes: "The apparent difference in susceptibility to CHD between the men of Crete and their counterparts of Corfu is particularly puzzling. In regard to the major risk factors of serum cholesterol and blood pressure, the men of Corfu should be slightly less prone to the disease than the men of Crete." I.e. the data is not saying what we want it to say.
- Italy: Crevalcore had twice as many deaths (both in total and from CHD) to those of Montegiorgio, despite the same cholesterol level (201.6mg/dl vs. 201.3mg/dl for Crevalcore and Montegiorgio respectively). This pattern continued with Crevalcore experiencing up to one and a half times as many deaths as Montegiorgio, at 5, 10, 15, 20 and 25 year follow ups.

So, five hand picked cohorts and three hand picked countries don't even support the weak relationship asserted, let alone causation.

The single biggest piece of counter evidence, which was available at the time of the study and is still relevant today, is that women worldwide have higher cholesterol levels than men and substantially lower incidence of heart disease.

Remember Blackburn's dismissal ..."we did not consider involving women because of the great rarity of cardiac events among them." So, half the world's population undermine this asserted relationship in one stroke. How can a hypothesis gain so much credence when half the evidence at the outset refutes its validity?

Dr. Malcolm Kendrick, in the brilliant book *The Great Cholesterol Con,*[137] provides additional evidence to undermine the proposed cholesterol/CHD relationship. Kendrick analysed the World Health Organisation MONICA study (an abbreviation of sorts from "Monitoring Trends In Cardiovascular Disease"). He noted that Switzerland has the highest cholesterol levels of any country in the world and their heart disease rates are approximately one third of those in the UK. He plotted the cholesterol levels and heart disease rates for Russia, Spain, France, Poland, Italy, Denmark, Lithuania, Sweden, UK, Belgium, Czech Republic, Germany, Iceland and Switzerland (listed in ascending order of average cholesterol levels in each country) and the chart looks like a random scatter diagram. There is no apparent relationship between the two variables whatsoever, let alone a clear association, let alone a proven causation. Kendrick also added in Australian Aboriginals as a comparator group. This is a particularly important group to include, as they have the lowest cholesterol level of any population studied and they have a heart disease rate approximately 30 times that in France and about 15 times that in the UK. Although the data available to Kendrick was not available to Keys, the countries were and the high meat and dairy consumption in Austria, France and Switzerland is likely only to have declined from Keys to Kendrick.

When not even Keys' own hand picked countries and cohorts can prove an association, when half the world's population kills the assertion in one fell swoop, when the World Health Organisation's own data doesn't demonstrate an association – again – let alone a causation, how on earth has this hypothesis become folk lore?

2) Cholesterol tends to be directly related to saturated fat.

Just using the data from the Seven Countries Study, is there any counter evidence to the notion that cholesterol tends to be related to saturated fat? Yes there is. Crevalcore (Italy) was alleged to have a higher saturated fat content diet than Montegiorgio (Italy), but there is no discernible differential in cholesterol levels. Greece with reported lower saturated fat intake than Italy should have lower cholesterol levels, but levels are, in fact, higher. In figures S9 and S10 in the summary volume of *Circulation*, both Japan and Yugoslavia were claimed to have 7% of men with cholesterol levels over 250mg/dl and yet Yugoslavia was claimed to have over three times the calories coming from saturated fat in the diet as Japan. Yugoslavia and Italy are then claimed to have the same amount of calories coming from saturated fat (10%) and yet Italy has twice the percentage of men with cholesterol levels over 250mg/dl than Yugoslavia.

I can drive a bus through these figures and this is despite the fact that Keys picked the countries, Keys picked the cohorts, Keys picked the demarcations (I can only assume picking the percentage of men with cholesterol levels over 250mg/dl was more favourable for his conclusions than absolute numbers) and, therefore, all the opportunity to prove his point is there.

Again, we don't need to be constrained by the Seven Countries Study to see if cholesterol tends to be directly related to saturated fat. Outside the study, if we turn to the Framingham Heart Study, the longest running diet, cholesterol, heart epidemiological study in the world, the director of that study, Dr. William Castelli said in 1992: "In Framingham, (Massachusetts), the more saturated fat one ate, the more cholesterol one ate, the *more calories one ate*, the lower the person's serum cholesterol."[138] (original emphasis).

The BBC Horizon programme, about The Atkins Diet (August 2004), interviewed Dr. Gary Foster who had recently led a study comparing the Atkins diet with the standard USA government low fat advice of the time.[139] The programme wanted to see if the Atkins diet were more effective for weight loss and, in the words of the programme transcript, they wanted to test "The scientists' biggest criticism of the diet was that the high fat would lead to high cholesterol which would clog the arteries and kill."[140] (Please note this example of typical media language on the subject of fat).

This was an important and probably overdue study. As Foster noted "Despite the popularity of the low-carbohydrate, high-protein, high-fat (Atkins) diet, no randomized, controlled trials have evaluated its efficacy". Foster and his team set out to rectify this and randomly assigned 43 women and 20 men to either the Atkins diet or a low-fat diet, for a one year duration.[141] The Atkins diet started with a carbohydrate intake limited to 20g per day for two weeks and the group following this diet were given a copy of *Dr. Atkins' New Diet Revolution* to follow thereafter.[142] The low-fat group followed *The LEARN Program for Weight Management*,[143] which was consistent with the dietary recommendations provided by the registered dietitian for the study and with the American food pyramid. The women in the latter group were allowed 1,200-1,500 calories a day, the men 1,500-1,800. The intake was designed to be approximately 60% carbohydrate, 25% fat and 15% protein. The calorie intake in the Atkins group was *not* limited.

Noting that "adherence was poor and attrition was high in both groups" (although a higher proportion of the low carbohydrate group managed to stay on the diet), the conclusions were that "subjects on the low-carbohydrate diet had lost more weight than subjects on the conventional diet". They had, in fact, lost twice as much. At three months the Atkins group had lost, on average (mean) 6.8% of their body weight vs. 2.7% for the low-fat group. At six months the comparator numbers were 7.0% vs. 3.2% of body weight. The difference at 12 months was described as *not* significant, but I'm not sure the slimmer group would have been so dismissive. At 12 months the Atkins group had lost, on average, 4.4% of their body weight vs. 2.5% for the low-fat group.

Turning to cholesterol, the programme's interview of Foster recorded him saying "My first reaction was could this be, this doesn't make a lot of sense. Not only were there no bad effects of the diet in terms of cholesterol, but actually there were quite positive ones." Triglyceride readings for the Atkins group showed an 18.7% *fall* at three months, compared with a 1.1% *rise* for the low-fat group. This was sustained with the 12 month readings showing a 17% fall vs. a 0.7% rise for the low-fat group. That means, even if the low-fat group results had fallen by 0.7%, the Atkins reduction would still have been 24 times greater.

The journal notes that the study was funded by the National Institutes of Health. Taubes notes in a question and answer session, in one of his presentations featured on YouTube, that no further funding was offered after the results of this study were published. "If you want to do a study that you think can show that this (government recommended) diet is unhealthy, you won't get funding. Not from the NIH, not from the American Heart association."[144]

3) CHD is as closely related to saturated fat as it is to cholesterol.

Actually, I could concede this one because it would still prove nothing. We have already undermined the relationship between CHD and cholesterol and cholesterol and saturated fat. As we have shown in (1) CHD is not consistently related to cholesterol and therefore if, as Keys asserts, CHD is as closely related to saturated fat, as it is to cholesterol, it is not closely related to either.

However, just for completeness, let us provide the evidence against this assertion from the study itself. In Figure S10, in the summary volume of *Circulation,* we find the following:

- Japan has higher estimated coronary heart disease (CHD) incidence than Greece with under half the saturated fat intake (as a percentage of calorie intake);
- Yugoslavia and Italy are then claimed to have the same number of calories coming from saturated fat (10%) and yet Italy has twice the CHD incidence of Yugoslavia;
- The Netherlands has higher saturated fat intake (as a percentage of calorie intake) than the USA, but lower CHD incidence, by some margin.

I could stop there because just one contradictory example would negate the claim that CHD is closely related to saturated fat. However, let not more brilliant work by Dr. Malcolm Kendrick go to waste. Kendrick did two *Seven Country Studies* of his own. He analysed the World Health Organisation data again (the MONICA information was from 1998, or within two years of this date if 1998 were not available) and his first seven countries were those with the *lowest* consumption of saturated fat. These were Georgia, Tajikistan, Azerbaijan, Moldova, Croatia, Macedonia and the Ukraine. Kendrick's second seven countries were those with the *highest* consumption of saturated fat. These were Austria, Finland, Belgium, Iceland, Netherlands, Switzerland and France. Every single one of the seven countries with the lowest consumption of saturated fat had significantly higher heart disease than every single one of the countries with the highest consumption of saturated fat. This concludes the exact opposite of the Keys' Seven Countries assertion. Does Kendrick go on to assert that *high* saturated fat consumption causes *low* heart disease and *low* saturated fat consumption causes *high* heart disease. Of course he doesn't. He is too sensible and responsible to do so.

The Seven Countries Study – 25-years on

More than 15 years after America changed its diet advice and precisely 10 years after the UK did the same, the 1993 *European Journal of Epidemiology* published a 25-year follow-up of the Seven Countries Study.[145]

This is when it gets interesting because the strength of the asserted relationship between cholesterol and heart disease (still only in seven hand picked countries, please remember) is finally quantified. Keys claimed that the linear correlation coefficient between cholesterol (mg/dl) at entry to the study and coronary heart disease (CHD) death rates at 25 years was **0.72**. This was presented as 'we can predict heart disease over a 25 year period from knowing what cholesterol levels are at the start of the period.'

I took the original data in this journal and validated the correlation as 0.72. This confirmed that Keys had used the standard (Pearson) correlation coefficient method of calculation:

$$r = \frac{n\sum xy - (\sum x)(\sum y)}{\sqrt{n(\sum x^2) - (\sum x)^2}\ \sqrt{n(\sum y^2) - (\sum y)^2}}$$

While repeating the correlation to test Keys' methodology, I happened to notice that death rates worsened the further north countries were in Europe. So I then ran a correlation with an alternative 'risk factor'. I found that, using a far more easily available 'risk factor', I would have been able to 'predict' CHD deaths with a correlation coefficient of **0.93** at cohort level and **0.96** at a country level.

That 'risk factor' is latitude.

I did the arithmetic mean for the latitudes of cohorts to represent the mean latitude for the country. I did the death rate in two different ways – arithmetic mean and weighted mean for the number of participants in each cohort. The correlation was **0.96** for both methods.

I then repeated this correlation analysis at the cohort level and found a correlation coefficient of **0.93**.

Keys used his correlation of 0.72 as a predictive tool. He asserted that this correlation meant that he could predict CHD death rates from the cholesterol levels at the start of the study. Correlation is not intended to be used in this way. The correlation coefficient indicates whether or not there is a relationship between two variables and the correlation coefficient squared indicates the strength of that relationship. The strength of the relationship, r^2, for cholesterol is 0.52 and the strength of the relationship for latitude is 0.86 at the cohort level and 0.92 at the country level. The strength of the relationship can be used as an indicator of how much can be explained by the linear relationship. Latitude explains about 90% of the observed relationship; cholesterol explains as much as it doesn't: 50%. This is notwithstanding the fact that Keys handpicked the countries in the first place and please don't forget that none of this says anything about causation – only association.

Keys did not need to do any blood tests, employ numerous medics across numerous medical centres and follow up 12,770 men with invasive tests at five-year intervals. He just needed to ask the men for their address at the start of the study and he could have 'predicted' heart disease with far greater accuracy than that afforded by his own assumed predictor of cholesterol.

I must admit I was as excited as a researcher can be upon discovering this. It is difficult to describe what it is like to have an idea, input the data, and press the recalculation button and to see a number in excess of 0.9 pop up. Not only does it make a mockery of the conclusion reached by Keys, but it actually has much logic. It provides an excellent example of the logical error number (3) listed in the introduction to this chapter. This is the notion that two things can be observed at the same time, but that they can be explained by something else completely different.

What my correlation of 0.93-0.96 says is that the Seven Countries Study produced an almost perfect association between latitude and CHD deaths. The further the cohort/country was away from the equator, the greater the incidence of CHD deaths. The closer the cohort/country was to the equator, the lower the incidence of CHD deaths. Can this explain Keys' observation of any kind of relationship between cholesterol and heart disease? Yes it can.

Vitamin D can be ingested and it can be made from skin cholesterol. Natural sunlight hitting cholesterol in our skin cell membranes turns the cholesterol into vitamin D. With reduced sunlight, in countries further away from the equator, there is reduced sunlight to turn cholesterol into vitamin D. This would logically leave more cholesterol in the body and higher cholesterol levels in areas where heart disease was found to be higher. However, the cholesterol level is in no way a cause of heart disease – it is simply a factor observed at the same time.

Dr. Robert Scragg, Associate Professor in Epidemiology at the University of Auckland, New Zealand, first proposed back in December 1981 that vitamin D deficiency plays a role in cardiovascular disease.[146] Keys could have discovered this first, had he run the latitude correlation and worked through the implications.

There is a more sinister issue here. Vitamin D is found exclusively in animal products and requires cholesterol for its synthesis. If people follow the current advice to avoid natural animal products (meat, eggs, dairy products etc) because of their supposed saturated fat content (or, even more pointlessly, because of their cholesterol content), people will reduce their intake of vitamin D and, if Scragg, is right, they will *increase* their risk of heart disease. Far too little thought was given, at so many different levels, to the implications of being wrong when we changed our dietary advice.

The Seven Countries Study – dietary analysis

It is important at this stage to look at what Keys actually meant by saturated fat in the Seven Countries Study.

As we are going to see in Chapter Twelve, most of the time when government and health organisations talk about saturated fat, they are in fact talking about processed carbohydrates. Is this a recent mistake or did Keys do the same?

"Volume XVII The Diet" of the study goes into detail about how the diets of the men were analysed – some by replicating the intake of a small sample of the men from each cohort and then analysing the breakdown of this in a laboratory. The USA railroad intake was done by questionnaire alone based on the men's recollection of what they had eaten the day before (notoriously unreliable). This information was then analysed by "trained dietitians" (I'm nervous already) and then protein, fat and carbohydrate content were "estimated". This is the key wording to note: "The check list, aimed particularly at sources of fat, included milk, eggs, butter, cheese, cake, ice cream and so on." So, processed carbohydrates – cake and ice cream as the listed examples – have been assumed to be saturated fat for the Seven Countries Study. Did Keys know that eggs are 63% *unsaturated* fat? Did Keys know, or care, that whole, real milk is just 3-4% fat and a third of this *unsaturated*?

In "Volume XVII The Diet" there is remarkably little mention of the composition of each country's diet, let alone that of each cohort. We can only glean slightly more from the individual volumes of each part of the study (I've been through each one):

- In "Volume IV USA Railroad employees", there is no information at all on diet, food intake or fat in this volume.

- "Volume V Dalmatia" is mentioned in the same sentence as "*olive oil*" and "*fish*". Slavonia is noted for a diet with "animal fat, especially pork fat", "meats and poultry in greater abundance than Dalmatia". Interestingly, 20% of calories in the diet of Dalmatia came from alcohol. For Slavonia, 8% of the dietary calories came from alcohol. These were the only mentions of diet, food intake or fat in the whole of Volume V.

- "Volume VI Finland": no description of diet was provided, other than the passing comment "butterfat was a prominent item." That tells me that bread, and likely cake, were prominent items. People don't eat butter on its own.

- "Volume VII Rural Italy": "The cuisine of Bologna and Modena is the richest of the regional cuisines of Italy, it is loaded with saturated fatty acids and cholesterol from butter, cream, meats, and eggs; the whole region in which Crevalcore is located is known as Emilia la grassa, 'Emilia the fat land.' It was expected, then, that the diet of the men of Crevalcore would be of the type that promotes high levels of cholesterol in blood. Actually, repeated dietary surveys on subsamples of the cohort of Crevalcore showed an average of only 27% of calories from total fats and only 15% of calories from fats of animal origin (Fidanza et al. 1964)."

"Actually, the diet of Crevalcore proved to be not so different from the diet of Montegiorgio. The average of surveys in three different seasons in Montegiorgio showed 25% of total calories from total fats and 16% of calories from fats of animal origin (Fidanza et al. 1964)."

This is exactly as written in Volume VII. Fidanza is one of the writers of this volume – the others being Vittorio Puddu, Bruno Imbimbo, Alessandro Menotti and Ancel Keys. So the Seven Countries dietary evidence, for two cohorts in Italy, appeared to rely upon a 1964 report from one of the writers.

Have the fats from animal origin simply been assumed to be saturated fat? Why are eggs and meat, which are predominantly *unsaturated* fat grouped together with butter and cream – which are still one third *unsaturated* fat?

- "Volume VIII Zutphen": there is only one reference to diet: "Finally, in regard to the nutrient composition of the diet, the data on the U.S. railroad men are not very precise, but the Americans seemed to be more like the Zutphen men than any other cohort in respect to total fats, kinds of fatty acids, etc. "

- "Volume IX The Greek islands of Crete and Corfu": *Crete* "This is the classic land of the olive tree, and its main produce, olive oil, continues to be a dominant item of the diet, as it has for at least four thousand years. Olive oil earns some cash too, but its importance is that it provides a third or more of the calories in the local diet." Corfu: "In regard to the diet, the only obvious difference between the two populations is a somewhat higher intake of fat in Crete, a difference entirely accounted for by olive oil."

As we demonstrate in Chapter Twelve, olive oil has nine times the saturated fat of pork. Was Keys aware of this? Please also note the repeatedly casual use of the word "fat", not always qualified with the word "saturated".

- "Volume X Japan": "Dietary data indicated that the low serum cholesterol levels observed were largely explained by the extremely low-fat diet, averaging only some 10% of calories from total fats." Tanushimaru: "The diet of Tanushimaru is typical of rural areas of central and southern Japan; it is dominated by rice, soybean products, vegetables in great variety, fish and seafood, very little fat, and very little dairy produce."

I will add, and virtually no processed carbohydrates – no cake, bread, biscuits, confectionery, ice cream and so on, but the mention and importance of the *absence* of certain foods is as lacking in this study as the *presence* of specifics on other foods.

Ushibuka: "At sea the fishermen subsist on rice and large quantities of fish, mostly raw, together with some condiments and pickled vegetables. On shore too the diet is basically similar except for more vegetables and the use of a good deal of cooked as well as fresh fish and seafood…it is surprising to find that they have an average daily intake of one to two or more kg of fish, shell fish, crustacea, octopus, and the like."

- In "Volume XI Railroad men of Italy", there is no mention of diet or fat intake at all.

- In "Volume XII Three cohorts in Serbia", there is no mention of diet or fat intake at all.

One would have to conclude, from looking at all the volumes of the Seven Countries Study, that this does not qualify as a robust dietary study. All the volumes go through the preselected variables (smoking, sedentary behaviour, weight, skin fold, blood pressure and cholesterol) and try to relate these to incidence of CHD. Dietary fat was one of the preselected variables but there is negligible mention of food, diet and dietary fat in the 1970 report write ups, let alone robust tables and analysis. What is written is anecdotal and more suited to a travel guide than to a study that changed the course of public health diet advice.

In the most comprehensive write up of the Study – "Seven Countries: a multivariate analysis of death and coronary heart disease", (1980), Keys notes the following "The fact that the incidence of coronary heart disease was significantly correlated with the average percentage of calories from sucrose in the diets is explained by the inter correlation of sucrose with saturated fat." (I am indebted to Dr. Robert Lustig for finding this key passage).[147]

We have here a clear acknowledgement of the precise foods being accused of causing heart disease. Foods containing saturated fat and sucrose are, with one exception, processed foods. There is no sucrose in meat/fish/eggs and natural animal foods. The only real food that could conceivably contain both sucrose and saturated fat would be a fruit with a fat content. Avocado and olives are the only two that fall into this category. Avocados contain 2.1 grams of saturated fat per 100 grams of product and 60 milligrams of sucrose. Olives have saturated fat, but no sucrose. Unless the Seven Countries Study was a study of the impact of avocado consumption in seven countries, we can safely assume that the accepted correlation between sucrose and saturated fat confirms that the saturated fat recorded in the Seven Countries Study was, in fact, processed food. If the study did provide any possible associations between diet and heart disease, these associations were between processed food and heart disease and not real fat, found in real food, and heart disease.

Had the Seven Countries Study concluded that smoking were the key risk factor, Americans (it was, after all, the end goal of the study to save Americans from heart disease) could have been given clear rationale to stop smoking. Had the key risk factor been sedentary behaviour, steps could be taken to get Americans more active. Had the key risk factor been weight, Americans could have been advised to lose weight and so on. I suggest that it was *unacceptable* for such a long and expensive study, with so much promise, to conclude that the only possible association was with cholesterol – something made by the body – and therefore not something that Americans could do anything about. Unless, of course, it could be alleged that dietary fat causes cholesterol, causes heart disease and then Americans can be told to eat the sandwich, but leave the cheese. Of course, what Americans should have been told, if the Seven Countries Study concluded anything, is to move as close to the equator as possible.

It is very interesting to note that, in the 25-year follow up article, published in the *European Journal of Epidemiology*, the word "fat" does not appear once. That bears repeating – in the 6,000 word report, 25-years on from the study that changed public health diet advice 180 degrees, fat no longer warranted a single mention. The damage had already been done.

Logic and the first rule of holes

Earlier in this chapter, we summarised the three assertions, made by Keys in 1970, as follows:

1) Coronary heart disease (CHD) tends to be directly related to serum cholesterol;
2) Serum cholesterol tends to be directly related to saturated fat as a proportion of the diet;
3) CHD is as closely related to saturated fat as it is cholesterol.

Please remember that even before the Seven Countries Study Keys tried, and failed, to prove that cholesterol consumption causes heart disease. This was followed by the attempt to prove that saturated fat consumption causes heart disease. This also failed, so the argument became that blood cholesterol levels cause heart disease and saturated fat consumption causes heart disease through blood cholesterol, (although the cholesterol consumed alongside the saturated fat plays no part). I like playing with logic as much as anyone, but I cannot see a basis for A causing C through B if there is no consistent association between A and C in the first place. If bathing and singing are not even associated, then having a duck in the bath is not going to make any difference.

The first rule of holes says – when you're in a hole, stop digging. The variables that were subsequently introduced, as the first rule of holes was ignored, were monounsaturated fat, LDL and HDL and even the ratio of HDL to total cholesterol. (Please remember that there was no mention of monounsaturated fat in the entire summary of the original *Circulation* 20 volumes and that the only mention of polyunsaturated fat was that it was unrelated).

So what do we know?

Saturated fat does *not* have a consistent association with CHD, let alone proven causation (see Georgia, Tajikistan, Azerbaijan, Moldova, Croatia, Macedonia, Ukraine, Austria, Finland, Belgium, Iceland, Netherlands, Switzerland and France and likely more).

I have seen no evidence that monounsaturated fat has a consistent inverse association with CHD, let alone proven inverse causation. The best web site to use is pubmed.org. This has over 19 million citations for biomedical articles. Enter "monounsaturated fat and heart disease" and 239 articles appear. That's 0.00125% of available articles that are concerned with this supposedly critical topic. When you see "A comparison of the fat composition and prices of margarines between 2002 and 2006, when new Canadian labelling regulations came into effect,"[148] on the first page, you realise that very few of even these 239 articles are trying to assert that monounsaturated fat will save the world from heart disease.

The best articles to devote attention to are those that review evidence from other articles. The most recent example of such an exercise was published in the *American Journal for Clinical Nutrition* in 2009.[149] As a researcher, I still don't take any article as fact. I see first if it concludes what we are trying to test – in this case that monounsaturated fat protects against heart disease – and then test the methodology and conclusions if it does. Thankfully, there is rarely a need to review a full article, as I have yet to find the article that even claims this protection in the first place. This article is no exception. This one, interestingly, does the test that should be done to review the impact of different fats on heart disease. Correctly, they review the studies where one type of fat has been exchanged for another type of fat. Less usefully they looked at studies where the same type of fat had been exchanged for a different macronutrient – carbohydrate. The latter tells us as much about the presence of carbohydrate, as it does about the absence of fat, if it tells us anything at all.

The authors declare their belief system from the start, as the opening sentence of the abstract (summary) is "Saturated fatty acid (SFA) intake increases plasma LDL-cholesterol concentrations; therefore, intake should be reduced to prevent coronary heart disease." All the unproven associations asserted as a direct causation, followed by a solution, in just one sentence. (Keys would have been proud). The aim of the article is to see if monounsaturated fats, or polyunsaturated fats, or carbohydrates, should replace saturated fat in the diet. The 16 authors conclude that polyunsaturated fats are the ones that will save us from heart disease (Keys would have been less proud at this stage). They state categorically in the summary of the whole article: "MUFA intake was not associated with CHD". For MUFA read monounsaturated fat and CHD is coronary heart disease.

There is not even a Seven Countries Study with a single table showing the higher the population intake of monounsaturated fat the lower the incidence of heart disease and the lower the intake of monounsaturated fat the higher the incidence of heart disease. And why pick monounsaturated fat? Why not the other whole macronutrients – protein and carbohydrate – rather than a particular type of one macronutrient? Why not processed food, white flour and sugar and substances that we have been eating massively more of in the recent years during which we have observed massively more heart disease? Why not exercise (sorry that was dismissed); smoking (also dismissed); weight (also dismissed). Why not stress? climate? work-life balance? having a wonderful family and community network? loving your occupation? being in a fulfilling and happy relationship, proximity to the equator etc? What was the obsession with fat and then subsections of fat when total fat failed to serve as an explanation.

It is only natural to wonder what the obsession was for Keys to try to prove that dietary fat causes heart disease. Kendrick quotes an extract from Henry Blackburn's diaries on the University of Minnesota website. Blackburn's Seven Country diaries are very open and informative and I have referred to them often.[150] However, the particular reference quoted by Kendrick no longer appears to be part of the diary entries. Hence, we are indebted to Kendrick for capturing it for posterity.

"In 1954, the fledgling World Health Organization called its first Expert Committee on the Pathogenesis of Atherosclerosis to consider the burgeoning epidemic of coronary disease and heart attacks. Several medical leaders of the time were assembled in Geneva: Paul Dudley White of Boston, Gunnar Björk of Stockholm, Noboru Kimura of Japan, George Pickering of Oxford, Ancel Keys of Minnesota, and others. As reported by Pickering, the discussion was lively, tending to tangents and tirades.

"Ancel Keys was in good form – outspoken, quick, typically blunt. When, at this critical conference, he posed with such assurance his dietary hypothesis of coronary heart disease, he was ill-prepared for the indignant reaction of some.

"George Pickering, recently named Knight of the Realm by Queen Elizabeth, interrupted Keys' peroration. He put it something along these lines: 'Tell us, Professor Keys, if you would be so kind, what is the single best piece of evidence you can cite in support of your thesis about diet and coronary heart disease?'

"Keys, ordinarily quick on the draw, was taken aback. Rarely, of course, is there ever a 'single best piece of evidence' supporting any theory. Theory is developed from a body of evidence and varied sources. This is particularly true in regard to the many facets of lifestyle that relate to disease. It is the totality and congruity of evidence that leads to a theory – and to inference of causation.

"Keys fell headlong into the trap. He proceeded to cite a piece of evidence. Sir George and the assembled peers were easily able to diminish this single piece of evidence, and did so. And by then it was too late to recover – for Keys to summon the total evidence in a constructive, convincing argument.

"My theory is that Keys was so stung by this event that he left the Geneva meeting intent on gathering the definitive evidence to establish or refute the diet-Heart Theory. Out of this singular, moving, personal experience – so my theory goes – came the challenge, the motivation, and eventually, the implementation of the Seven Countries Study." Henry Blackburn.

So in his best friend's own words, Keys was humiliated and presumably keen on revenge. Well the Seven Countries Study certainly left a legacy.

There is one final part about which I need to concern myself. Notwithstanding the fact that there is no consistent association, let alone proven causation, between fat (any kind) and heart disease, we need to dismiss the notion that this causation can somehow happen via a third party – cholesterol. And, as we have already dismissed the simple route of serum (total) cholesterol, we have the products of the first rule of holes being ignored – LDL and HDL.

So, let's do a bit of discrete mathematics. Let us see if there is any logical way in which cholesterol can provide a 'flip switch' in the middle to provide a consistent association between saturated fat and CHD. 'H' indicates high in Table 8 and 'L' indicates Low. Fat will be any fat that may give the desired result at the next stage (I'm trying to be fair here). Let us look at all the theoretical combinations (assuming that all are practically possible) to see if we can even establish the *possibility* of an association between fat and CHD involving LDL and/or HDL:

There are 16 different permutations of H and L across the four variables Fat, LDL, HDL and CHD. In four of the permutations, fat will be high and CHD will be high and LDL and HDL can be L/L, H/H, H/L and L/H in between. (This is the example represented by the USA in the Seven Countries Study). We need to assume for this exercise that LDL is 'bad' cholesterol and HDL is 'good' cholesterol. (At the end of this chapter we will see that LDL and HDL are not even cholesterol, let alone bad or good, but, for now, let not the facts get in the way of the story).

In option 1, HDL must determine the outcome and, it being low must outweigh LDL being low and cause heart disease. In option 2 LDL would have to determine the outcome and it being high must outweigh HDL being high and cause heart disease. Option 3 is the commonly used argument – High LDL and Low HDL and heart disease. Option 4 is the opposite – Low LDL and High HDL and heart disease.

You can see that the same four options could exist for high fat intake and low heart disease (France et al); low fat intake and high heart disease (Georgia et al) and low fat intake and low heart disease (Japan in the Seven Countries Study).

Table 8: Possible permutations for fat, LDL, HDL and CHD:

Option	Fat	LDL	HDL	CHD	Example
1	H	L	L	H	USA
2	H	H	H	H	USA
3	H	H	L	H	USA
4	H	L	H	H	USA
5	H	H	H	L	France et al
6	H	L	L	L	France et al
7	H	L	H	L	France et al
8	H	H	L	L	France et al
9	L	L	L	H	Georgia et al
10	L	H	H	H	Georgia et al
11	L	H	L	H	Georgia et al
12	L	L	H	H	Georgia et al
13	L	H	H	L	Japan
14	L	L	L	L	Japan

| 15 | L | L | H | L | Japan |
| 16 | L | H | L | L | Japan |

For high fat intake to cause high heart disease through cholesterol, there has to be a consistent association between fat and LDL or HDL (or both) and CHD. I am not aware that the heart/cholesterol hypothesis has ever suggested that high fat intake causes low LDL (causes low heart disease) or that low fat intake causes high LDL (causes high heart disease). Hence we can discard the permutations of high fat and low LDL and vice versa to leave:

Table 9: Possible permutations for fat, LDL, HDL and CHD (excluding high fat/low LDL and vice versa):

Option	Fat	LDL	HDL	CHD	Example
2	H	H	H	H	USA
3	H	H	L	H	USA
5	H	H	H	L	France et al
8	H	H	L	L	France et al
9	L	L	L	H	Georgia et al
12	L	L	H	H	Georgia et al
14	L	L	L	L	Japan
15	L	L	H	L	Japan

Similarly, I am not aware that the heart/cholesterol hypothesis has ever suggested that high LDL and low HDL causes low heart disease or that low LDL and high HDL causes high heart disease. Hence we can discard options 8 and 12 to leave:

Table 10: Possible permutations for fat, LDL, HDL and CHD (excluding options rejected by the heart/cholesterol hypothesis):

Option	Fat	LDL	HDL	CHD	Example
2	H	H	H	H	USA
3	H	H	L	H	USA
5	H	H	H	L	France et al
9	L	L	L	H	Georgia et al
14	L	L	L	L	Japan
15	L	L	H	L	Japan

The two interesting options are 2 and 14 – where all measures are high or all measures are low. However, options 5 and 9 undermine these. If fat, LDL and HDL are all high, we cannot say that this is consistently associated with (let alone causes) high heart disease, as it isn't with France and many other countries. If fat, LDL and HDL are all low, we cannot say that this is consistently associated with low heart disease, as it isn't with Georgia and many other countries.

Removing 2 and 14 to leave 3, 5, 9 and 15, we still have all four permutations of USA, France et al, Georgia et al and Japan.

Table 11: The four possible permutations for fat, LDL, HDL and CHD:

Option	Fat	LDL	HDL	CHD	Example
3	H	H	L	H	USA
5	H	H	H	L	France et al
9	L	L	L	H	Georgia et al
15	L	L	H	L	Japan

The logic then becomes:

- It is theoretically possible that fat and LDL can be associated;
- It is theoretically possible that HDL and CHD can be inversely associated;
- LDL and CHD can *not* be consistently associated, as every permutation exists. Hence LDL can *not* be a predictor of heart disease;
- Fat and HDL can *not* be consistently associated, as every permutation exists. Hence fat can *not* be a predictor of heart disease directly, or through HDL.

So dietary fat cannot predict, let alone cause, heart disease either directly or indirectly through total cholesterol or indirectly through some assumed components of cholesterol.

If you still haven't given up, the only option remaining is the ratio of LDL to HDL and/or the ratio of HDL to total cholesterol. Using the above scenarios 3, 5, 9 and 15 and replacing the H/L for LDL/HDL for the USA National Cholesterol Education Programme (NCEP) guidelines for high and low cholesterol levels[151] (hence – we are working in mg/dL for now – but the ratio would be the same for mmol/L), we find:[xxvi]

Table 12: Ratios of LDL/HDL in the remaining permutations:

Option	Fat	LDL	HDL	CHD	LDL/HDL
3	H	160	40	H (USA)	4.0
5	H	160	60	L (France)	2.7
9	L	100	40	H (Georgia)	2.5
15	L	100	60	L (Japan)	1.7

This still can't explain the four permutations observed and, of course, logically it wouldn't as the base relationships don't hold in the first place, so

---

[xxvi] The NCEP defines high LDL as 160 mg/dL and low LDL as 100 mg/dL. They define high HDL as 60 mg/dL and low HDL as 40 mg/dL. Please note that I don't accept any of these figures as evidence based or healthy targets – I am using them for the purposes of the exercise, not to give them credence.

derivatives of those variables will not hold. (You may like to look at the National Cholesterol Education Programme guidelines in full. The information for Americans presented as 'education', without evidence, is quite shocking).

I will address the ratio of HDL and total cholesterol in the 'post-amble' to this chapter, as we need to know a bit more about cholesterol and how cholesterol blood tests actually work, before covering this. Suffice to say at this stage, any ratio between HDL and total cholesterol actually presents a circular reference, as these two measures are used to estimate the other readings that we are given in our blood test results.

The problem is that because fat and CHD have no consistent association to start with, any 'flip switch' in the middle cannot have a consistent association through any added link in the chain. If A is not consistently associated with C, then A cannot be consistently associated with B *and* B consistently associated with C. If people in the bath don't always sing, then, as I've said before, having a duck in the bath, even a good duck or a bad duck, is not going to change matters.

All I care about at this point, as an obesity researcher, is that fat is fully exonerated of all charges. Saturated fat doesn't predict/cause (whatever) CHD and, if saturated fat does predict/cause (whatever) LDL, the four logical options cannot consistently predict/cause (whatever) heart disease. If HDL does predict/cause (whatever) heart disease, the four logical options cannot have fat as a predictor of HDL.

I could actually bow out here, given that saturated fat does not predict/cause heart disease. However...

'Post-amble' – cholesterol

...This chapter started with cholesterol and it seems appropriate to end with the same topic. As an obesity researcher, my only need to enter the debate on cholesterol was to remove any argument against people eating real food. (Interestingly, cholesterol is *only* found in real food). We must return to eating food as nature provides it, to cure the obesity epidemic, and therefore we need to negate the counter argument that one gets – there is fat (and cholesterol) in animal foods (provided by nature) and they are going to kill us. (I do wonder, even given the persuasive skills of Ancel Keys, how we ever got into such an absurd mindset. Do we really think that nature would put anything in real food to kill us, let alone in the same foods that contain all the vital nutrients that sustain life?)

Having been drawn into the cholesterol debate, to understand and overcome the rationale for the current dietary advice, I have been so shocked by some of the findings that I do want to share five observations before moving on. Cholesterol also remains important to the chapters that follow on fat and carbohydrate, so we can't ignore it from hereon in anyway:

1) Cholesterol is a vital substance in the human body. We would die without it. Here are the key critical functions that it performs:

- Cholesterol builds and maintains the integrity of the cell walls. Every cell in our body is covered by a membrane made largely of cholesterol, fat and protein. Membranes are porous structures, not solid walls, letting nutrients and hormones in while keeping waste and toxins out. If cholesterol were removed from cell membranes they would literally explode from their internal water pressure. Human beings are simply not viable without cholesterol.
- Cholesterol plays a vital role in hormone production. Steroid hormones can be grouped into five categories by the receptors to which they bind: glucocorticoids; mineral corticoids; androgens; estrogens; and progestagens. (Vitamin D derivatives are seen as a sixth hormone system, but we will discuss this separately). Glucocorticoids help to regulate blood glucose levels and without cortisone, for example, the body could not cope with stress. Mineral corticoids regulate minerals, such as calcium, and they help to regulate blood pressure (the mineral corticoid, aldosterone, regulates sodium and water levels). The sex hormones and therefore the entire human reproductive system are totally dependent on cholesterol. Hence, not only would humans die without cholesterol, the human race would die out.
- Cholesterol is vital for digestion. The human body uses cholesterol to synthesise bile acids. Without cholesterol-rich, bile salts, the human body could not absorb essential fatty acids or the fat soluble vitamins (A, D, E and K) and serious, even life threatening, deficiencies could develop. (It is interesting, therefore, that nature puts cholesterol in virtually every food that contains fat – providing a digestion mechanism in tandem).
- Cholesterol is abundant in the tissue of the brain and nervous system and is critical for the brain and memory functions. Even though the brain is only 2% of the body's weight, it contains approximately 25% of the body's cholesterol. Myelin (which we read more about in Chapter Twelve) covers nerve axons to help conduct the electrical impulses that make movement, sensation, thinking, learning, and remembering possible. Myelin is over one fifth cholesterol by weight. One of the key reasons that we need to spend approximately one third of our lives sleeping is to give the body time to produce cholesterol, repair cells and perform other essential maintenance.
- Cholesterol is also critical for bones and for all the roles performed by vitamin D. Vitamin D is best known for its role in calcium and phosphorus metabolism, and thus bone health, but we are continually learning more about potential additional health benefits of vitamin D from mental health to immune health. Vitamin D can be ingested (and is, interestingly again, found in foods high in cholesterol) and it can be made from skin cholesterol. As we noted in our latitude observation in the Seven Countries Study, sunlight hitting cholesterol in skin cell membranes turns the cholesterol into vitamin D. Modern 'health' advice to avoid the sun, take cholesterol-lowering drugs, eat a low cholesterol diet – combined with there not even being a recommended dietary allowance for vitamin D – is undoubtedly contributing to avoidable modern illness.

When you read in detail the life essential role of cholesterol in the human body, through cell viability to hormones to digestion to the central nervous system and the skeletal system, it is impossible not to question the efficacy of our widespread prescription of statins – drugs that stop the body from producing the cholesterol that the body was designed to produce.

The following diagram represents a simplified flow chart for the complicated process by which the body makes cholesterol.

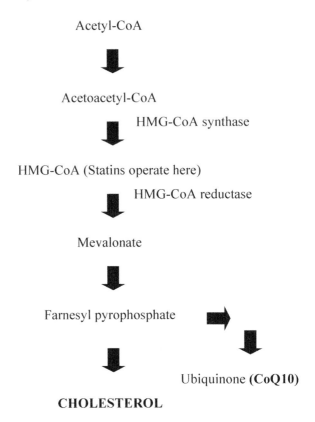

Figure 4: A simplified flow chart to show key steps in the process by which the body makes cholesterol.

The three important things to note about this diagram are:

a) The fundamental building block for the production of cholesterol, Acetyl CoA, is produced during carbohydrate metabolism (we will see how in Chapter Thirteen). So why are carbohydrates not accused of raising cholesterol levels?

b) The step in the process from HMG (3-hydroxy-3-methyl-glutaryl) CoA to mevalonate requires an enzyme – HMG-CoA reductase. Statins inhibit this enzyme. This is why statins have the formal name of HMG-CoA reductase inhibitors. This is quite a key distinction – statins do not work by lowering cholesterol *per se*. They stop the body from producing cholesterol i.e. they stop the body doing what it is designed to do. Hence, we should consider the possibility that the impact that statins do appear to have on men with existing heart disease (the evidence is not pervasive outside this group) could be the result of a different action, with cholesterol lowering as a side effect. An unfortunate side effect I would suggest.

c) Statins operate 'upstream' of Coenzyme Q10 (CoQ10) production and have been found to decrease the body's synthesis of CoQ10 by approximately 40%.[152] CoQ10 is also called "ubiquinone", from the word "ubiquitous" meaning "present everywhere". That's a good description of CoQ10, as it is found in virtually all cell membranes. CoQ10 is a critical component in the production of ATP, the body's form of energy and a term that we will come across in carbohydrate metabolism in Chapter Thirteen. Hence CoQ10 is particularly concentrated in those organs that have the highest energy requirements – the brain, heart and liver. The vital roles played by both cholesterol and CoQ10 in the body help explain why the side effects of statins can be unpleasant at best and serious at worst. Such side effects include energy loss, muscle pain, muscle weakness, even muscle wasting and memory loss, amongst other undesirable symptoms.

"First do no harm" – can we really be sure that we are following the Hippocratic oath during the administration of statins?

2) Cholesterol is cholesterol. It is not good or bad.

The chemical formula for cholesterol is $C_{27}H_{46}O$. There is no molecular formula for a good version or a bad version and we must stop using such erroneous and emotive terminology. What differs is the *carrier* of the cholesterol – the lipoprotein.

Lipoproteins are microscopic bodies found in our blood stream. We can think of lipoproteins as tiny 'taxi cabs' travelling round the blood stream acting as transporters. They are needed because the vital substances fat and cholesterol are not water soluble, so they cannot exist freely in blood. The lipoproteins, therefore, carry fat and cholesterol around the body to perform their critical tasks.

There are many different sized lipoproteins. The largest lipoproteins are called chylomicrons. It would be logical for them to be called extremely low density lipoproteins (ELDL's), but they aren't. The next largest are very low density lipoproteins (VLDL's), which are often called triglycerides, also somewhat unhelpfully. There is a lipoprotein called intermediate density lipoprotein (IDL), which is rarely talked about. However, given the obsession with positioning cholesterol as 'deadlier than Hannibal Lecter', it can only be a matter of time before this also features in medical journals. Then we have the much more widely known low density lipoprotein (LDL), erroneously known as 'bad' cholesterol and high density lipoprotein (HDL), equally erroneously known as 'good' cholesterol.

If one chylomicron lipoprotein were the size of a football, then one VLDL would be about the size of a large orange, one IDL would be about the size of an apricot, one LDL about the size of a plum and one HDL about the size of a small grape. You can see where the notion of density comes from – the smaller the lipoprotein, the more dense/tightly packed the contents and hence the smallest lipoprotein (HDL) is high density and the largest lipoprotein (chylomicron) is the one that should, logically, be called extremely low density lipoprotein.

Since I am hoping that this book can lead to heated agreement, before we move on from LDL, please note the following:

- The means by which dietary fat (and cholesterol) are transported into the blood stream, to play their vital roles in reaching and nourishing all our bodily cells, was first established by Michael Brown and Joseph Goldstein in the 1980's[153] and was recognised in them being awarded the Nobel Prize in Physiology or Medicine (1985). Their work informs us that chylomicrons are formed in the intestine, as a result of digestion, and chylomicrons are the transport mechanism for taking dietary fat (and cholesterol) from the digestive system into the blood stream and from there to the different parts of the body. Dietary fat is not turned into LDL – certainly not directly and many would argue not at all.
- VLDL's, also called triglycerides, are made by the liver and these lipoproteins leave the liver with a composition of approximately 50% triglyceride, 22% cholesterol, 18% phospholipids and 10% protein. As the VLDL's encounter lipoprotein lipase (LPL), they are hydrolysed (broken down) and glycerol and fatty acids are released. The VLDL's become intermediate density lipoproteins (IDL's) with a composition of approximately 31% triglyceride, 29% cholesterol, 22% phospholipids and 18% protein. These are hydrolysed further by hepatic lipase to become low density lipoproteins (LDL's) – with a composition of approximately 8% triglyceride, 45% cholesterol, 22% phospholipids and 25% protein.[154] The liver doesn't make LDL. LDL is a residue of IDL, which is a residue of VLDL.

So, even if you think that LDL is harmful in some way, the key question is – since LDL is a remnant of VLDL (through IDL), what determines VLDL? The answer is – carbohydrates (we will show how in Chapter Thirteen). The Horizon 2004 Atkins study, referred to earlier in this chapter, presented the carbohydrate/triglyceride connection as something of a surprise, but we have known this since the time of the Seven Countries Study.

In 1958, John Gofman reported that it was carbohydrates that raised VLDL and only by restricting carbohydrates could VLDL be lowered.[155] Gary Taubes gathers the ensuing evidence extremely well and I highly recommend the chapter "Triglycerides and Cholesterol", from *The Diet Delusion*. To mention just two other key players at the time of Gofman: Pete Ahrens had come to the same conclusion in 1955, studying triglycerides (i.e. VLDL). Margaret Albrink was working in parallel and she and Ahrens presented their respective papers at a meeting of the Association of American Physicians in New Jersey in May 1961. Both reported that elevated triglyceride levels were associated with an increased risk of heart disease and that low-fat, high-carbohydrate diets raised triglycerides. The timing could not have been worse for them, as the American Heart Association had just endorsed the Keys' hypothesis. Tragically, now that we realise that Keys had been referring to processed carbohydrates and not real fat in real food, these strands could have come together in heated agreement at the time. I hope that we can agree now – albeit 50 years and an obesity epidemic later.

There is a final point to note under lipoproteins – Kendrick presents a compelling case that we should not be tempted to try to keep the 'LDL is bad' view alive by trying to make a connection between carbohydrates -> VLDL-> IDL -> LDL path. "There is absolutely no connection whatsoever between the VLDL level and the LDL level," he states. In much the same way that the body regulates protein and blood glucose levels, "LDL receptors" remove LDL at whatever rate is necessary to keep LDL levels constant. VLDL levels can rise and fall rapidly (and do so after a meal, which is why cholesterol tests require fasting beforehand). LDL levels, however, may change over months, but not hours. Kendrick asserts "All of this, by the way, is known by researchers who specialise in lipids."[xxvii]

3) The body makes cholesterol.

Let us return to one of my opening belief statements – I do not believe that, in normal circumstances, the body will make a substance that will kill us. I do believe that there are illnesses, i.e. abnormal circumstances, which, by definition, defy the norm. Cystic fibrosis, for example, is a condition where the body produces excess mucous, making it difficult for the person to digest food and breathe. This is a genetic condition and those suffering the condition have a life expectancy of barely one third of the average. Familial hypercholesterolemia is similarly a genetic condition caused by a gene defect on chromosome 19. The defect makes the body unable to remove LDL from the bloodstream, resulting in consistently high levels of LDL. Both conditions are not 'normal.' Both conditions are rare. One in 7,225 people in the UK have cystic fibrosis[156] and one in 500 people (a non UK specific estimate) have

---

[xxvii] What may be important is not LDL per se but a) the LDL receptor/clearing mechanism, which is known to be deficient in people with familial hypercholesterolemia and b) the *size* of the LDL particles. Since 1994, an association has been noted between higher triglyceride levels and higher levels of smaller, denser LDL particles and lower triglyceride levels and higher levels of the larger, less dense LDL (http://www.lbl.gov/Science-Articles/Archive/cholesterol-particles.html).

familial hypercholesterolemia. (One in fourteen people in the UK are taking statins).[157]

I do think that our current consumption of processed food, carbohydrates particularly, is *abnormal*. I do think that this could be having a profound effect on body measurements – it is on blood glucose, so why not blood lipoprotein measurements. I differ, however, on the recommended course of action. I would rather stop people eating processed food than administer powerful drugs, like statins, to try to overcome the effects. If someone is self harming, we should try to stop this, rather than putting a plaster on the cuts.

Human breast milk contains significant quantities of cholesterol.[158] I assume that it would not do so if cholesterol were in any way a harmful substance.

Given that cholesterol is such a crucial substance for every cell and nerve ending in the body – and that the brain is largely comprised of cholesterol, it is vital that the body continues to manufacture cholesterol so reliably. If a person's cholesterol levels remain relatively high (either for them, or relative to a genuine 'norm'), after a period of eating how we have evolved to eat, there is likely to be a sound reason for this.

In 2006, I had a blood test as part of a routine annual health check up and the results showed elevated white blood cells. The doctor explained that I must have an infection, as my body was producing extra white blood cells to fight that infection. How daft it would have been for the doctor to conclude – you have raised white blood cells, which have *caused* an infection? So why would the doctor say that raised cholesterol is a cause of something rather than seeing this as a sign that the body has made 'extra' for a reason.

If we have an operation, there is a lot of cell repair needed, so we need more cholesterol. Pregnant women have 'high' cholesterol levels – presumably to make a healthy baby. If we consider all the functions that cholesterol performs, the body having a special requirement for any one of these should result in the body producing more cholesterol – just the same as the body needing more white blood cells to fight infection. The 'raised' cholesterol level is then a symptom of something else, not a cause. Doctors may wish to look for what the body is trying to tell us – not merely try to 'end the conversation'.

4) The standard blood cholesterol test does not measure LDL – it estimates it. I did not know that.

The fasting blood cholesterol test is the traditional way to measure the level of LDL, but it doesn't measure LDL directly. We can only measure total cholesterol and HDL with the standard blood test and Triglycerides (VLDL) and LDL are together assumed to account for the difference. The estimation is refined further using the Friedewald equation (named after William Friedewald, who developed it). This uses the fact that VLDL is 22% cholesterol to establish the equation:

Total cholesterol = LDL + HDL + Triglycerides/5 which leads to:

LDL = Total cholesterol – HDL – Triglycerides/5.[159]

You can also now see the problem with trying to assert any meaningful relationship between HDL and total cholesterol. Total cholesterol/HDL = LDL/HDL + 1 + Triglycerides/5HDL and we have one equation, with four variables, only two of which can be measured. We need at least one more equation or known variable, to avoid circular references.

As the November 2004 Harvard medical school publications note, "You have to fast for about 12 hours before the test because triglyceride levels can shoot up 20%-30% after a meal, which would throw off the equation. Alcohol also causes a triglyceride surge, so you shouldn't drink alcohol for 24 hours before a fasting cholesterol test." They also caution "At a triglyceride level of about 250 or higher, the Friedewald equation becomes less reliable because dividing triglycerides by a factor of 5 provides a less accurate estimate of VLDL."

These complications and inaccuracies aside, the fact that LDL is estimated means that:

- All other things being equal, LDL will rise if a) total cholesterol rises and/or b) if HDL falls and/or if c) VLDL falls.
- All other things being equal, LDL will fall if a) total cholesterol falls and/or b) if HDL rises and/or if c) VLDL rises.

No wonder an inverse association is observed between LDL and HDL – it is by definition. More surprising is that a fall in VLDL (triglycerides), which would be welcomed by doctors, would be accompanied by an automatic increase in LDL, all other things being equal, which would not be welcomed by doctors. There was me thinking this was scientific.

5) And finally, if cholesterol is found at the scene – did it commit the crime?

We accuse cholesterol of causing atherosclerotic plaques because we may find lipoproteins alongside such plaques. As we will see in Chapter Twelve, analysis of plaques shows them to be comprised primarily of polyunsaturated fats. Given that fat and cholesterol particles are travelling around the blood stream in lipoproteins, if anything causes a lesion along the endothelial wall (the lining of an artery), it is virtually guaranteed that some lipoproteins will get caught by this lesion. (If we have a broken nail, anything that comes into contact with the rough edge will 'snag' or get caught). This also supports the 'small dense LDL's are the main problems' theory, as the smaller particles are the ones most likely to get caught. This means that lipoproteins will be at the scene of the crime, but it doesn't mean that they caused the crime. The best analogy I can think of here is that we would never allege that police commit all crime – and yet they are always found at the scene of the crime.

Chapter Nine

What did we change our advice to?

"There are lies, damn lies and statistics", Mark Twain.

The USA

Have you ever wondered why you constantly hear "one in three people die from heart disease" and yet you don't lose one third of your friends and family every year? The USA death rate from all causes for 2006 was 0.78%.[160] That means 777 people, per 100,000 residents of the population, died in 2006. Death certificates recorded 200 of these deaths as heart disease. So 0.2% of the USA population died from heart disease in 2006. If you have 500 friends, you are likely to lose one of them to heart disease during a year. If most of your friends are female, heart disease is so weighted towards males that you could have 620 female friends, or 405 male friends, with the same risk of losing one friend during a year. That's still one lost friend too many, but there is also an age dimension to consider. You would need to know 166,667 children aged 5-14 to have a likelihood of one dying from heart disease (which would in turn most likely be a rare hereditary condition) and yet, if you know 100 people aged 85 and over, 22 of them are likely to have heart disease on their death certificate over the next year.

In 1950, staying with the same American data, the death rate from all causes was 1.45%. Hence, this has been virtually halved with advances in medical treatment. (I would argue that, had we maintained our natural eating heritage *and* advanced our treatment options in the way that we have, death rates could have been reduced further still). Of these 1,446 deaths per 100,000 people, 589 (41%) were recorded as heart disease. This is interesting *per se* as the World Health Organisation was only formed in 1948 and heart disease was a little recognised condition before then. By 1960, the death rate had fallen to 1.34% with 42% of those deaths recorded as heart related.

In 1970, the year that the Seven Countries Study was published, the overall death rate had fallen further to 1.22% and heart deaths had fallen to 40% of these. This could be interpreted as fewer than six people in 1,000 were dying from heart disease, or four in ten – depending on lies and statistics. The four in ten positioning provides the context for the impetus for change that preceded the 1977 *Dietary Goals for the United States* announced by Senator George S. McGovern, chair of the Senate Nutrition Committee.

It is worth noting that the conclusions from the 1970 Keys' study were all that were available at the time when America changed its dietary advice in

1977. The data from the 25-year follow up (which no longer mentioned fat) was not available until 1993. Other studies, not least by Keys and his disciples, were continuing to assert the relationship between saturated fat and heart disease and cholesterol and heart disease and saturated fat and cholesterol (without actually explaining how any of this could happen biochemically). However, it is not unreasonable to assert that America changed its entire public health dietary advice on the basis that some people had been observed bathing and singing and some people had been observed not bathing and not singing. And there wasn't much more evidence than that.

Another point worth noting is that, on the flimsy proposal that CHD, cholesterol and dietary fat "tend to be related" in some of a few hand-picked observations, even if this may have had any relevance for a handful of people in a thousand, the dietary advice was changed for everyone. There were 203 million Americans in 1970; 226 million by 1980[161] and the *Dietary Goals for the United States* were mandated for the whole population.[162] The report summary states: "The major objective of the report is to identify 'risk factors' in the American diet and ways to reduce them in order to minimize their harmful effects on health." The dietary goals recommended were:

1) "Increase carbohydrate consumption to account for 55 to 60% of calorie intake;
2) "Reduce overall fat consumption from 40% to about 30% of calorie intake;
3) "Reduce saturated fat consumption to account for about 10% of total calorie intake; and balance with poly-unsaturated and monounsaturated fats, which should account for about 10% of energy intake each;
4) "Reduce cholesterol consumption to about 300 mg a day;
5) "Reduce sugar consumption by almost 40% to account for about 15% of total energy intake;
6) "Reduce salt consumption by about 50 to 85% to approximately three grams per day."

While triglycerides/VLDL are hopefully still fresh in our minds, from the post-amble on cholesterol at the end of the last chapter, we should pause here to note a study done by Elizabeth Parks in 2001 entitled "Effect of dietary carbohydrate on triglyceride metabolism in humans". The study concluded: "When the content of dietary carbohydrate is elevated above the level typically consumed (>55% of energy), blood concentrations of triglycerides rise. This phenomenon, known as carbohydrate-induced hypertriglyceridemia, is paradoxical because the increase in dietary carbohydrate usually comes at the expense of dietary fat. Thus, when the content of the carbohydrate in the diet is increased, fat in the diet is reduced, but the content of fat (triglycerides) in the blood rises."[163]

Only those (although they are the majority) who think that dietary fat "tends to be related to cholesterol" may consider this paradoxical. To those who have looked at carbohydrate metabolism and made the connection between Acetyl CoA being the first step of the cholesterol making process, there is no paradox.

Please note the level at which carbohydrate-induced hypertriglyceridemia (so well known that it has its own terminology) is inevitable, rather than paradoxical – described by Parks as "above the level typically consumed (>55% of energy)". Yet, what was the first guideline for Americans? "Increase carbohydrate consumption to account for 55 to 60% of calorie intake." Americans were thus told to eat more of the macronutrient that raises triglycerides in a supposed attempt to reduce triglyceride/cholesterol levels. Just as we saw with the tobacco industry, I would not rule out class action suits one day being issued to seek compensation for the advice that has been given out, proven to be wrong and yet continues to be reiterated.

The *Dietary Goals for the United States* formed the basis for the 1980 *Dietary Guidelines for Americans,* which have been republished every five years since 1980.[164] The 1980 publication, jointly written by the United States Department of Agriculture and the United States Department of Health, Education and Welfare, had seven dietary guidelines as follows:

1) Eat a variety of food;
2) Maintain ideal weight;
3) Avoid too much fat, saturated fat and cholesterol;
4) Eat foods with adequate starch and fiber;
5) Avoid too much sugar;
6) Avoid too much sodium;
7) If you drink, do so in moderation.

This 1980 document is worth reading in full. It starts with a good first guideline "Eat a variety of food" and a very good explanation as to why: "You need about 40 different nutrients to stay healthy. These include vitamins and minerals, as well as amino acids (from proteins), essential fatty acids (from vegetable oils and animal fats), and sources of energy (calories from carbohydrates, proteins and fats). These nutrients are in the foods you normally eat." The food choice suggestion is also good: "Select foods each day from each of several major groups: for example, fruits and vegetables; cereals, breads and grains; meats, poultry, eggs and fish; dry peas and beans... and milk, cheese and yoghurt." The food groups would be better listed in order of nutritional value. The document emphasises "fruits and vegetables are excellent sources of vitamins", but, as we will see when we review five-a-day, animal foods are the ones that are unbeatable nutritionally.

The guidelines are honest in their acceptance of the debate that was raging at the time, as the Keys' view had strong opposition from the outset: "There is controversy about what recommendations are appropriate for healthy Americans." The document goes on to use the strongest word that Keys used "tend": "Populations like ours with diets high in saturated fats and cholesterol *tend* to have high blood cholesterol levels," (my emphasis). The inference to epidemiology confirms that the Seven Countries Study was the clear foundation for the new guidelines.

Obesity, albeit still in single figures in the USA at the time, was becoming a sufficient concern to have "maintain ideal weight" as the second key guideline. The document noted: ""Obesity is associated with high blood pressure, increased levels of blood fats (triglycerides) and cholesterol and the most common type of diabetes. All of these in turn are associated with increased risks of heart attacks and strokes." That's a more sensible implied causation – obesity as the route and other conditions following.

Guidelines (3) and (4) come together with the comment "If you limit your fat intake, you should increase your calories from carbohydrates to supply your body's energy needs". This is interesting for two reasons:

- If you believe the calorie theory, there is a contradiction in the notion that we need to 'keep our energy up' while obesity is rising.
- The same reason is given by the UK for the advice to switch to carbohydrates (not surprising as the UK just followed the USA). The global change in dietary advice was *not* issued because we suddenly discovered carbohydrates to have some health benefits not previously known. The advice to "eat foods with starch and fiber" is the outcome of a) thinking that fat is bad and b) then realising that there is only one other macronutrient that can take its place (protein is in everything other than sucrose or pure oils and eating protein without the fat provided by nature is not natural or healthy).

The reason given for avoiding sugar is "The major health hazard from eating too much sugar is tooth decay (dental caries)." It is only natural to wonder about the lobbying power of the sugar industry when this one criticism is shortly followed by "Contrary to widespread opinion, too much sugar in your diet does not seem to cause diabetes. There is also no convincing evidence that sugar causes heart attacks or blood vessel diseases." This is supposed to be the launch of healthy eating guidelines for Americans, not a defence document for the least nutritious 'food' that humans consume. There was also no convincing evidence at the time (and nor has there been since) that saturated fat causes heart attacks, but that didn't stop the damnation of this macronutrient. I also find myself wondering – if sugar can erode the strongest substance in the human body – tooth enamel – are we certain that it can *not* cause damage to the lining of blood vessels?

The document acknowledges "Estimates indicate that Americans use on the average more than 130 pounds of sugars and sweeteners a year". That represented (at the time) up to 625 calories per day per average American with no nutrition being provided. Why do the guidelines not make the connection between this and obesity or this and the fact that the average American would have needed to get the 40 different nutrients after having consumed all these empty calories? For 625 calories per day to be consumed *and* for the 1977 guideline of sugar representing 15% of total energy intake to be achieved, Americans would need to be eating 4,166 calories per day.

This should have been a concern to the authors of the document, as they believe the calorie formula. There is a pure quotation of the calorie formula in the 1980 guidelines for Americans: "A pound of body fat contains 3500 calories. To lose 1 pound of fat, you will need to burn 3500 calories more than you consume. If you burn 500 calories more a day than you consume, you will lose 1 pound of fat a week."

The UK

The UK lagged a few years behind the USA, but the British change was first slipped in to a discussion paper called *Proposals for nutritional guidelines for health education in Britain* – prepared for the National Advisory Committee on Nutrition Education (NACNE) by an ad hoc working party under the chairmanship of Professor Philip James.[xxviii]

The report was 40 pages long and had some very interesting information within – not least a bar diagram on P21, taken from Newbrun (1982),[165] showing a virtual mirror correlation between sugar consumed and Decayed/Missing/Filled (DMF) teeth in children aged 11-12 in countries from China to Columbia to west Germany to Australia to Ecuador.

The two real nuggets in the report, however, were the following statements:

- "The previous nutritional advice in the UK to limit the intake of all carbohydrates as a means of weight control now runs counter to current thinking and contrary to the present proposals for a nutrition education policy for the population as a whole…" and
- "The problem then becomes one of achieving both a reduction in fat intake to 30% of total energy and a fall in saturated fatty acid intake to 10%."

As stated in the opening pages of this book: "And so started the obesity epidemic". This discussion paper led to the policy paper *Diet and Cardiovascular Disease* from the Department for Health and Social Security, as it was then. As this was presented by the Committee on Medical Aspects of Food Policy, it became known as the COMA report (1984).[166] Its impact has been nothing short of catastrophic.

Although it has long been out of print, I managed to procure a copy and have read it with much interest. It is referenced repeatedly by the Food Standards Agency in their rationale for their current advice. Here are the recommendations to the general public – in the order that they are presented in the report – the first point is emboldened covering almost half the first page of the recommendations:

1) "The consumption of saturated fatty acids* and of fat in the United Kingdom should be decreased. There are no specific recommendations for change in the consumption of polyunsaturated and monounsaturated fatty acids, but to facilitate the recommendation for saturated fatty acids* we recommend that the ratio of polyunsaturated fatty acids to saturated fatty acids* (the P/S ratio) may be increased to approximately 0.45. The intakes recommended are

---

[xxviii] Professor W.P.T. James is currently the president for the International Association for the Study of Obesity and has been an outstanding contributor to the field of obesity for much of his life.

15 per cent of food energy for saturated fatty acids* and 35 per cent of food energy for total fat". (Clause 2.1.1.3 tells us that the panel would have liked total fat intake lower, at 30%, but recognised that this was a step too far for the UK at the time).

The '*' is explained as "inclusive of trans fatty acids". So, throughout the 30 page report, "saturated fatty acids" and "trans fatty acids" are grouped together as equally evil.

The recommendation that there shall be a P/S ratio and that the number should be 0.45 is as inexplicable as it is innovative. The historical P/S ratio was calculated in the report. In 1959 it was 0.17, in 1969 it was 0.19 and in 1979 it was 0.22. The report was therefore recommending that the UK more than double the historical ratio between two types of fat. No reason for this was given.

I can only find one real food (as provided by nature) that has a ratio of 0.45 polyunsaturated fat to saturated fat. There may be some man-made foods with a ratio of 0.45 polyunsaturated to some combination of saturated fat and trans fats, but my personal view is that trans fats should be banned and I refuse to investigate (and by implication give credence to) man-made substances containing any amount of trans fats. The real food with the 'magic' 0.45 ratio of polyunsaturated to saturated fat is the humble egg. Of the 10 grams of fat per 100 grams of egg (100 grams would be a couple of eggs), 37% is saturated, 46% is monounsaturated and 17% is polyunsaturated. Hence, if you struggle with maths, ensure that eggs are the only food you consume containing fat and you will meet the 0.45 target. Sadly, 37% of your fat intake would be saturated and you would thus fail on another of the triple simultaneous equations – the proportion of fat that is saturated.

If you try to get your P/S ratio met in another way, it gets complicated. Or, shall I say impossible? If you eat 100 grams of chicken, you have the same percentage of saturated fat as polyunsaturated (and monounsaturated – all at one third), so you have clocked up a P/S ratio of 100%. Should you then have 100 grams of coconut oil, with a P/S ratio of 2% to try to redress the balance? No is the answer. Because of the amount of fat in coconut oil (100%) vs. 10% in chicken, you actually need to have 0.44 grams of coconut oil with 100 grams of chicken to achieve your specified P/S ratio. Where does that leave the other two measures? I don't know and I don't care.

You end up with a heck of a simultaneous equation puzzle if you try to design even one day's eating plan to achieve all of the following: 35% of food energy in fat; 15% of food energy in saturated/trans fats; a ratio of 0.45 for saturated/trans fats to polyunsaturated fats; salt intake to be reduced from 7-10 grams a day (as it was then); increased carbohydrate intake (cereals, bread, fruit) without increased sucrose, glucose and fructose intake (cereals, bread and fruit of course either are, or break down into, sucrose, glucose and fructose). Don't forget: don't smoke; don't drink too much; take regular exercise and be the right weight.

Could we make our dietary advice any more complicated? What about just "eat real food"?

2) The second recommendation merely reinforces the asterix (*). "Trans fatty acids should be regarded as equivalent to saturated fatty acids".[xxix]

This is irresponsible and indefensible. Saturated fat occurs naturally in the majority of foods on the planet (even in brown rice, porridge oats and avocados, as examples). Trans fats also occur naturally in the milk and body fat of ruminants (grazing animals such as cattle and sheep), but this is not widely known and is rarely, if ever, what is being referred to. When we mention trans fats, we mean the unnatural, manmade, substances where some rather serious alterations have been made to real foods, like vegetable oil, to make them solid at room temperature. At the time of the COMA report, trans fats were invariably made by hydrogenation – literally adding hydrogen atoms in the food manufacturing process. Subsequently, alternative methods of making trans fats have been found, but they still remain a product for which we have no physiological need and without which, surely, we must be healthier. Real fats, found in real food, on the other hand are vital for every aspect of human health.

The consequences of this connection are still being seen over twenty five years later. A statement from the Margarine & Spreads Association, released by Nexus Public Relations on 18 January 2010, stated: "Following on from a report that the UK Faculty of Public Health has demanded a ban on trans fats in the UK, the Margarine and Spreads Association would like to draw your attention to the following facts: Experts have concluded that most people in the UK are eating well within the recommended limits[xxx] for TFAs, so it is believed that there is no major dietary concern. Instead, people should be more wary about the amounts of saturated fat in their diets. Saturated fat intake is being overlooked by many as a health issue, yet it too is responsible for raising the levels of 'bad' cholesterol, which can lead to coronary heart disease. Today sees the launch of Phase 2 of a Food Standards Agency campaign to encourage people to cut their saturated fat intake. The Committee on Medical Aspects of Food and Nutrition Policy (COMA) set a daily recommended value (DRV) of <11% of daily energy intake for saturated fat, but current consumption is at 13%. That means that, on average, we are eating 17% too much saturated fat each day." (The reference given as evidence by the Margarine & Spreads Association is placed as a footnote – the COMA report). (TFA's are trans fatty acids).

[xxix] This is actually somewhat ironic, as trans fats can be monounsaturated or polyunsaturated but *never* saturated fats. Saturated fats have no double bonds and can therefore never display a *trans-* configuration.

[xxx] This is the reference as it appears in the statement from the Margarine and Spreads Association The Committee on Medical Aspects of Food and Nutrition Policy (COMA has been replaced by the Scientific Advisory Committee on Nutrition (SACN).

We can't move on without looking more at trans fats in more detail. It really is inexcusable for a public health document to discuss real fats found in real food in the same sentence as man-made hydrogenated fats.

There is a wealth of evidence in diet and nutrition journals worldwide on the dangers of trans fats: "On a per-calorie basis, trans fats appear to increase the risk of CHD more than any other macronutrient, conferring a substantially increased risk at low levels of consumption (1 to 3 percent of total energy intake). In a meta-analysis of four prospective cohort studies involving nearly 140,000 subjects, a 2 percent increase in energy intake from trans fatty acids was associated with a 23 percent increase in the incidence of CHD."[167]

In a study conducted in Australia,[168] scientists collated dietary information and fat biopsy samples from 79 people who had just had a first heart attack. The researchers compared this with similar information and biopsy samples from 167 people without heart problems. The outcome of the study was: "We conclude that TFAs in adipose tissue are associated with an increased risk of coronary artery disease and rapidly disappear from adipose tissue when not included in margarines."

For more information, the web site www.bantransfats.com is highly recommended, as are many other sites, with similar aims, to be found on the internet. A cessation of the connection between man-made trans fats and nature's saturated fat is long overdue. I find the behaviour of the UK Food Standards Agency (FSA) consistently remarkable in that they continually attack saturated fat and we hardly hear a whisper about trans fats. Could this be because of successful lobbying of the food industry and/or the fact that the FSA has a representative from Unilever (margarine producers) on the board? For whatever reason, the FSA loses respect and credibility for attacking a substance found naturally in real food and virtually ignoring products that will partially hydrogenate human beings.

3) Recommendation three simply says "There are no specific recommendations about the dietary intake of cholesterol". The panel goes on to say "current intake is not excessive and evidence for an influence of this level of intake on blood cholesterol is inconclusive." i.e. we have no evidence that consuming cholesterol impacts cholesterol levels and cholesterol consumption is not high anyway.

4) "The panel recommends that intake of simple sugars (sucrose, glucose and fructose) should not be increased further." Professor John Yudkin noted that UK sugar consumption was "about 100 pounds a year" at the time of writing his book (1972).[169] Unlike the American Dietary Guidelines, the UK recommended no reduction in this intake – only that it should not increase further.

This clause also gave another example of saturated fat taking the blame for refined carbohydrates: "Certain foods containing these sugars may also contribute saturated fatty acids (e.g. cakes, biscuits)".

5) Recommendation five is more in line with the USA advice, which also addressed alcohol. This recommendation says "An excessive intake of alcohol is to be avoided on more general health grounds".

6) "The panel recommends that the dietary intake of common salt should not be increased further." The only point I wish to make here is that, if we eat real food, we don't have to worry about salt – nature puts sodium and potassium naturally in the correct balance.

7) "The panel sees advantages in compensating for a reduced fat intake with increased fibre-rich carbohydrates (e.g. bread, cereals, fruit, vegetables,) provided that this can be achieved without increasing total intake of common salt or simple sugars." There is no mention of what these advantages could be. (We will see in the next chapter that this position has not been reviewed since). Notice also how the "without increasing total intake of common salt of simple sugars" has been lost along the way. I would hope that the COMA committee would be horrified to see the white flour and sugar dominating the 'eatwell' plate.

8) The eighth recommendation is "Obesity should be avoided in adults and children by a combination of appropriate food intake and regular exercise". Easier said than done, but at least the word 'appropriate; could cover what food is eaten and not just how much.

   There is a table in the report (3.3), which presents the Ministry of Agriculture Fisheries and Food data for energy consumption per day for the average citizen. Using the energy (calorie) intake each year for the decade when obesity really started to take hold, the 1970's, and applying the 3,500 calorie formula, we would conclude that, all other things being equal, the average Briton should have lost two stone during just this decade. This supports the calculation in Chapter Seven that we should have been losing pounds per capita, during the period of the obesity epidemic.

The remaining recommendations include good advice like "don't smoke" and not such good advice with there being no specific recommendations on vitamin C, D and E intake and intake of selenium and magnesium – all assumed to be "adequate" in the UK diet.

All of the above summarises the recommendations to the general public. There is also a section on recommendations to "producers manufacturers and distributors of food and drink and caterers". Clause 2.4.1 is interesting to note, if only as an example of the power of the food industry. It recommended "simple (food) labelling codes" and yet in March 2010, 26 years later, the Food Standards Agency finally gave up their battle for traffic light labelling, in the face of overwhelming resistance from the food industry and Members of the European Parliament also rejected traffic light labelling in a vote on 17 June 2010. (I have a really simple food labelling policy – don't eat anything that needs a food label).

The 'evidence' for the recommendations is presented at the end and there are three things worthy of note:

1) We have confirmation that the UK advice, just as was the case with the USA advice, is based on the Seven Countries Study with the comment "comparisons between countries have shown a strong positive relationship between the proportion of dietary energy derived from saturated fatty acids and mortality from coronary heart disease." Chapter Eight showed that this has no evidence base.

2) Clause 4.1.4 asserts "Isocaloric and other dietary studies in man have shown that dietary saturated fatty acids increase plasma total cholesterol whereas dietary polyunsaturated fatty acids decrease plasma total cholesterol." We are in the evidence section of the report, but no evidence is provided for this statement (and Keys had recently concluded the contrary).

3) Clause 4.1.9 is quite something: "There has been no controlled clinical trial of the effect of decreasing dietary intake of saturated fatty acids on the incidence of coronary heart disease nor is it likely that such a trial will be undertaken." You may like to read that again if you thought that we have in any way proven that saturated fat consumption has anything whatsoever to do with heart disease. We had not even done the study at the time we changed our advice and we have still not done the study since. In Chapter Eleven, you will see this exact phrase repeated by the FSA 26 years later.

Interestingly fibre gets only the briefest of mentions in the USA and UK advice and, both times, it is in the context of advising carbohydrate consumption. The USA advised "Eat foods with adequate starch and fiber" and the UK recommends "fibre-rich carbohydrates". Fibre's importance has been inflated over the years since the initial changes in dietary advice. I suggest that this is because the notion that fibre might be good has been beneficial for the food industry. It has spawned bran and fibre cereals, snack bars and other products that we managed to survive without for tens of thousands of years.

Denis Burkitt (1911-1993) was the key proponent of fibre, even writing a book in 1979 called *Don't Forget Fibre in Your Diet.*[170] Burkitt was a British surgeon who served with the Royal Army Medical Corps during the Second World War. He continued his medical service in Africa after the war and noticed the distinct lack of 'modern' disease in 'underdeveloped' countries. Burkitt concluded, quite bizarrely in my view, that the *absence* of fibre in the western diet was to blame. Not the *presence* of things like drugs, smoking, pollution, stress, processed food, and so on, but the *absence* of fibre. Just as Keys concluded that it was the absence of fat that was good (not the presence of refined carbohydrates that was bad), so Burkitt made the same mistake. I suggest that the issue is not lack of fibre, but the excess of non-fibrous, refined carbohydrates. Surely the presence of modern processed food is more important than the absence of something that is not even digestible. The obesity epidemic is not the result of things that we are not eating; it is the result of the modern processed foods that we are.

Please note that, although the *Dietary Goals for the United States* mentioned monounsaturated fat, neither the *Dietary Guidelines for Americans* nor the COMA report made any recommendations or claims for monounsaturated fat. The *Dietary Guidelines for Americans* did not even contain one reference to the term monounsaturated fat. There is a useful summary table tracing the revisions of the *Dietary Guidelines for Americans* from 1980 to 2000, with the revised advice published every five years.[171] Monounsaturated fat is not mentioned here either. It will be useful to remember this when we come on to our current dietary advice.

Chapter Ten

What is our current diet advice?

USA

The *Dietary Guidelines for Americans*[172] have been published jointly by the Department of Health and Human Services (HHS) and the United States Department of Agriculture (USDA), every five years since 1980. The Guidelines are intended to provide advice for people aged two years and older about how good dietary habits can promote health and reduce risk of major chronic diseases. The guidelines serve as the basis for federal food and nutrition education programs. The recommendations below are from the 2005 report.

The key recommendations for weight management are:[173]

- "To maintain body weight in a healthy range, balance calories from foods and beverages with calories expended;
- "To prevent gradual weight gain over time, make small decreases in food and beverage calories and increase physical activity."

This means that the American public health bodies subscribe to the over simplification "energy in equals energy out", based on the misapplication of thermodynamics that we have already detailed.

The key recommendations for carbohydrates are:[174]

- "Choose fibre-rich fruits, vegetables, and whole grains often;
- "Choose and prepare foods and beverages with little added sugars or caloric sweeteners;
- "Reduce the incidence of dental caries by practicing good oral hygiene and consuming sugar- and starch-containing foods and beverages less frequently."

I have to make two comments on point (3) before moving on. First, recommendation (1) can be summarised as eat starch often and recommendation (3) says don't eat starch often. Which is it to be American advisors? Secondly, it is interesting that the only caution made in relation to sugar is that it increases dental caries i.e. it rots your teeth. This is also the only criticism that the UK Food Standards Agency makes about sugar – more on this later.

The key recommendations for fats are:[175]

- "Consume less than 10 percent of calories from saturated fatty acids and less than 300 mg/day of cholesterol, and keep trans fatty acid consumption as low as possible;
- "Keep total fat intake between 20 to 35 percent of calories, with most fats coming from sources of polyunsaturated and monounsaturated fatty acids, such as fish, nuts, and vegetable oils;
- "When selecting and preparing meat, poultry, dry beans, and milk or milk products, make choices that are lean, low-fat, or fat-free."

We should note here that the *Dietary Guidelines for Americans* (2000) stated: "Aim for a total fat intake of no more than 30 percent of calories, as recommended in previous editions of the Guidelines." Hence the guidelines changed in 2005 – removing the upper limit on total fat intake as a percentage of energy intake. Why? As Dariush Mozaffarian noted in chapter 48 of Braunwald's Heart Disease[176] "... evidence has demonstrated convincingly that the proportion of energy consumed from total fat has no appreciable effect on CHD... Based on these multiple lines of evidence for no effect, both the United States Department of Agriculture (USDA) and the American Heart Association (AHA) have dropped prior recommendations to maintain total fat intake <30% energy". How similar this is to the UK change of position on cholesterol, which was slipped in with no major announcement, sparing the blushes of public health advisors, but proving useless as a public health message in the process.

The key recommendations for fruit and vegetables are:[177]

- "Consume a sufficient amount of fruits and vegetables while staying within energy needs. Two cups of fruit and two and a half cups of vegetables per day are recommended for a reference 2,000-calorie intake, with higher or lower amounts depending on the calorie level;
- "Choose a variety of fruits and vegetables each day. In particular, select from all five vegetable subgroups (dark green, orange, legumes, starchy vegetables, and other vegetables) several times a week."

Just as the UK has the 'eatwell' plate, the USA has the USDA food pyramid. This is also updated every five years, but the 1992 original pyramid can still be found on much of the USA packaging. This lists advised servings of different food groups as follows:

- Bread, cereal, rice & pasta 6-11 servings a day;
- Vegetables 3-5 servings a day;
- Fruit 2-4 servings a day;
- Milk, yoghurt & cheese 2-3 servings a day;
- Meat, poultry, fish, dry beans, eggs & nuts 2-3 servings a day;
- Fats, oils & sweets "use sparingly".

The updated food pyramid is now called *My Pyramid* and it reflects feedback that consumers found 'servings' too vague. There are also allegations that the pyramid has been changed to reflect lobbying from different food groups.

For a 2,000 calorie a day diet, the following amounts are recommended:

- 6 ounces of grains every day;
- 2.5 cups of vegetables every day;
- 2 cups of fruit every day;
- 3 cups of low-fat or fat-free milk every day;
- 5.5 ounces of low-fat or lean meat, fish, beans, peas, nuts & seeds.

In both the original and updated pyramids, carbohydrates form the overwhelming majority of the diet and every single food eaten can contain carbohydrate and therefore require insulin to be released. In the updated pyramid, as an example, grains, vegetables and fruits are primarily carbohydrates. Dairy products have a carbohydrate content and, if the consumer chooses bean, pea, nut and seed options from the last group, all of these contain insulin raising carbohydrates (albeit 'good' carbohydrates). The only zero carbohydrate groups are meat and fish (eggs have virtually no carbohydrate content), but these do not have to be consumed as part of this 'ideal' American diet.

Michelle Obama launched a key initiative on 9 February 2010 to address childhood obesity, called "Let's Move!"[178] "Let's Move!" has an ambitious and critical goal: to solve the epidemic of childhood obesity within a generation. Michelle Obama is one of the few people in the world who could impact the obesity epidemic. She is in a high enough position of power to change direction, set new strategies and to transform the obesity epidemic in the United States and from there the world. Absolutely tragically, it would appear that the "Let's Move!" initiative meets the definition of insanity – it thinks that something different will result from repeating the same thing.

The initiative has four themes:

1) Helping parents make healthy food choices (through improved nutritional information). Example of initiatives include the Food and Drug Administration reviewing food labelling and "the nation's beverage industry are taking steps to provide clearly visible information about calories on the front of their products, as well as on vending machines and soda fountains." The food pyramid remains the key dietary advice tool – this will be promoted even more to ensure that all Americans know to base their meals on carbohydrates. I hope that, by the end of Part Three of this book, you are horrified by the current consumption of carbohydrate, let alone the prospect of any more.

2) Healthier schools – in recognition that children get a proportion of their food intake at school. The dietary guidelines here will, unsurprisingly, be no different. There will be a menu planner for 'healthy' school meals, which provides tips on serving more carbohydrate and less saturated and trans fats

in school menus. Trans fats should be banned, but leave nature's real fats alone – saturated or unsaturated.

3) Physical Activity – this is a great thing for children to adopt on a regular basis. However, as will be set out in Chapter Fourteen, obesity is magnitudes more about what we put in to our bodies than it is about what we try to do. Plus – if children glug fizzy soft drinks while out playing, or after activity, or satiate the inevitable hunger resulting from exercise with consumption of fast food, they would be better off not having done the exercise to drive such food and drink intake in the first place.

4) Access to affordable healthy food – this part of the initiative would be valuable if the healthy eating advice were good in the first place. I completely agree that we cannot hope to solve an obesity epidemic when a bag of salad leaves can cost more than a dozen cookies. "Let's Move!" says that, as part of the President's proposed Financial Year 2011 budget, $400 million a year will be allocated to a new program – the Healthy Food Financing Initiative. The money is intended for things like – bringing grocery stores to underserved areas and to help convenience stores carry healthier food options. The last thing that people in remote parts of America need is better access to grocery stores. Plus, it is all very well having healthier options (whatever these are considered to be) in convenience stores – but, lower income families will still buy processed food if it is cheaper. Finally, with a population of 309 million people, this budget equates to $1.30 per citizen. If we could guarantee that the money only went to the 23 million people, identified by the initiative as being low income neighbourhoods, that's $17.40 each, per year.

The Washington Post reported the story on 10 February 2010 and announced that a new foundation was being set up to support the initiative: *Partnership for a Healthier America*. Its members include the Kellogg's Foundation – you'll be seeing much more of Kellogg's in Chapter Fifteen. You will also see revenues of over $400 *billion* generated by the small number of sponsors of the American Dietetic Association – the organisation driving dietary advice across America. The government has made available $400 *million*. What chance does Mother Nature have to argue the case for her food being healthier against this kind of funding?

I take no pleasure from being able to critique this initiative so easily. This is a complete tragedy and the biggest lost opportunity in the obesity epidemic to date. I wrote to the First Lady on 28 January 2010 (the press release came out early) sharing the graph presented in the introduction to this book with the clear kink in all but one trend during the period 1976-1980. This was when American dietary advice changed with the dictat to avoid fat and eat carbohydrates. Childhood obesity, the prime target for Michelle Obama, has increased from around 3% to nearer 20% since this dietary change. I begged the First Lady to lead America back to eating food as provided by nature and not food as provided by food manufacturers. I have received no response.

Australia

The dietary guidelines for Australians are set by the National Health and Medical Research Council (NHMRC).[179] The current version was published in 2003. Like the USA guidelines, the Australian guidelines have the aim of promoting the potential benefits of healthy eating to reduce the risk of diet-related disease and also to improve the community's health and wellbeing. The Australian government has been providing nutrition advice for more than 75 years. The 2003 document is the third edition of the Dietary Guidelines for Australian Adults. The second edition was published in 1992. The NHMRC has also published Dietary Guidelines for Children and Adolescents and the Dietary Guidelines for Older Australians was published in 1999.

The summary of advice is as follows:
1) Enjoy a wide variety of nutritious foods:
- Eat plenty of vegetables, legumes and fruits;
- Eat plenty of cereals (including breads, rice, pasta and noodles), preferably whole grain;
- Include lean meat, fish, poultry and/or alternatives;
- Include milks, yoghurts, cheeses and/or alternatives. Reduced-fat varieties should be chosen, where possible;
- Drink plenty of water.

2) Take care to:
- Limit saturated fat and moderate total fat intake;
- Choose foods low in salt;
- Limit your alcohol intake if you choose to drink;
- Consume only moderate amounts of sugars and foods containing added sugars.

3) Prevent weight gain: be physically active and eat according to your energy needs. Later on in the report, the following quite specific reference to obesity is made: "All successful treatments involve some form of lifestyle change affecting energy intake (food) or energy expenditure (physical activity), or both."

So Australia also thinks that weight is about energy in and out and that humans need to eat less and/or do more. Australia also wants its citizens to limit saturated fat and total fat intake and to eat plenty of carbohydrate (grains, vegetables, fruits, cereals) and lean meat/fish plays a small part in the recommended 'healthy' diet and, again, carbohydrate/protein alternatives (beans, pulses etc) to meat/fish are welcome.

The Australian Guide to healthy eating[180] looks remarkably similar to the UK 'eatwell' plate. The amounts of each food group to be consumed are very specifically documented for the Australian plate:

Pregnant women, breastfeeding women, women over the age of 60, men over the age of 60 all have individual and specific recommendations. Let us look at the standard advice for women aged 19-60 (not pregnant or breastfeeding) and men aged 19-60:

	Women 19-60	Men 19-60
Cereals/grains	4-9 servings	6-12
Vegetables	5	5
Fruit	2	2
Dairy	2	2
Lean meat/fish/pulses	1	1
"Extra foods" (Junk basically)	0-2	0-3

Sample serves are:

- Cereals/grains – 1 serving would be 2 slices (60 grams) bread, 1 cup cooked rice, pasta or noodles;
- Vegetables – 1 serving would be 75 grams cooked vegetables, 1 cup salad vegetables, 1 small potato;
- Fruit – 1 serving would be 1 medium piece (150 grams) of fruit, 1 cup diced pieces or canned fruit, 1 cup fruit juice;
- Dairy – 1 serving would be 1 cup (250 millilitres) fresh milk, 2 slices (40 grams) cheese, 1 small carton (200 grams) yoghurt;
- Lean meat/fish/pulses – 1 serving would be 65-100 grams cooked meat or chicken, 80-120 grams cooked fish fillet, 2 small eggs, 1 cup cooked pulses.

So, an Australian woman, following this optimally healthy eating advice, could eat 12 slices of bread, three cups of pasta, five small potatoes, two cups of fruit juice, a cup of cooked beans and two servings of junk food every day. This is a staggering amount and proportion of carbohydrate.

P39 of the NHMRC report actually spells out how to ensure that Australian citizens consume this evolutionary unprecedented level of carbohydrate:

- "Consume breads with each meal;
- Regularly use rice, couscous, pasta or noodles to accompany hot dishes;
- Eat breakfast cereals daily;[xxxi]
- Include whole grain cereals as extenders to soups and casseroles;
- Use oats in crumble toppings on desserts;
- Choose grain-based snacks such as low-fat cereal bars, muffins and popcorn."

In June 2008, a report entitled Australia's Future 'Fat Bomb', from Melbourne's Baker IDI Heart and Diabetes Institute, was presented at the

---

[xxxi] The Commonwealth Scientific and Industrial Research Organisation (CSIRO) is the national government body for scientific research in Australia. They have published a well known and widely read "Healthy Heart Programme". Kellogg's Guardian cereal is a regular feature in the diet – such government endorsed carbohydrate advice must be welcomed by makers of (sugary) cereals.

Federal Government's inquiry into obesity. The report's lead author was Professor Simon Stewart.

The report announced that Australia had officially become the fattest nation in the world, with more than nine million adults classified as obese or overweight. The figures in the report showed that four million Australians, 26% of the adult population, were obese compared to an estimated 25% of Americans. A further five million Australians were classified as overweight. This report noted the stark realisation, that Australians outweighing Americans, means that Australia is facing a future "fat bomb" that could cause 123,000 premature deaths over the next two decades.

I think that the Melbourne study had some statistics wrong for America, as all statistics I have seen place America firmly at the top of the world obesity table. However, Australia undoubtedly has a significant obesity problem and, having seen some of the impactful press releases like *Bum Nation: Australia the fattest on earth,*[181] it wouldn't have hurt Australia to have the data presented in this way to try to shock people into action. The trouble is that if Australians follow their own government advice, particular this astonishing 'how to eat more carbohydrate at every opportunity throughout the day' advice, they will continue to close the gap with America with obesity increasing, not declining.

UK – The advice

So now we turn to the UK. I am going to use the UK as an example to go into in some detail, as it is the easiest country for me to get the most data. This still has complete relevance to the USA and Australia because the three key areas we will be looking at (eat less fat, eat more carbohydrates and the fruit and vegetable advice) are so similar across these 'developed' nations and the findings hold in each region.

Whether this is a sign of democracy or bureaucracy, the UK doesn't have a single source of authoritative advice. There is a plethora of (public) healthy eating advice, which is aimed at trying to create a calorie deficit by getting us to eat less and/or do more. I analysed just four different official sources of such advice:

- The Food Standards Agency (FSA) eight tips for eating well;[182]
- The British Nutrition Foundation (BNF) eight guidelines for a healthy diet;[183]
- The National Health Service (NHS) *Change4Life* campaign;[184]
- The Department of Health (DoH) *Healthy Weight Healthy Lives.*[185]

Across just these four sources of advice, we find the following:

- Three have eight tips (not the same eight tips); the fourth has five tips;
- There are 18 different messages across the four sources of advice;
- 14 messages are not repeated (i.e. they are unique to one source of advice);
- Only one message is similar in each of the tips, but the words differ each time. Messages on activity can be found in the FSA, NHS and Department of Health tips and the second part of the FSA tip "Get active and try to be a

healthy weight" is repeated in the British Nutrition Foundation message "Eat the right amount to be a healthy weight".

Can you imagine giving a blue chip company this as a marketing brief? You are required to communicate with the whole of the UK. Do so from at least four different departments. Deliver 18 messages in total – four messages are to be repeated in some way, but use different words every time and then make 14 different messages unique to the campaigns of one particular department.

Table 13: UK Government dietary messages in more than one campaign (the numbers refer to the message number in each campaign):

FSA	BNF	NHS	DoH
1. Base your meals on starchy foods	4. Eat plenty of foods rich in starch and fibre		
2. Eat lots of fruit and vegetables	5. Eat plenty of fruit and vegetables	5. 5 a day	
4. Cut down on saturated fat and sugar	6. Don't eat too many foods that contain a lot of fat. 7. Don't have sugary foods and drinks too often	4. Cut back fat 8. Sugar swaps	
6. Get active and try to be a healthy weight	3. Eat the right amount to be a healthy weight	6. 60 active minutes 1. Up & About	3. Building physical activity into our lives

Table 14: UK Government dietary messages in only one campaign:

FSA	BNF	NHS	DoH
3. Eat more fish	1. Enjoy your food	2. Meal time – make time for 3 meals a day	1. The healthy growth and development of children
5. Try to eat less salt	2. Eat a variety of different foods	3. Snack check – limit snacking	2. Promoting healthier food choices
7. Drink plenty of water	8. If you drink alcohol, drink sensibly	7. Me size meals – kids portions	4. Creating incentives for better health
8. Don't skip breakfast			5. Personalised advice and support

UK – Have we been following the current advice?

The FSA tips seem to be the most practical and measurable, so let us look at how the UK has been doing against the FSA's first four tips. The first four are the ones that are more relevant to weight loss. Tip 6, "Try to be a healthy weight", cannot practically serve as a weight loss tip. (It would be like a 'how to be a good footballer' manual saying 'try to be a good footballer').

We can use the Ministry of Agriculture, Fisheries and Food (MAFF) National Food Survey to evaluate UK food consumption from 1974-2000. (As we noted in Chapter Seven, this period was chosen as it is the longest with consistent data in the past fifty years).

Table 15: Increases and decreases in UK food consumption between 1974 and 2000:

National Food Survey	Difference (1974 to 2000)	Ratio of 2000 over 1974
DOWN		
Bread	-24%	0.76
Eggs	-57%	0.43
Fat – all	-41%	0.59
Fat – butter	-76%	0.24
Fresh potatoes	-46%	0.54
Meat – all carcase meat	-40%	0.60
Milk – whole	-75%	0.25
Preserves	-54%	0.46
Sugar	-72%	0.28
Vegetables – all	-19%	0.81
Vegetables – Fresh green	-32%	0.68
UP		
Alcoholic drinks (Note 1)	+41%	1.41
Cheese	+ 5%	1.05
Confectionery (Note 1)	+25%	1.25
Fish	+16%	1.16
Fruit – fresh	+49%	1.49
Fruit – other and fruit products	+119%	2.19
Ice cream and ice cream products	+183%	2.83
Meat – other meat products	+18%	1.18
Milk – other milk and cream	+553%	6.53
Other cereals and cereal products	+16%	1.16
Processed potatoes	+185%	2.85
Soft drinks (Note 2)	+443%	5.43
Vegetables – other fresh	+26%	1.26
Vegetables – processed	+36%	1.36

Note 1 – data for 1992 – 2000 only
Note 2 – date for 1975 – 2000 only

The National Food Survey data shows that, for the FSA tips 1-4:

Tip 1 "Base your meals on starchy foods": Many people won't even know what starch is. However, the large category *Other cereals or cereal products* is up, as is processed potatoes – all starchy foods. Bread and fresh potatoes are down and I would argue that not all starch is the same and that we are better off eating real, fresh potatoes than processed ones and (whole-meal) bread rather than sugary cereals. So, two 'poor' starch categories have increased, one 'good' starch category has declined and one mixed category (some of the bread will be refined and some whole-meal) has declined.

Tip 2 "Eat lots of fruit and vegetables": The statistics show that fresh fruit consumption has increased 50%. Other fruit and fruit products (i.e. processed fruit) has more than doubled. Processed vegetables and non green fresh vegetables have all increased. The only category where consumption has fallen is fresh green vegetables. So, overall, another box ticked here.

Tip 3 "Eat more fish": More than what? More than a vegetarian? More than an Eskimo? We eat 16% more fish in 2000, than we did in 1974, so we'll assume we've done well here.

Tip 4 "Cut down on saturated fat and sugar": We've done well on the first one and ostensibly well on the second. The data in the National Food Survey is extremely comprehensive, to the point of including detail on both macro and micronutrients. The information on macronutrients says that we consumed 51.7 grams per person per day of saturated fat in 1975 and 28.1 grams in 1999. The food examples in the table support this – all fat, butter, meat, whole milk and eggs – real foods and sources of saturated fat – are down. Dramatically in some cases – we eat half the number of eggs that we used to and one fifth of the butter and whole milk.

Sugar is deceptive – on the survey line for sugar alone, we have reduced our consumption significantly (to about one fifth of what it was). However, World Health Organisation statistics show that we consume approximately 1.6 pounds of sugar per person per week in the UK[186] and we know from the National Food Survey that buying bags of sugar for the household has declined. What has happened, therefore, is that sugar is now hidden in almost every processed food we can buy – from the obvious ones like biscuits, cakes and sweets to less obvious products like tins of vegetables, soups, packaged hams and virtually every manufactured food.

We would have to conclude, from looking at what we have been told to do and what we have done over the years between 1974 and 2000 that we have done very well. We have eaten far fewer calories. Our consumption of saturated fat has almost halved and our consumption of carbohydrate (starchy foods, fruit etc) has gone up. So, have we been rewarded for all this hard work with healthy, slim bodies? Quite the contrary – obesity has increased nearly ten fold during this time. On the evidence of *what* we have been eating, during the period in which obesity has increased so dramatically, dietary fat is fully exonerated from any role in the obesity epidemic and starchy foods are firmly on trial.

UK – The 'eatwell' plate

There is one piece of advice that appears to be common to UK public health advice and it can be found on the walls of hospitals, surgeries, clinics and even schools across the UK. The 'eatwell' plate was launched at a press release on Sunday 16 September 2007.[187] It is described in the British Nutrition Foundation video on YouTube as the "healthy eating model for the UK" – suitable for young or old, vegetarian or not and for any ethnic group.

It replaced *The Balance of Good Health*, which was launched by the UK Department of Health in 1994 and was also a picture of a segmented plate. In April 2000, responsibility for the Balance of Good Health (BOGH) diagram and concept passed to the newly formed Food Standards Agency. The FSA web site details the differences between the two plates. The BOGH title was seen as "unfriendly" and "lacking in emotion"[188] and so the title and some colours on the plate rim changed. Food groups were renamed. For example "bread, other cereals and potatoes" became "bread, rice, potatoes, pasta (and other starchy foods)". May I suggest that a marketing company made a lot of money making the plate more "friendly" and "emotional", but, to all intents and purposes, what we know as the 'eatwell' plate has been around since 1994.

On 10 August 2009 I wrote to the Food Standards Agency and asked where the eight tips for eating well came from and I asked where the proportions for the 'eatwell' plate came from and what the rationale was for the proportions. The response was that the calculation of segment size was determined as follows:

- The calculations are based on the model average diet which was developed by the Ministry of Agriculture, Fisheries and Food (MAFF) for COMA.
- The weight of food in each group, with the exception of fluids, was calculated.
- The weights of fluids (e.g. milk and fruit juice) were halved before being added to the rest of the foods in milk and dairy and fruits and vegetables respectively. "The reason for doing this is that these fluids contain a high proportion of water and are used in large quantities in the diet."
- The weight of all foods was then totalled. Portion size data was obtained from MAFF (from the national household food survey) and was converted into amounts to be consumed on a weekly basis.
- As a percentage of the total of this, the five food groups were comprised as follows:

Starchy foods (bread, potatoes, pasta, cereals etc)	33%
Fruit and vegetables	33%
Milk and Dairy products	15%
Non dairy protein (meat, fish, eggs, beans etc)	12%
Foods high in fat and sugar	8%

(101% due to rounding)

(Please note the vague use of the term "fat" once more). Despite the fact that the plate seems to be about a visual estimate of proportions, weight is clearly the important factor in the detailed explanation. So, I did an interesting calculation. I started with 100 grams of starchy foods and then calculated the weight of the other categories, to maintain the proposed proportions. The weight of fruit and vegetables would also be 100 grams; milk and dairy would be 45 grams; there would be 36 grams of non dairy protein and 24 grams of foods high in fat and sugar. I estimated the calorie averages for 100 grams of each of these food groups as 333, 42, 183, 188 and 595 respectively.[xxxii] This would give the estimated calorie values (for each of these weights) of 333, 42, 83, 68 and 144 respectively. If these are then scaled up in proportion for a 2,000 calorie a day diet, the five groups end up with 993, 125, 248, 204 and 430 calories respectively. The numbers will vary for each person's interpretation of the plate, but you can see how one third of intake in the form of starchy foods can represent half of calorie intake and another third from fruit and vegetables just 6% of energy. The supposedly smallest segment, being so energy dense, can form a perhaps unanticipated 21% of calorie intake.

I did the above calculation for interest and to show the law of unintended consequences, not because I want to legitimise the 'eatwell' plate in any way. I consider it to be an appalling proposal for healthy eating advice. Please do look up the diagram on line and see for yourself the products we are being encouraged to eat.[189] The "Starchy foods" segment features a box of cornflakes – not Kellogg's branded on the 'eatwell' plate, but Kellogg's branded on my version of the *Balance of Good Health* plate from the National Obesity Forum conference, which I attended in October 2004. Even without branding, the starchy foods segment on the 'eatwell' plate also features Weetabix cereal, white pasta, white rice, white bagels, white bread and other refined carbohydrates.

The fruit and vegetable segment makes no distinction between fruit (we will see the problem with fructose in Chapter Thirteen) and vegetables. The poster also features dried fruit, fruit juice, tins of vegetables (often containing sucrose) and other fruit and vegetables, which are not in the form that nature delivers them.

The non dairy protein can all be consumed in carbohydrate form – and presumably is by vegans and mostly will be by vegetarians. This section has baked beans prominently shown at the front (not branded) and tins of chick peas and kidney beans are also in the segment. There is no caution to look out for the sugar and salt added into many such tinned products.

The dairy section also contains carbohydrate. As a rule of thumb, dairy contains approximately 5% carbohydrate levels. The (likely) sugared yoghurts in this segment will be even higher in carbohydrate levels and sugar content.

The final segment is astonishing – 8% of our weight intake for foods high in fat and sugar, which becomes over 20% of our calorie/energy intake. The products featured include a can of cola, sponge cake, Battenberg cake, sweets, biscuits, pies, pastries, chocolate and crisps alongside what looks to be sunflower oil and butter – surely two real and good foods.

[xxxii] I keep a database of common foods, derived from the USDA nutrition database. I averaged all my sample foods for each of the five categories: starchy foods averaged 333 calories; fruit and vegetables 42; milk and dairy 183; meat, fish, eggs, beans 188 and foods high in fat and sugar 595 calories (all per 100 grams).

Each of the five segments therefore features carbohydrate, to a greater or lesser extent. Every food consumed, as recommended by this "model of healthy eating" can have an impact on insulin. Add to this the often heard advice "Graze – eat little and often" and you can see how our government advice is keeping UK citizens in a fat storing, not a fat burning, environment all day long. It is no wonder that insulin sensitivity and insulin resistance are becoming increasingly commonplace, as the human pancreas has never before had to cope with this quantity or frequency of carbohydrate, let alone this poor quality of carbohydrate.

Americans, please don't feel deprived by not having this plate. You have your food pyramid, as we saw earlier in this chapter. This has been updated in the most recent *Dietary Guidelines for Americans* (2005) and, the latest guidelines for a woman aged 19-30 are to consume: six ounces of grains (approximately 600 calories); two and a half cups of vegetables; two cups of fruit; six teaspoons of oil/equivalents; three cups of milk/dairy equivalents and five and a half ounces of meat/beans. The pyramid doesn't have the 'junk' segment, which the 'eatwell' plate does. However, the latest American food pyramid allows for discretionary calories. The mypyramid.gov web site gives an example of someone with a 'calorie budget' of 2,000 calories a day needing 1,735 calories for essential nutrients (this just shows the poor nutrient content of grains, fruits and vegetables relative to meat, fish and eggs). The guide works out for the person "Then you have 265 discretionary calories left. You may use these on 'luxury' versions of the foods in each group, such as higher fat meat or sweetened cereal. Or, you can spend them on sweets, sauces, or beverages". So our American friends can have 13% of their intake in the form of junk, under government advice. The UK is only supposed to have 8% – but we do have sugar and flour in abundance in the other segments – so we are getting our fair share of empty and low nutrient calories.

The Food Standards Agency will no doubt say that this segment is supposed to imply no more than 8% of intake in the form of junk food, but this, of course, is not how it has been adopted by the food industry. The UK Nutella web site justifies its recommendation for Nutella for breakfast by saying "The Food Standards Agency 'Eatwell plate', states that both sugar and fat are acceptable in appropriate quantities as part of a balanced diet."[190] The nutritional information lists 8.3 grams of sugar, per 15 grams of product, giving a sugar content of 55% for Nutella.

The Nutella USA nutrition page[191] leads with a picture of Nutella spread on bread with a glass of orange juice and states "The ideal balanced Nutella breakfast, as pictured here, is close to the breakfast recommended by the 2005 dietary guidelines for Americans." Two tablespoons of Nutella contains 200 calories and 22 grams of carbohydrate (21 grams of which is sugar). How can the American government recommend this, as a way to start the day, in an obese nation?

UK – What are we currently eating?

Let us go back to the Household Food Survey and look in detail at what we are currently eating and how this has changed. This is where we will use the 2008 Family Food Survey,[192] as the most up to date data available.

I have analysed the 2008 Family Food Survey in the same way that I did the 1974-2000 National Food Survey. The comprehensive reports caution against comparisons between the pre-2000 National Food Surveys and the post-2000 Family Food Surveys. However, the 2008 report notes "Since 1974 it is estimated that average energy intake has dropped by 29% after adjusting for changes in methodology", so the weight should have been falling off us.

The closest we have to a comparator with the National Food Survey is the detailed list of household foods consumed per average person in the UK per day. For the 2008 Family Food Survey, this accounted for 2,027 calories, broken down in useful detail into 24 categories from fish to biscuits. The top category consumed – accounting for over 10% of the calorie intake of the day – was "other cereal products". This includes cereals, pasta, pizza, rice puddings, frozen cakes and pastries (non-frozen cakes & pastries have their own separate category), cake and pudding mixes.

The second most consumed category was bread. Then other meat and meat products – where we find 75% of this category is processed meat including more carbohydrates – pies, pasties, sausage rolls, puddings and so on.

Precisely one third of our average calorie consumption comes from these three food categories. In total I calculated that 1,536 calories were from processed food sources and 491 were from real food. The real food sources were: 147 calories from milk, cheese, eggs and real dairy products; 126 calories from all real meat and fish; 116 from fresh potatoes, vegetables and fruit; 89 from real fats (olive oil, butter etc) and just 13 from whole grains. And the government wants us to eat less fat, cheese, meat, dairy products and so on. How successful and powerful must a food industry be to have this kind of market dominance over nature and to still have governments telling us to "Base our meals on starchy foods."

In the excellent BBC Television Programme *Who made me fat?*,[193] Rebecca Wilcox, calculated her daily intake of sugar. Wilcox represents a typical dieter – she admits "keeping the weight off pretty much dominates my life" and her processed food intake is very typical of a weight watcher. She has: a calorie counted cereal for breakfast (Kellogg's Start) with cranberry juice; a calorie counted cereal bar for morning snack; beans on (whole wheat) toast for lunch; another cereal bar mid afternoon; skinless chicken breasts with brown rice and a ready made sauce for dinner, followed by fat-free yoghurt. Her sugar intake added up to 167 grams – substantially more than the UK per capita estimate of 100 grams of sugar per day. By the law of averages, someone must be eating my share and we may have discovered who. Wilcox was visibly shocked and closed the experiment with the words "I'm eating healthy food – I thought."

Chapter Eleven

Have we reviewed the U-turn?

Evidence since the Seven Countries Study

When I wrote to the UK Food Standards Agency (FSA) in August 2009, and asked why their number one piece of dietary advice is "Base your meals on starchy foods", their reply was:

"Diets high in fat are *associated* with increased risk of cardiovascular disease (CVD), therefore it was recommended that people reduce their fat intake. It was advised that starchy carbohydrates should replace the reduction in fat as an energy source" (my emphasis). (Please note the use of the word fat and not saturated fat or any specific type of fat).

So, just as when the original advice was set in the COMA report of 1984, we don't advise people to base their meals on starchy foods because we know this to be beneficial for obesity, heart disease, cancer, diabetes and other modern illnesses. We simply went along with the idea that diets high in fat are associated with increased risk of heart disease (thank you for not saying caused by, FSA, but that's what the developed world has been led to believe). Never mind that there is not even a consistent association, let alone causation. We observed some incidences of people in the bath singing, so we associated bathing with singing and therefore issued a directive to stop bathing in the hope that it would stop singing. Never mind, also, that there is no evidence for any benefit from eating carbohydrate – just – people have got to eat something and if it's not fat, it has to be carbohydrate.

In 1981, in the heart journal *Atherosclerosis*, an article was published describing 246 factors that had been identified in different studies as having an influence in heart disease. The UK and USA public would be forgiven for thinking that there are only two – (saturated) fat and cholesterol. Ironically, neither of these has been proven.

Extremely worryingly, the letter I received from the FSA also stated that "SACN, which has now replaced COMA, is currently reviewing the evidence of carbohydrate on cardio-metabolic health." (SACN stands for Scientific Advisory Committee on Nutrition). This was not news to me, as I have seen invitations to comment on this review as part of a general consultation. It's just a bit late, 25 years on, to start looking at whether switching to a high-carbohydrate diet could be a factor in cardio-metabolic health. Personally, I have no doubt that a high-carbohydrate diet, especially the modern refined carbohydrate diet, *does* have a detrimental effect on cardio-metabolic, and most other aspects of, health. I am curious to see what public health bodies recommend that we eat when they discover that carbohydrates are bad for us, if they continue to maintain the view that fats are bad for us – protein is in virtually everything, so protein (in real food anyway) has to be part of a carbohydrate and/or a fat based food.

In the same letter to the Food Standards Agency I asked "What is the evidence for beneficial effects of reducing saturated fat intake on the risk of developing heart disease?" The reply I got was:

"The best evidence for beneficial effects of reducing saturated fat intake on risk of developing heart disease comes from randomised controlled dietary trials". The single journal, which the FSA offered as evidence for our absolute instruction to reduce saturated fat, was Stewart Truswell, *Australia NZ Journal of Medicine* 1994.[194] So, I procured a copy of this journal and dissected it.

The FSA letter set the scene by stating "the ideal controlled dietary trial for prevention of heart disease (a long-term intervention trial with differing levels of saturated fatty acids and measuring coronary disease endpoints) has not yet been done and it is unlikely ever to be done, due to huge cost and compliance and ethical issues." The UK's own Food Standards Agency, with 2,300 references to fat on their website, admits that the trial to demonstrate that saturated fat causes heart disease has not even been done, let alone proven. And, it is unlikely ever to be done. Please note the "due to ethical" issues bit. This may be interpreted as 'we can't do a trial because the people avoiding saturated fat would live and those eating it would die and this cannot be ethical.' Never mind that we switched the entire diet advice for the developed world 180 degrees on the back of one man's flimsy study. We appear to have no ethics when it comes to encouraging humans to eat a diet completely alien to that which we have consumed for over 3.5 million years and yet we think that meat or eggs might have people dying in the thousands.

The Truswell abstract (summary) opened with virtually identical words to the Food Standards Agency (FSA): "The perfect randomised controlled dietary prevention trial of coronary heart disease has never been done."

The main article also opened with the words "It has been accepted by experienced coronary disease researchers that the perfect controlled dietary trial for prevention of coronary heart disease (CHD) has not yet been done and we are unlikely ever to see it done." "Huge cost and compliance are major problems, but on top of these a large trial may no longer be ethical." I genuinely wonder how many people, who have been brainwashed into thinking that they should eat a tasteless, low-fat (by definition high-carbohydrate) diet, are aware that there is no proof for the fat/heart assertion – the study has not even been done.

May I suggest that the definitive study of dietary fat and heart disease can never, and will never, be done – not because of any ethics involved, but because the epidemiology of populations and the macronutrient composition of food would make such a study virtually impossible. The necessary study (to justify having put saturated fat in jail) would involve a long term dietary study (at least five years) where saturated fat was swapped out for one type of fat only (e.g.

saturated fat out and monounsaturated fat in). The diet would have to maintain carbohydrate, fat and protein, in the precise amounts and proportions as were being consumed at the start of the study (virtually impossible alone to achieve) and not change this intake throughout the course of the study. All other variables would also need to be maintained precisely during the study and certainly all those that could impact on heart disease: general health; weight; exercise; occupation; work life balance; family and marital situation; smoking; location; lifestyle and so on. This is why the study is not likely to be done. Such a study would still only tell us about the relative merits of saturated fat vs. monounsaturated fat and not about either alone. We just need to apply a bit of (not so) common sense – the notion that real fat, found in real food, kills humans, in evolutionary terms alone, is preposterous.

Back to the journal – Truswell says "The best we can do is to look at all the trials together", so this is what he does. He reviews 14 trials, which had disease or death as the end point. Three of the trials had a sub set to them, so technically there are 17 to review. There is another classic comment in the introduction: "the failure to see a reduction in total deaths was disappointing" i.e. we were a bit gutted that more people eating the 'normal' diet didn't die relative to the others eating our fat adjusted diets.

This paper is important to analyse in some detail, as it represents the entire evidence presented by the FSA to justify why we are told to avoid saturated fat. Here is a summary table of the 17 studies in the paper. In what follows, the type of study (column 4) is either Primary (P) or Secondary (S) and Dietary (D) or Multi-factorial (M). Primary studies have been done on the population as a whole. Secondary studies are those done on people already known to be at risk of heart disease. Table 16 is for total deaths – we can look at coronary heart disease deaths alone if there are any relevant dietary studies left, once we have gone through them:

Table 16: Participants and total deaths in the studies reviewed by Truswell.

	Study	People	Type	Years	Deaths Interv- ention	Deaths Control
A	Research Committee (1965)	264	SD	3	20	24
B	Rose (1965)	52	SD	2	5	1
C	MRC Soybean Oil (1968)	393	SD	3.4	28	31
D	Dayton (1969)	846	PD	7	174	177
E	Leren, Oslo (1970)	412	SD	5+	101	108
F	Helsinki men (1972)	1,900	PD	12	188	217
	Helsinki women (1972)	2,836	PD	12	415	465
G	Woodhill, Sydney (1978)	458	SD	5	39	28
H	Kallio (1979)	375	SM	3	41	56
J	WHO (*) (1985)	57,460	PM	6	1,250	1,261
K	Oslo diet & smoking (1986)	1,232	PM	5	19	31
L	DART fat advice (1989)	2,033	SD	2	111	113
	DART fish advice (1989)	2,033	SD	2	94	130
M	Frantz Minnesota men (1989)	4,393	PD	1	158	153
	Frantz Minnesota women (1989)	4,664	PD	1	111	95
N	MRFIT (1990)	12,866	PM	7	496	537
P	Singh (1992)	406	SD	1	21	38
	TOTAL	92,623			3,271	3,465

The 17 studies together include 92,623 people. However, the World Health Organisation study (J in the table)[195] alone accounted for 57,460 of these people – 62% of the overall number of people; so, the Truswell article is predominantly a review of one study. Plus this study, along with three others, is a multi-factorial study – they are not dietary studies – and therefore must be disregarded.

A basic scientific principle is that a valid experiment must be what is called a control experiment i.e. it must change one variable at a time. Only then can the impact of that variable be determined. As an example, the MRFIT study[196] (N in the table) actually stands for "Multiple Risk Factor Intervention Trial" i.e. we are going to intervene with many risk factors and see what happens. That's an interesting thing to do, but it tells us nothing about any of the factors in isolation. If I stop smoking, change my diet, lose weight, take a hypertension drug and diuretics (to reduce water retention) and if I then feel better – what has had any impact, let alone the most impact? Not only must individual factors be able to be isolated, any two factors must be able to be considered together e.g. if 10 people change their diet and some lose weight and others don't, we need to be able to look at those who changed their diet and lost weight vs. those who changed their diet and didn't lose weight. Then we can see the impact of combinations of variables as well as isolated variables.

In MRFIT, one of the most famous and often quoted studies in the heart disease arena, 6,428 men were in the intervention group and 6,438 in the control group. All the subjects were men aged 35 to 57 and they were selected for the study because they had one, or more, of three health conditions considered risk factors for heart disease: hypertension, hypercholesterolemia and cigarette smoking.

The interventions included: antihypertensive drugs; diuretic drugs; smoking cessation and dietary changes. That's a lot of variables all changing at once. If the intervention group did show a beneficial difference, following this cocktail of measures, all that could be implied would be – if a person with one or more of three health conditions, which are considered to be heart disease risk factors, takes antihypertensive drugs *and* diuretic drugs *and* stops smoking *and* makes dietary changes (*and*, presumably there will be indirect factors such as reduced water retention, reduced blood pressure, weight reduction, reduced strain on lungs etc) *and* all other things remain equal (location, income, stress, family and marital situation, other health factors and conditions and so on), there would appear to be an association between one, or a combination of, these interventions and coronary heart disease. We still cannot claim causation, let alone what has caused what. Given that this would be the best possible conclusion we could reach – why would a study such as this ever be started? Surely we need to know specifics?

The JAMA 1982 article about the MRFIT study[197] noted: "Over an average follow-up period of seven years… Total mortality rates were 41.2 per 1,000 (in the intervention group) and 40.4 per 1,000 (in the control group)." I.e. 264 men died in total in the intervention group and 260 died in the control group. Notwithstanding the fact that this study needs to be dismissed from the FSA 'evidence', because it is not a dietary study, I wanted to share this information to show that the seven year study data published at the time showed slightly more deaths in the intervention group. Although 264 vs. 260 is not statistically significant, whichever way round it were, how did the seven year data apparently change so much in a report eight years later in 1990 i.e. the source for study N in the table?

The other multi factorial studies, H, J and K also need to be excluded for the same reasons. They have no relevance in any assertion that dietary fat causes heart disease, for the same reason that nothing can be isolated as an association, let alone causation.

Before we discard J, however, there are some interesting general comments to make about this study. It is by far the largest study in Truswell's paper, accounting for 62% of the number of people in the 17 studies together. Of the 57,460 people involved, 30,489 were in the intervention group and 26,971 were in the control group. 1,325 died in the intervention group and 1,186 died in the control group. The study had one more intervention than MRFIT. The European collaborative study included: a 'cholesterol lowering diet'; smoking control; management of weight; drug intervention for blood pressure and exercise. (Please note that the notion "cholesterol lowering diet" is something of a tautology – the study is trying to see if diet has an impact on heart disease. We know that the body makes cholesterol and eating cholesterol has no impact on cholesterol levels *per se*. Hence by claiming that one intervention is a cholesterol lowering diet, it must be being assumed that dietary fat influences heart disease through cholesterol and yet this is what the study is allegedly setting out to investigate). Allowing for the fact that the intervention and control groups were of different size, we can compare them directly by calculating deaths per 1,000 people in each group. This results in the deaths in the intervention group being 4.35 people per 1,000 and deaths in the control group being 4.4 people per 1,000. This has no statistical significance whatsoever and yet was the largest study by a margin *and* a study with five different intervention strategies.

This six year study, therefore, should have concluded that none of five factors appeared to have any association with total mortality. The data for coronary heart disease (CHD) deaths (from the original journal – not presented in Truswell's summary) was that 428 people died in the intervention group and 398 in the control group. When this is adjusted to account for more people being in the intervention group, we find that 1.5% of the intervention group died of CHD and 1.4% of the control group died of CHD. Had both groups been evenly populated i.e. 28,730 people in each group, using these ratios, 424 in the intervention group would have died of CHD vs. 403 in the control group. Did the study *cause* the people supposedly being helped (the intervention group) to die? I would not suggest that for one minute, but the opposite is quite frequently asserted. As I was writing this book, the Chief Medical Officer for England, Sir Liam Donaldson, wrote in his 2009 annual report "…a 30% reduction in animal product consumption would save the equivalent of 175,000 healthy years of life every year." Where is the evidence for such an assertion? What does Donaldson think that homo sapiens and our ancestors have been eating for 3.5 million years – cornflakes?

So, H, J, K and N need to be dismissed, as they are multi factorial studies and, to be fair, noted by Truswell as such. A and C were also multi factorial studies, and noted in the text as such, but not in the table. A and C were dietary change and weight reduction studies so these are also not control studies, as we would not be able to say if any results were attributable to dietary changes, or to weight loss, or some combination of both. A was a low-fat diet with increased fish intake advised. Depending on the type of fish consumed, study A could be both trying to reduce and increase fat intake at the same time – the specific dietary claim would need to be clarified. A and C should be excluded, as we can make no conclusion about the impact of whatever the dietary change was planned to achieve.

Truswell himself actually suggests that the Helsinki (F) data be removed "because there is some uncertainty over which numbers to use." This study has been widely attacked on many grounds – the main two being the fact that a crossover trial is an inappropriate way to study a condition with a long incubation period. There is no way of telling that any occurrences in one period were the result of the circumstances in that period, or in the period before. Any deaths at the start of the crossover phase would almost certainly be linked to health in the previous period and render the allocation of that death to the current period inappropriate. The Finnish Mental Hospital was the only trial done on a crossover basis and has been discarded as often as it has been quoted. The second key criticism is that this study was not a controlled trial. In an editorial in *The Lancet* (November 1972) John Rivers and Professor Yudkin noted that the sugar consumption varied by almost 50% between the trial periods. This led the lead author of the Finnish study, Osmo Turpeinen to respond in the December issue of The Lancet confirming that the variations in sugar intake were "regrettable" and admitting that the hospitals in each 'side' of the study had been given freedom in dietary matters outside the prescribed fat composition. I concur with Truswell, therefore, that this study also needs to be discarded.

What this Finnish study was trying to do was to replace saturated fat with vegetable oil. That it failed to hold anything else constant is clearly "regrettable". What is interesting is that the three other studies trying to achieve the same, which did hold as many other factors constant as possible, actually concluded the opposite. The Rose et al corn oil trial (Study B in the table – 1965), the Woodhill Sydney (Study G – 1978) and a study that, for some reason Truswell chose to ignore, the Anti-Coronary Club Trial (1966), all had more deaths in the intervention group than the control group. The data for Studies B and G is in Truswell's table. In study B, I could be harsh and say that five times as many people died in the intervention group as in the control group. This is true, but only one died in the control group and five in the intervention group. In study G, 39 people died in the intervention group and 28 in the control group, from a study of 458 people. In the Anti-Coronary Club Trial, the first report in February 1966[198] suggested that the 'prudent' diet may have substantial benefit. In November, later that year, the Anti-Coronary Club Trial team published a follow up report where it was noted that 26 members of the intervention group died compared with only six whose diet was not considered 'prudent.'[199]

Interestingly, upon reading the text in Truswell, we learn that B was a three way trial (corn oil, olive oil and a control group) and that Truswell only included the corn oil and the control in his table. I can only conclude from this that olive oil did no better than the control, which is interesting, as this would imply that another 'unfavourable' study has been excluded. Other than being too small (52 people) and too short (two years), B has some small relevance as a dietary study.

The final study that needs to be removed is P – the article text notes that, in this study, butter was replaced by unsaturated oils while simultaneously intakes of eggs and meat were reduced. This will have the effect of increasing *unsaturated* fat on the one hand and reducing it on the other. Singh may not have been aware of the fat composition of different foods – I have yet to meet a doctor or dietitian who knows the fat composition of meat or eggs i.e. that they are primarily monounsaturated fat and with a reasonable measure of polyunsaturated fat.

Taubes notes that there are seven studies looking at the impact of dietary fat on heart disease and they are all epidemiological (arguably with the exception of Helsinki).[200] This means that they have all the problems, which we have already raised: they are selective, rather than comprehensive; they are studies of association not causation; even where an association is observed, an alternative explanation may be involved in causation and they can never be control experiments, as so many other variables are changing at the same time.

Taubes' seven are: the longest and possibly most renowned of all – The Framingham Heart Study (1950+); Western Electric Company (1957); Keys' Seven Countries Study (1970); Anti Coronary Club Trial (1962); Dayton (1969); Helsinki (1972) and Minnesota (1989). Truswell only included the last three of these. Remember from Chapter Eight, one of the most definitive quotations from the Framingham Study was made by Dr. William Castelli 1992 when he said "In Framingham, Mass, the more saturated fat one ate, the more cholesterol one ate, the *more calories one ate*, the lower the person's serum cholesterol." The Western Electric study had fewer deaths in the high fat than the low-fat group. Keys we have already reviewed extensively and the Anti Coronary Club Trial had over four times as many deaths in the intervention group as in the control group. I share this to state that Truswell has not included all available and relevant studies and to insinuate that rather more *unfavourable* studies have been omitted. This is additionally unfair, as Truswell attacks Uffe Ravnskov in the journal for incomplete citation of available information in one of his articles.

Truswell's conclusion from the article is that the total 3,271 deaths in the intervention group vs. the 3,465 deaths in the control group show that "for total deaths the ratio of intervention/control in all 17 trials is 0.94 and for coronary events the pooled odds ratio is 0.87."

If we exclude the multi-factorial studies (H, J, K and N), as we can conclude nothing specifically about diet from these, we are left with 13 studies, four of which had more deaths in the intervention group, seven of which had more deaths in the control group and two of which were of negligible difference. Of the seven that had more deaths in the control group, two of these were studies A and C, where weight reduction effectively made the studies multi-factorial. Although these together only had seven more deaths in the control than the intervention group (hardly significant), excluding these two studies would make the deaths higher in the intervention group on four occasions and deaths higher in the control group on five occasions. Removing the Helsinki study, as Truswell actually advises, renders all remaining numbers meaningless, as there is then not even a weak association apparent in either the intervention or the control group. Finally, the removal of Study P, (from which we cannot even conclude if fat content, let alone composition, increased or decreased), leaves the following: B, D, E, G, L (2) and M (2) – eight studies in total. In these eight studies, there were more deaths in the intervention group than the control group four times and more in the control group than the intervention group four times. Additionally, two of the occasions where the control group apparently had more deaths were virtually negligible: In study D there were 174 deaths in the intervention group and 177 in the control group and in Study L (fat advice) there were 111 deaths in the intervention group and 113 in the control group. Neither of these is statistically significant.

Of these eight studies that remain, if we then look at heart disease deaths, five of the studies had more deaths in the control group and three in the intervention group. That's without including other available studies, as Taubes documented, which Truswell left out.

There is another fundamental and quite remarkable thing to note. In this entire journal, which represents the sole evidence offered by the FSA for their instruction to avoid saturated fat and, allegedly, the summary of all available dietary evidence on the subject of fat and heart disease (although we know that this is not the case), there is actually no firm conclusion in the article about fat generally, fat specifically, saturated fat, monounsaturated fat and/or polyunsaturated fat. Truswell notes "The dietary advice differed." "In most (studies) however, the dietary prescription was a reduced saturated fat and cholesterol intake with partial replacement by polyunsaturated oils."

We know that cholesterol intake has no impact on cholesterol levels, which leaves reduced saturated fat and partial replacement by polyunsaturated oils. Was overall fat reduced therefore? ("partial replacement") Were calories reduced therefore? By how much was saturated fat reduced and by how much were polyunsaturated oils increased? Notwithstanding the fact that as many studies showed more deaths in the intervention group as in the control group, how can such a vehement condemnation of saturated fat come from such non existent 'evidence'? My guess is that extremely busy doctors don't have time to question everything and rely upon supposedly independent organisations, such as the Food Standards Agency (FSA), to have robust and unquestionable evidence. I sincerely hope that this book makes our front line health professionals, who are in a unique position to make a difference to the obesity epidemic, question the public health position and come to their own conclusion about nature's food vs. processed food.

It is critical to remember that all of this is merely about trying to establish an association. As with the Seven Countries Study, even if Truswell's analysis of other studies did establish a clear association (which it doesn't), this says nothing about causation (either way round) and nothing about any other factors that could be involved in any observed association and it says nothing about all the data not included, which could conclude to the contrary (i.e. the people in the bath and/or singing that we didn't include).

For the FSA to be relying on this, as the definitive study to issue "eat less fat" orders, can only be described as negligent.

We also need to address the central theme in Truswell. Truswell assumes that cholesterol causes heart disease. He actually thinks that total cholesterol causes heart disease. He mentions HDL once, and LDL once, so he really is still digging the first hole. Indeed, he says "If there were no worthy difference in plasma cholesterol, there is no reason to expect any reduction of CHD or deaths." This means that Truswell believes that fat (he's not even specific about the type) causes heart disease via cholesterol because of his statement that if cholesterol doesn't go down there is no reason to expect heart disease will go down. So Truswell believes that A causes C through B – please see Chapter Eight.

The importance placed by Truswell on the benefits of reducing cholesterol is at complete odds with the major studies in the world on cholesterol and overall mortality. Hence, even if Truswell could have shown that lower cholesterol *causes* lower heart disease (and he hasn't even established a consistent association), the major studies of cholesterol and mortality alone conclude that the lower one's cholesterol, the higher the risk of overall mortality.

Cholesterol and mortality

The Honolulu Study[201] was a 20 year study of cholesterol levels and mortality in 3,572 Japanese American men. The study concluded that "Only the group with low cholesterol concentration at both examinations had a significant association with mortality". The authors went on "We have been unable to explain our results". (I.e. we were expecting lower cholesterol to equal lower mortality, not the other way round). All credit to the team for their honest reporting of these unexpected results and their final statement in the abstract: "These data cast doubt on the scientific justification for lowering cholesterol to very low concentrations (<4·65 mmol/L) in elderly people."

Framingham similarly concluded that "There is a direct association between falling cholesterol levels over the first 14 years and mortality over the following 18 years (11% overall and 14% CVD death rate increase per 1 mg/dL per year drop in cholesterol levels)."[202] Kendrick does a clever calculation on this quotation and translates this into – a reduction in cholesterol from 5 to 4 mmol/L would increase your risk of dying by 400%.

Elaine Meilahn reported in Circulation (2005) "In 1990, an NIH (National Institutes of Health) conference concluded from a meta-analysis of 19 studies that men and, to a lesser extent, women with a total serum cholesterol level below 4.2 mmol/L exhibited about a 10% to 20% excess total mortality compared with those with a cholesterol level between 4.2 and 5.2 mmol/L. Specifically, excess causes of death included cancer (primarily lung and hematopoietic), respiratory and digestive disease, violent death (suicide and trauma), and hemorrhagic stroke."[203]

If you want more evidence for the connection between low cholesterol levels and increased mortality, I recommend Kendrick's comprehensive sample of references[204] and Dr. Natasha Campbell Mc-Bride's *Put your heart in your mouth*.[205] Just reading the list in Chapter Eight of this book, detailing the vital importance of cholesterol to the entire functioning of the human body, is enough for me for this to be common sense.

The average cholesterol levels for England were reported by the National Health Service (NHS) as 5.5 mmol/L for men and 5.6 mmol/L for women.[206] The NHS further noted that "two out of three adults have a total cholesterol level of 5mmol/L or above". I found the BBC statement of the position statistically implausible: "The average total cholesterol level in the UK is 5.5mmol/l for men and 5.6mmol/l for women, which is above a normal level."[207] What is the average, if not the norm? Even if we get into the detail of the mean, median and mode, surely the average for a data group defines normal for that data group. The notion that an actual norm is somehow abnormal – because it has been decreed to be as such, makes no sense. The normal distribution curve sets a norm by definition. For us to declare the actual cholesterol norm to be abnormal, is not normal in itself. This would be like suddenly declaring normal blood pressure to be 100/60 and not the normal distribution norm of 120/80, because we picked the number and declared it to be so.

In the *Western Journal of Medicine*, (May 2002) Thomas Samaras and Harold Elrick posed the question "Height, body size and longevity – is smaller better for the human body?"[208] The study took 100,000 males from six different ethnic populations – in the same city (California) to try to normalise other factors. The table had the following height orders (tallest first): African Americans; White Americans; Hispanics; Asian Indians; Chinese and Japanese (the first two groups were recorded as of equal average height – 70 inches). The age standardised death rates for all causes and coronary heart disease were included in the table. A clear pattern was immediately obvious. I calculated the correlation coefficients as 0.85 for height and CHD and 0.9 for height and all causes of death. What if we concluded that height were a cause of CHD (and all causes of death) and that we should therefore redefine the average height to declare the actual average of 69.7 inches (for all American men) to be abnormal. What if we picked an arbitrary new target 10% lower than the actual average (5.0mmol/L is approximately 10% below the actual cholesterol norm of 5.5mmol/L) and decreed that normal height should be approximately 63 inches. We could then stop the body from performing a normal bodily function (growth) by administering drugs to stop growth hormones from doing their job. I trust that this analogy disturbs you. The Chinese practice of foot binding – an artificial intervention in the normal development of the human body, to achieve an artificial 'norm' – was thankfully outlawed in the early twentieth century, but trying to reduce the normal cholesterol level continues.

Fat and heart disease

Just to return to the core subject of this chapter – does eating fat (any type other than trans fats) cause heart disease? Let us return to Braunwald's Heart Disease and Mozaffarian's excellent contributions in chapter 48: "In the 1960's and 1970's, ecologic (cross-national) studies and short term feeding trials evaluating single risk factors (e.g. total cholesterol levels) suggested that higher fat consumption, as a percentage of total energy (%E), increased CHD risk. But subsequent evidence has demonstrated convincingly that the proportion of energy consumed from total fat has no appreciable effect on CHD."[209]

Available to Mozaffarian at the time of writing were the results of the "Women's Health Initiative Randomized Controlled Dietary Modification Trial", published in 2006.[210] This was a large study of 48,835 post menopausal women, aged 50 to 79. Study enrolment occurred between 1993 and 1998 in 40 American clinical centres. The conclusion was "Over a mean of 8.1 years, a dietary intervention that reduced total fat intake and increased intakes of vegetables, fruits, and grains did not significantly reduce the risk of CHD, stroke, or CVD in postmenopausal women." This study is for total fat.

Mente et al's systematic review of the evidence supporting a causal link between dietary factors and coronary heart disease was also available (2009).[211] The objective of the review was to assess the strength of evidence available, "in a wealth of literature", supporting valid *associations* (my emphasis, i.e. not causation). The conclusion was "Insufficient evidence of association is present for... saturated and polyunsaturated fatty acids; total fat; linolenic acid; meat; eggs; and milk." I.e. not even an association between any of these factors and CHD, let alone causation. This study is for total fat, saturated fat, polyunsaturated fat and linolenic acid (omega-3 fat).

The most recent study available at the time of writing this book was from the March 2010 *American Journal of Clinical Nutrition*. The article was called "Meta-analysis of prospective cohort studies evaluating the association of saturated fat with cardiovascular disease", by Patty W Siri-Tarino, Qi Sun, Frank B Hu and Ronald M Krauss.[212] This study is for saturated fat.

The objective of the study was to summarise the evidence related to the *association* of dietary saturated fat with risk of coronary heart disease (CHD), stroke, and cardiovascular disease (CVD) in prospective epidemiologic studies. That means, in effect, this is an up-to-date version of Truswell's analysis – a study aimed at reviewing all the evidence available and drawing a conclusion. This study has the benefit of 16 years worth of evidence unavailable to Truswell and all the evidence that was available in 1994 – whether included by Truswell or not. This article reviewed twenty-one studies covering 347,747 people with the results: "During 5-23 y of follow-up of 347,747 subjects, 11,006 developed CHD or stroke. Intake of saturated fat was not associated with an increased risk of CHD, stroke, or CVD. Consideration of age, sex, and study quality did not change the results". The overall conclusion was "A meta-analysis of prospective epidemiologic studies showed that there is no significant evidence for concluding that dietary saturated fat is associated with an increased risk of CHD or CVD. More data are needed to elucidate whether CVD risks are likely to be influenced by the specific nutrients used to replace saturated fat."

That last sentence is important. It brings us, rather worryingly, full circle to the 'side note' in the FSA letter – "SACN, which has now replaced COMA, is currently reviewing the evidence of carbohydrate on cardio-metabolic health."

So, the current position in the latest review of all evidence available, including almost 350,000 people over a 5-23 year period, is that saturated fat is not even *associated* with coronary heart disease (CHD), stroke or cardio vascular disease (CVD). This review recommends more research into the nutrients that are replacing saturated fat – i.e. carbohydrates. Are we getting close to realising that our move away from real food (containing real fat as nature intends) to processed food (containing carbohydrates, processed fat and many new and unfamiliar ingredients) could have caused heart disease? Are we close to realising that not only has our move to an unprecedented level of carbohydrate and processed food led to an obesity epidemic, but, with ultimate irony, it has worsened the condition it was intended to prevent?

Closing comment

There are three facts that I can state without any fear of being proven wrong:

1) It has *not* been proven that saturated fat consumption causes heart disease;
2) It has *not* even been proven that there is a consistent association between saturated fat consumption and heart disease;
3) The definitive study to try to prove this has *not* been done and likely never will be.

None of the other adaptations of this accusation have been proven either – not for association, let alone causation – monounsaturated fats, polyunsaturated fats, ratios of polyunsaturated fats to saturated fats, swapping one real fat for another real fat. This is all just digging holes at best and lying to one's citizens at worst.

The most tragic observation of all is that we have been confusing fat and carbohydrate for over half a century. Had we done all of the work we have done with the clear distinction between real food and processed food, not by studying real fat, as found in processed food, we may well have found a powerful relationship between modern food and modern illness. We may then have given the right dietary advice to avoid the emerging modern substances and have avoided an explosion in obesity, diabetes, cancer and other modern illness.

The fact remains that our current diet advice (eat low fat/avoid saturated fat/base your meals on starchy foods) was never developed as, nor intended to be, an obesity strategy. It became an American healthy heart strategy (launched in January 1977), on the basis of one of the most biased and fundamentally flawed studies ever to determine public health advice. The UK then followed the USA in adopting this as universal dietary advice (not just for people deemed at risk of heart disease, but for everyone) and, over the past 26 years, from whence this came has long been forgotten.

The implications of this dramatic shift away from the natural animals (fat), which we and our ancestors have been consuming, since man walked upright, towards the man-made starches and sugars (carbohydrate), which we have been eating for the blink of an eye in evolutionary terms, are immense.

How can any modern illness, such as heart disease, not even recorded as a cause of death until 1948, be in any way related to food that nature has been providing for 3.5 million years? Equally, how can heart disease *not* be related to food that man has been providing in increasing quantities during the period in which we have gone from not recording heart disease as a cause of death, to recording it as the cause of one in three deaths.

As we will see in the next chapter – the issue is not fat vs. carbohydrate but real food vs. processed food. The study that can then be done, which is not even difficult in terms of macronutrient composition, is not fat vs. carbohydrates but real food vs. processed food. The intervention group would eat as nature intends us to eat and the control group are the rest of America, UK and Australia. They carry on eating processed food as food manufacturers intend us to eat. Recent history suggests that they then will carry on gaining weight and losing energy; gaining serious illness and losing years of life expectancy. Where is the balance of ethics now?

Chapter Twelve

"Eat less fat"

Introduction

We have been eating fat and cholesterol, found naturally in animals and animal by-products, since man first walked the planet. *Australopithecus Lucy* is believed to be the first upright ape/man – dating back approximately 3,500,000 years. If anything in animals were bad for us, let alone responsible for a killer disease, evolution tells us that we would have either a) died out or b) evolved to not need the 'fatal' substance. As there is no evidence of either (a) or (b), common sense alone tells us that we are quite safe eating animals and animal products.

It is useful, at this juncture, to get an expert view on our evolutionary diet. One of the best review articles I have found is Professor John Gowlett's "What actually was the Stone Age Diet?"[213] which uses fossil records and archaeological evidence to ascertain what our ancestors were eating. Gowlett goes back even further than *Australopithecus Lucy* and asserts "The broad outline of the evolutionary record is becoming increasingly clear: human ancestors diverged from the last common ape ancestor about 8-10 million years ago." Human DNA is most closely related to that of the chimpanzee, followed by the gorilla and then the orang-utans. I was interested to learn from this article that, while our ape ancestors did consume any fruit and vegetation that they could find, chimpanzees hunted monkeys and even baby antelope and baboons, thus refuting the notion that we are of vegetarian ancestry.[214]

Gowlett traces the major stages of dietary evolution, noting that the location of settlement was a major determinant of the diet consumed. What we now know to be Africa provided root vegetables and tubers in good measure. However, over the past two million years, as early human beings settled in more northern regions, including the arctic, there were increasing geographical areas where there was no choice but to eat meat.

A quick summary of historic periods will help with the next part: The Stone Age, also known as the Palaeolithic era, is the name given to the period between about 2.5 million and 20,000 years ago. It began with the earliest human-like behaviours of crude stone tool manufacture, and ended with modern human 'hunting and gathering' societies. (The Palaeolithic is the earliest archaeology; anything older is Palaeontology). Scholars traditionally divide the Palaeolithic period into three: The Early Stone Age/lower Palaeolithic period, which lasted between 2.5 million to 200,000 years ago; The Middle Stone Age/Middle Palaeolithic period, which is generally taken as the period between

200,000 to 45,000 years ago; and The Late Stone Age/Upper Palaeolithic era is estimated to have covered the period from 45,000 to 20,000 years ago.

There were some wonderfully named species between *Australopithecus Lucy* and Homo sapiens – as humans are known today. Homo erectus, (always gets a giggle in science lessons), was on earth from approximately 1.8 million years ago to approximately 300,000 years ago. Then we had Homo heidelbergensis (also known as Homo sapiens archaic) covering the period circa 600-500,000 to 200,000 – thereby overlapping Homo erectus and our most immediate ancestors – Homo neanderthalensis. Neanderthals, as they are more commonly known, are estimated to have evolved approximately 300-250,000 years ago. No definite specimens younger than 30,000 years ago have been found, although some remnant evidence from Gibraltar may suggest evidence of Neanderthals approximately 24,000 years ago. The Middle Palaeolithic period saw the emergence of the first anatomically modern Homo Sapiens (approximately 120,000 years ago). By the end of the Late Stone Age/Upper Palaeolithic era, only what we know to be modern humans were left and we were spread all over the planet.

History cannot agree on when fire was commonly used for warmth and cooking. The date options range from 1.5 to 0.5 million years ago. Meat can be consumed raw, but Peters et al estimated that approximately half the root vegetables and tubers in the African region would have been indigestible without cooking.[215] This means that animal foods would have needed to have been staple nutrition for several hundreds of thousands of years, even in areas with more abundant vegetation.

Gowlett states that "Stable isotope analyses of carbon and nitrogen in bone collagen now show Neanderthals to have been carnivores to a very high degree." Paleolithic cave art of Europe centres very heavily on the representation of animals. Gowlett notes for Europe: "There can be little doubt that the ancestors of most Europeans had such a meat-based diet for approximately 30,000 years of ice age (40,000-10,000 before present), some 1200 generations. From 10,000 years ago, climatic improvement led to warm-period hunting and gathering, probably involving larger components of roots and berries. Then farming came in, so that cereals and milk have been major products for the last 5000 years, or 200 generations."

So, history tells us that we have been carnivore/omnivores. Our survival has depended on us finding and consuming anything provided by nature. We would have consumed any berries, nuts and vegetation in the local environment. The provision of these would have been seasonal at best and virtually nonexistent in more northern regions of earth and completely non existent during the last ice age. Hence, it cannot be in doubt that we would have hunted and consumed any animals that we could catch. The idea that our ancestors would have trimmed the fat off meat is laughable and yet this is the advice that we give the generations of the twenty-first century.

What are fats?

Fats, commonly known as lipids, consist of a wide group of organic substances that are not soluble in water. In simple terms, fats are chains of carbon atoms (chemical symbol C) with hydrogen atoms attached (chemical symbol H) and they have a COOH group at one end (carbon, oxygen, oxygen and hydrogen). There are two groups of fats in which we have a nutritional interest – saturated and unsaturated. Within the unsaturated category, there are two further types – monounsaturated and polyunsaturated fats.

Saturated fats are the most stable fats (this is merely a statement about chemical structure). They have all available carbon bonds filled with (i.e. saturated with) hydrogen. Saturated fats are solid at room temperature. Interestingly, when our glycogen (storage form of glucose) capacity is full, the liver turns the excess glucose (from carbohydrates) into fat in the liver and it turns it into saturated fat. If saturated fat is bad for us, this could be the first example of the human body, in normal circumstances, trying to kill itself. Breast milk is also high in saturated fat, so did evolution also design us to kill our offspring? I have my own views on this; I'll let you develop yours.

Unsaturated fats, quite simply, have pairs of hydrogen atoms missing. Monounsaturated fats have one double bond in the form of two carbon atoms 'double-bonded' to each other and, therefore, lack two hydrogen atoms. Mono means one and hence, with monounsaturated fat, there is one double bond. Monounsaturated fats tend to be liquid at room temperature (but solid at fridge temperature) and are the next most stable fat. The best known monounsaturated fat is oleic acid, the main component of olive oil. Oleic acid is also found in the oils from almonds, pecans, cashews, peanuts and avocados.

On the web site "margarine.org.uk" (described on the site as "the mouthpiece of the margarine and spreads industry"), unsaturated fats are described as follows: "In unsaturated fats, some of the carbon atoms are joined to others by a double bond and, therefore, could accept more hydrogen atoms."[216] They could accept more hydrogen atoms. Isn't that just a wonderful way of saying they are missing some hydrogen atoms (and are therefore less stable)?

Normally poly means many, but, in the case of polyunsaturated fat, it can mean only two. Polyunsaturated fats have two or more pairs of double bonds and, therefore, lack four or more hydrogen atoms. Polyunsaturated fats are liquid at room and fridge temperature. The two polyunsaturated fats found most frequently in our food are double unsaturated linoleic acid, with two double bonds, also called omega-6; and triple unsaturated alpha-linolenic acid, with three double bonds, also called omega-3. (The omega number indicates the position of the first double bond. If the double bond is three carbon atoms along from the right hand end, this is an omega-3 fat. If it is six carbon atoms from the right hand end, this is an omega-6 fat. The logic comes from the Greek alphabet, which goes from Alpha to Omega – like we go from A to Z). Omega-3 and omega-6 fats are called "Essential Fatty Acids" because the body cannot make them, so it is essential that they are consumed.

It is not widely known that all fats and oils, whether of vegetable or animal origin, are a combination of saturated, monounsaturated and polyunsaturated fat. Coconut oil has the highest saturated fat content of all foods at 92% saturated, 6% monounsaturated and 2% polyunsaturated. Lard is 41% saturated, 47% monounsaturated and 12% polyunsaturated. Olive oil is 14% saturated fat, 75% monounsaturated and 11% polyunsaturated. The above are 100% fats, so we can usefully compare their composition as percentages. Butter has a significant water content and a trace of protein, so 100 grams of butter has 51 grams of saturated fat, 21 grams of monounsaturated fat and 3 grams of polyunsaturated fat.[217]

There is another relevant aspect of fat chemistry – fats can be classified according to their chain length, as well as their degree of saturation. Mary Enig and Sally Fallon Morell's book, *Know Your Fats,* is invaluable if you want to do as the title suggests:[218]

- Fats that have fewer than six carbon atoms are called short chain fatty acids (SCFA's). SCFA's are always saturated and include butyric acid (found mostly in butterfat from cows) and caproic acid (found mostly in butterfat from goats), as examples.
- Medium chain fatty acids (MCFAs) have 6-12 carbon atoms and are found mostly in butterfat and the tropical oils. Like the short chain fatty acids, these fats have antimicrobial properties; are absorbed directly for quick energy; and contribute to the health of the immune system.
- Long chain fatty acids (LCFAs) have 14-18 carbon atoms[xxxiii] and can be either saturated, monounsaturated or polyunsaturated. Lauric acid, palmitic acid and stearic acid are perhaps the best known examples of saturated long chain fatty acids, with 12, 16 and 18 carbons in their chains respectively. Oleic acid, mentioned above as the well known component of olive oil, is an 18 carbon chain monounsaturated fat. The two essential fats (omega-6 and omega-3) are also long chain, each 18 carbons in length. Another important long chain fatty acid is gamma-linolenic acid (GLA) which has 18 carbons and three double bonds. It is not 'essential', in that the body makes GLA out of omega-6 linoleic acid.
- Very long chain fatty acids (VLCFAs) have 20-24 carbon atoms. They tend to be highly unsaturated, with four, five or six double bonds. Some people can make these fatty acids from EFA's, but others, particularly those whose ancestors ate a lot of fish, lack the enzymes needed to produce them. These 'obligate carnivores' must obtain them from animal foods such as offal, egg yolks, butter and fish oils.

[xxxiii] The debate on categories starts here. Although it is widely agreed that SCFAs have fewer than six carbon atoms and MCFAs have 6-12; LCFAs have been classed as 12 plus carbons and VLCFAs as 22 plus. I follow the guidance of Enig and Fallon Morell and this is what is presented above.

What role does fat play in the human body?

After all the attacks on dietary fat, over the past fifty years, it is important to remind ourselves of the vital role that fat plays in the human body. Fats serve four key purposes:

1) They provide the essential fatty acids (EFA's);
2) They are the carriers of the fat soluble vitamins A, D, E and K;
3) They supply the most concentrated form of energy in our diets;
4) They help make our diets palatable. Food with little or no fat can be quite tasteless and sometimes difficult to digest.

Fats are crucial for every aspect of our wellbeing as they form the membrane (protective wall) that surrounds every cell in our bodies. Excluding water, our brains are approximately 60% fat (lipids in fact, including cholesterol).[219] Fats also play a crucial role in cushioning vital organs, as some people have tragically found out when fat (and lean tissue) has been lost suddenly on a very low calorie diet. Put simply, with the right fats and enough of them our cells are strong, without them they are weak and prone to attack.

Let us look at these four key roles in more detail.

1) Starting with the EFA's, good sources of the essential fats are as follows: omega-6 is provided by meat, eggs, avocado, nuts, whole grains and seeds and their oils (sunflower seeds, rapeseeds and pumpkin seeds as common examples). Omega-3 is found in meat, fish and fish oils – salmon, halibut, shark and swordfish being particularly valuable sources.

   Omega-6 deficiency may cause: growth retardation; eczema-like skin conditions; behavioural disturbances; arthritis-like conditions; liver and kidney degeneration; excessive water loss through the skin accompanied by thirst; drying up of glands; susceptibility to infections; wounds fail to heal; sterility in males; miscarriage in females; heart and circulatory problems; dry skin and hair; dry eyes and hair loss.

   Omega-3 deficiency may cause: growth retardation; dry skin; behavioural disturbances, tingling sensations in arms and legs; weakness; impairment of vision and learning ability; high blood pressure; sticky platelets; tissue inflammation; mental deterioration and low metabolic rate.

   Both lists present a compelling case for ensuring adequate consumption of essential fats.

2) Moving on to the four fat soluble vitamins – A, D, E and K. (We can become blasé about the role of vitamins and minerals in the body. It may be interesting to read the following lists with the mindset – would you personally like to have any, or all, of the following functions impaired and can you be sure that you eat the foods necessary to deliver these vital nutrients?)

- Vitamin A has many functions within the body. It is needed for our sight, cell function, skin, bones, growth, reproduction, blood formation and to fight infection. Vitamin A is particularly important for pregnant women and growing children. Deficiency in vitamin A can lead to: sight conditions generally and night blindness particularly; growth and reproductive impairment; increased susceptibility to infections; and rough, dry, scaly skin. Retinol is the pure form of vitamin A – the form used most easily and readily by the body. This makes for a memorable connection between retinol, the retina of the eye and the role vitamin A plays in sight.

There is much debate as to whether plants can provide adequate vitamin A, or whether it needs to be consumed in an animal product. We can say the following with certainty: a) only animal products contain retinol; b) plant sources of vitamin A come in the form of carotene, which requires conversion within the body into retinol; c) even with Beta-carotene, the carotene most easily converted into retinol, there is substantial loss such that the conversion ratio is at best 6:1 ("The accepted 6:1 equivalency of beta-carotene to preformed vitamin A must be challenged and re-examined in the context of dietary plants");[220] d) not every person is capable of converting carotene to retinol "Diabetics and those with poor thyroid function cannot make the conversion. Children make the conversion very poorly and infants not at all"[221] and e) carotenes are converted by the action of bile salts and very little bile reaches the intestine when a meal is low in fat. Our grandparents put butter on their vegetables for good reason. We can confidently assert, therefore, that animal food generally, and liver particularly, are the best sources of vitamin A.

- Vitamin D is critical for the absorption of calcium and phosphorus. Vitamin D is increasingly being studied in nutritional journals and its possible role in cancer prevention is being explored. Deficiency in vitamin D can lead to tooth decay, muscular weakness and a softening of the bones (rickets), which can cause bone fractures or poor healing of fractures.

Vitamin D is found naturally in oily fish (for example herring, halibut, catfish, salmon, mackerel and sardines) and unnaturally in fortified breakfast cereals. Vegetarians would need to eat 26 medium eggs each day (1,634 calories) to get 10 micrograms of vitamin D – considered an "adequate intake". Mushrooms, which have been exposed to sunlight, are the only conceivable option for vegans. Over two kilograms of such mushrooms would need to be sourced and eaten daily to deliver 10 micrograms of vitamin D. Ideally, but not an option for vegans, these would need to be consumed with butter to make them 'bio-available' to the body.

- Vitamin E is a generic term for a family of fat soluble vitamins active throughout the body. We are learning more about the different forms of vitamin E and more of them are being found to have unique functions. The key role of vitamin E is as an antioxidant. The oxygen that we need to breathe can make molecules overly reactive and this can damage cell structure. This imbalanced situation involving oxygen is called oxidative stress. Vitamin E helps prevent oxidative stress by working together with a group of nutrients (including vitamins B3, C and selenium) to prevent oxygen molecules from becoming too reactive. Vitamin E protects the skin (cells) in much the same way as it protects other cells. We hear little about the possible heart protection role of vitamin E, yet it acts as an anti-blood clotting agent and it maintains healthy blood vessels.

Deficiency in vitamin E can lead to dry skin, poor muscular and circulatory function, damage to red blood cells and blood vessels and an inability of the white blood cells to resist infection.

Vitamin E is found naturally in seeds, nuts and oils that derive from these. Hence, we don't need to eat animal foods to obtain vitamin E, but we do need to consume fats. Sunflower seeds are one of the best sources of vitamin E and they have 51 grams of fat per 100 grams of product.

- Vitamin K has a number of important functions, such as its role in blood clotting and wound healing. Vitamin K is very important for the health of our gut and it is being destroyed with the high modern consumption of anti-biotics, leaving humans prone to imbalance in the gut flora and concomitant illness. Deficiency in vitamin K complicates blood clotting and can manifest itself in nose bleeds, bleeding gums, heavy menstruation or even blood in the urine or stools. A propensity to bruise can also be a sign of vitamin K deficiency.

Vitamin K comes in two forms: K1 and K2. K1 is found in plants, green leafy vegetables particularly, and is also called phylloquinone. Vitamin K2 is found in animal foods. K2 is also known as menaquinone and comes in different forms – MK-4 through to MK-10 (the 'MK' comes from a phonetic abbreviation of MenaKwinone). Meat is a primary source of MK-4. Eggs and calcium rich hard cheese are particularly good sources of MK-7, 8 and 9. The Rotterdam Study[222] concluded: "Intake of menaquinone was inversely related to all-cause mortality and severe aortic calcification. Phylloquinone intake was not related to any of the outcomes. These findings suggest that an adequate intake of menaquinone could be important for CHD prevention." I share this as another example of the animal form of fat soluble vitamins being the most useful – in the context of current public health advice steering us away from these nutritious foods.

Two thoughts come to mind, after reviewing the critical importance of fat from a nutritional perspective. First, how can anyone who *knows* about nutrition put low fat and healthy diet in the same sentence? Secondly, how can anyone who *cares* about nutrition put orlistat in a human body? With this drug, the consumption of fat (soluble vitamins) needs to be restricted and the drug then works to prevent the digestion of approximately one quarter of the fat soluble vitamins that are eaten.[223] We are trying to stop people consuming vital nutrients and then trying to ensure that many consumed are flushed down the toilet. Orlistat has been available on prescription since 1998 (usual dose 120 milligrams). GlaxoSmithKline (GSK) was given a non prescription license for Alli (60 milligrams of orlistat) on 21 January 2009. Their press release said

"The centrally approved marketing authorisation means GSK can now introduce alli for adults with a BMI of 28 kg/m2 or more, in all 27 EU member countries."[224] Alli had already been available in the USA since June 2007 and was launched in the UK in April 2009. As for the conditions of licence, I took a two minute break from writing, to buy 42 Alli capsules for £21.99 from amazon.co.uk. No questions even possible, let alone asked. The tablets arrived within a couple of days. I'm over 18, but my BMI is under 21. I could have bought LIPObind, Bio-synergy CLA, fat blockers, fat binders, carb blockers, metabolism boosters, appetite suppressants – you name it. Where do we draw the line on trying to stop nutrition being absorbed by the human body? Why not avoid the risk of soiled underwear and bed sheets and have doctors issue "A guide to bulimia: How to purge the food that you eat"?

3) The fact that fat supplies the most concentrated form of energy in our diets is used against this macronutrient in today's modern, obese environment. It is argued in our calorie obsessed world that we should avoid fat because of its calorie content. There are two ironies here:

a) Man would not be here today without the energy supplied by fat (predominantly from animals, but also from nuts) during evolution and particularly during the ice age and in regions of the earth where vegetation was not available. At 80-90% water and containing only approximately four calories per gram, humans would simply not have been able to get enough vegetation to survive. (If any ancient berry approximated to, say, a wild strawberry in nutritional content, Neanderthals would have needed over three kilograms of berries to provide 1,000 calories).

b) The second irony is that fat cannot make us fat – only carbohydrate can do this. The glycerol backbone, which turns fat particles into a triglyceride (the form in which adipose tissue is stored), is produced in the presence of glucose and insulin – the environment created following the consumption of carbohydrate.

4) In this carbohydrate consuming/calorie avoiding world, we have lost the awareness of the palatability and unique satiety of fat. 100 grams of a well known brand of cereal, marketed to slimmers, contains rice, wheat (whole wheat, wheat flour), sugar, wheat gluten, defatted wheat germ, dried skimmed milk, salt, barley malt flavouring, and a number of added vitamins to give the product nutritional value. This brand has 76 grams of carbohydrate and 379 calories per 100 grams of product. Most people could eat 100 grams of this with relative ease. (I work with people who commonly binge on cereal). Try to eat 300 grams of "pork chop, boneless, raw lean and fat" – calculated by the USDA database as having slightly fewer calories than the cereal and no carbohydrate content. It will be substantially more filling, and therefore more difficult, to eat the meat than the cereal.

I hope that a short story may help bring the body's need for fat to life. I have a rating system for movie films. I like to be Entertained, Educated and

Emotionally stimulated. The rare film that ticks all three 'E's' in good measure can be a great film. Lorenzo's Oil (1992 Nick Nolte, Susan Sarandon) is a great film. I recommend watching it for all three reasons, but you may understand more about the chemistry of fats after enjoying that film, than you will trying to read biochemistry books.[xxxiv]

It is based on a true story about a boy called Lorenzo who suffered the rare, inherited condition, ALD (Adrenoleukodystrophy), which affects approximately one in 20,000 males (genetically, only boys get the most severe form of the disease). ALD sufferers are missing an essential protein and this protein is needed to carry an enzyme which is used to break down very long chain fatty acids (VLCFAs). ALD progressively attacks the myelin sheath (the 'insulation' around nerves). Without myelin, nerves are not able to conduct an impulse, which leads to increasing disability. Unfortunately the body can not make myelin, so the disorder can only worsen. The condition leads to progressive brain damage, failure of the adrenal glands and death at a young age.

Lorenzo's parents were Augusto and Michaela Odone. As of June 2010, Augusto was still alive and has been awarded an honorary PhD for his work. Michaela died in 2000 – before Lorenzo who died in 2008, a day after his thirtieth birthday. These parents were quite literally remarkable. When told that Lorenzo (then aged six) would not reach his ninth birthday they refused to accept that nothing could be done. They ended up inventing something that became known as Lorenzo's oil. At the simplest level, this oil was a combination of an extract from olive oil and an extract from rapeseed oil.[xxxv] It proved successful in normalising the accumulation of the VLCFAs in the brain, thereby halting the progression of the disease. The oil doesn't cure the condition (there is no Hollywood happy ending), but it did prolong Lorenzo's life and the credits at the end of the film noted that Lorenzo had regained some sight and was learning to use a computer. The credits also showed other young boys, who had been substantially helped by Lorenzo's oil, the results being best in the pre-symptomatic stage where the onslaught of the nerve degeneration can be deferred and slowed, although not avoided completely. Many were teenagers – an age that they had never been expected to reach.

The most interesting message in the film for us is that, once ALD was diagnosed, Lorenzo was put on a virtually fat-free diet by the doctors, but was also advised to avoid some quite unusual foods such as apple skins, spinach, olive oil and peanuts. The doctors said that these were sources of VLCFAs and these should be removed from the diet because Lorenzo would not be able to handle these fats in his food. When Lorenzo was placed on this diet, his blood lipid measurements started to rise. The Odones concluded that the body must be

---

[xxxiv] If you do watch the film, my only criticism is that saturated fat is presented as the 'baddie' and unsaturated fat as the 'goodie'. Lorenzo was far more intelligent – he knew that the "boo-boo" was the 'baddie' and saturated fat is just saturated fat.

[xxxv] Oleic acid (unsaturated C18) was the long chain fatty acid part of the oil and erucic acid (unsaturated C22) was the very long chain fatty acid part of the oil. The former from olive oil, the latter from rapeseed oil.

making fat in the absence of fat being ingested and so started their quest to see if there could be a fat that Lorenzo could ingest that would not make things worse and would stop his body effectively producing its own fat. That they even thought of this as an idea is a credit to them, that they actually worked out the chemistry for what such a substance needed to be is a triumph. The final hurdle was perhaps the most difficult – they approached a hundred companies before an elderly British chemist took on the project, working for Croda International. Lorenzo's oil then became available – that was the happy ending.

We know that carbohydrate (via insulin) facilitates the storage of fat. We know that stored carbohydrate, glycogen, is turned into fat if not needed by the body within approximately 24 hours. The story of Lorenzo should inspire scientists to investigate further the biochemical response to very low-fat diets. There are plenty of low-fat consumers to study in the world of dieting.

It is interesting to search for a daily requirement figure for fat. You will find maximum guidelines – not minimum. There appears to be no minimum set, and yet we have just summarised the many different and vital roles played by fat within the human body. The maximum daily guidelines for the USA are not to exceed 20-35% of calories from all fat and to consume less than 10% from saturated fat. For the UK, the government instructions are not to have more than 35% of total calories in the form of fat and not to exceed 11% for saturated fat. Presumably both governments would be happy if USA and UK citizens consumed no animal products or nuts whatsoever (real sources of saturated fat)? These are nature's staple real foods for human beings and the sources of energy that sustained the population until today. Many people, women particularly, are living on virtually fat-free diets and this cannot be healthy and must deny them access to this critically important macronutrient.

What is the government position on fat?

We have covered the history of the damnation of fat at length, so we will just recap here the current government position on fat:

- "Eating a diet high in saturated fat can raise the level of cholesterol in your blood. This increases your chance of developing heart disease." (UK Food Standards Agency – FSA).[225]
- "Eating a lot of saturated fat can increase the cholesterol in your blood. High levels of cholesterol can increase your risk of: a heart attack, stroke, and narrowed arteries (atherosclerosis). Cholesterol is a type of fat that your liver makes from the fatty food that you eat." (UK National Health Service – NHS).[226]
- "High intake of saturated fats, trans fats, and cholesterol increases the risk of unhealthy blood lipid levels, which, in turn, may increase the risk of coronary heart disease." (*Dietary Guidelines for Americans* 2005).[227]
- "Saturated fats increase the risk of cardiovascular disease by raising the 'bad' cholesterol in your blood." (Australian Government "Measure Up campaign").[228]

These are bold statements, when the study to review these assertions has not even been done.

Turning now to monounsaturated fat, as we saw in Chapter Eight, a 2009 systematic review of the relationship between monounsaturated fat (MUFA) and coronary heart disease (CHD) concluded: "MUFA intake was not associated with CHD". Yet, the UK National Health Service tells us: "Monounsaturated fats can lower bad cholesterol, while maintaining good cholesterol. Polyunsaturated fats reduce total cholesterol."[229]

In the 2005 *Dietary Guidelines for Americans*, no such claims are made for monounsaturated and/or polyunsaturated fat. The only references made to these fats are in the context of "Keep total fat intake between 20 to 35 percent of calories, with most fats coming from sources of polyunsaturated and monounsaturated fatty acids."[230]

Hopefully, by now, you are starting to read government statements on saturated and unsaturated fat (and cholesterol) with far more critical evaluation and seeing the errors, inconsistencies and misleading information endemic in our public health advice.

Let us have a common sense check at this point. Anyone who knows the macronutrient composition of meat would laugh out loud at the absurdity of thinking that saturated fat is trying to cause heart disease while monounsaturated fat is simultaneously trying to protect against it. I cannot find one meat on the planet with more saturated than *unsaturated* fat. Surely no sensible person can really believe that, of the small part of their steak that is fat, 45% of this is trying to kill them and 51% is trying to save them – no doubt helped by the 4% polyunsaturated fat backup?[231] The fat in "goose, domesticated, meat and skin, raw" is 57% monounsaturated, 31% saturated and 12% polyunsaturated. This has 34 grams of fat per 100 grams, so is a much better source of fat overall than steak, which can be as low as 7% fat.[232]

Then chicken breast (the white meat we are told to eat more of) has identical proportions of saturated, monounsaturated and polyunsaturated fat (33% of each), so how can we eat this and increase our intake of monounsaturated fat while simultaneously decreasing our intake of saturated fat. Did you know that lentils have equal proportions of saturated and monounsaturated fat? (Albeit in a very small total fat content).

Nature puts macronutrients, let alone fat, in real foods in quite an interesting way. Protein is in virtually everything from lettuce to lamb. Other foods then tend to fall into 'things from faces' which are fat/proteins or 'things from trees and the ground', which are carbohydrate/proteins. The former group comprises zero carbohydrate foods (meat, fish), virtually zero carbohydrate foods (eggs) and low carbohydrate foods (dairy products). The latter group includes fruit, vegetables and whole grains (remember this is all about real food as nature delivers it, not processed food as manufacturers deliver it). Rarely does nature put all three macronutrients in good measure in a food (nuts, whole milk and avocados being three notable exceptions).

170

Nature puts fat in real foods in a similarly interesting way. In 100 grams of pork chop (USDA reference – pork chop, boneless, raw, lean and fat), there is no carbohydrate, 21 grams of protein and 4.2 grams of fat. The rest is water (75%). Of the 4.2 grams of fat, 1.5 grams are saturated and 2.7 grams are unsaturated. The (very small) part of this pork chop that is fat is 47% monounsaturated fat, 40% saturated and 13% polyunsaturated fat. If dietitians know this, why are they not telling us? Dare I suggest that it doesn't fit with the advice 'don't have bacon for breakfast – have a (Kellogg's) (sugary) cereal instead'?

We are told to eat oily fish – mackerel is one of the oiliest fishes and, of the 14 grams of fat per 100 grams of mackerel (much higher in fat overall than the common meats, pork and beef), 45% is monounsaturated and 27% is saturated (the rest is polyunsaturated fat, which is high in fish generally). So, 100 grams of the oily fish we are supposed to eat has more saturated fat than beef or pork. Olives have a similar level of saturated fat to the beef example above. For the finale, olive oil (the alleged reason why Mediterraneans have the healthiest diet on the planet) has 13.8 grams of saturated fat per 100 grams. So, olive oil has nine times the saturated fat level of our pork chop, lean and fat, above.

There was an advert on UK television in 2009 made by the Food Standards Agency. The advert showed a jug of, what can only be described as, gunge being taken out of a fridge and poured down the plug hole in a kitchen sink and getting stuck in the U-Bend of the drainage system. The advert had the deep voice-over, designed to scare the life out of you, saying: "Certain foods are high in saturated fat. This is the average amount of saturated fat a person consumes in a month. If you eat too much of this, then, over time fatty deposits could build up in your arteries and this increases your risk of heart disease. If saturated fat can clog this pipe, imagine what it's doing to yours."[233]

Where do I start on how outrageous and erroneous this advert is? (I complained to the Advertising Standards Authority, but I didn't see the advert early enough and I was 'out of time' for a valid complaint to be investigated). First of all, we eat food, we don't intravenously inject it. The visual implication that we are pouring gunge directly into our arteries is ridiculous and ignorant and it is deeply troubling that the UK Food Standards Agency appears to have no understanding of the human digestive system. Secondly, saturated fat is solid at room temperature, let alone at fridge temperature, so there is no way it could be poured down a sink, as the advert manages to achieve. You would struggle to get solidified (saturated) fat down the plug hole, even scraping and pushing with a knife – as we all did in student days, before we owned our own homes. Thirdly, there is no pump or even gravity in a U-Bend. Sinks do block – plumbers make a living from such inconveniences, but not only do we not inject food into our arteries, there is a pump mechanism around the body (the heart, blood and circulatory system) to ensure regular movement of nutrients in our blood stream to all parts of the body.

Let us see what does happen when we eat pure fat. Examples of pure fat are oils – olive oil, sunflower oil, coconut oil etc – all other foods that contain fat also have protein. Let us assume that we have just consumed some coconut oil – this has the highest saturated fat content of any food, at 92%, so this will serve as a good approximation to saturated fat. (The remainder of coconut oil is unsaturated fat – mono and poly). The oil passes from our mouth very quickly into the pharynx (the part of the throat that goes from behind the nose to the start of the oesophagus) and then into the oesophagus (the muscular tube through which food travels from the mouth to the stomach). From there it goes into the stomach (the main area for food 'short-term' storage and digestion of protein and carbohydrate). Fat is not digested until it passes from the stomach into the small intestine (where almost all nutrients are absorbed) and, from there, it passes into the large intestine (the main function of which is to transport waste out of the body and to absorb water from the waste before it leaves). So, our coconut oil has quite a journey through our digestive system and we haven't yet started to describe how it can go anywhere near our arteries.

In Chapter Eight we learned that chylomicrons are formed in the intestine, as a result of digestion, and chylomicrons are the transport mechanism for taking dietary fat (and cholesterol) from the digestive system into the blood stream and from there to the different parts of the body to do their vital work. As any young biology student will know, arteries pump blood around the body from the heart. There is no artery to take dietary fat away from the intestines.

The chain length of fatty acids determines how they are transported out of the digestive system. If a fatty acid has fewer than 12 carbon atoms, it will "probably travel through the portal vein that connects directly to the liver. If the fatty acid is a more typical long-chain variety, it must be reformed into a triglyceride and enter circulation via the lymphatic system."[234]

Coconut oil has eight saturated fats, a monounsaturated fat and a polyunsaturated fat.[235] The main saturated fats are lauric, myristic and palmitic fatty acids, with 12, 14 and 16 carbons in their respective chains. Three of the saturated fatty acids in coconut oil have fewer than 12 carbon atoms, so they go in the portal vein to the liver. (The liver is the body's main metabolic organ and it prepares absorbed nutrients for use by the rest of the body. The liver plays a critical role as gatekeeper to the body and it gets the first chance to detoxify any harmful bodies that could threaten any other vital organs – not that anything in real food is harmful in normal circumstances). The five longer chain saturated fats and the unsaturated fats are packaged into chylomicrons, released into the lymphatic system and they glide from there into the blood stream.

So, our coconut oil has not been injected into our arteries. It has not gone into any arteries through any less invasive route. It has gone on a normal digestive process journey, probably taking a few hours for fat, still without going into an artery. Yet, the vast majority of UK citizens, thanks to the irresponsibility of the Food Standards Agency now have a vision in their heads that eating any dietary fat is going to clog up their arteries.

Here is another thought: if a juggernaut were travelling round a country's transport system – which roads would clog up first? The minor roads – the country lanes would actually be impassable. The motorways would continue to run freely if a large vehicle were moving along one lane. So where is the logic that says fat travelling round the blood stream (and remember it is not freely travelling around the blood stream – it is in the lipoprotein 'taxis') will clog up the arteries and only the arteries? Veins never clog and yet surely they would clog first, not least the portal vein, if fat did block the blood stream in the way that the FSA would have us believe.

Finally, the FSA does not appear to have read the journals that I have, where the composition of aortic plaques has been examined. (The aorta is the largest artery in the body and not one we want to get blocked up). Writing in *The Lancet* in 1994,[236] Felton et al compared the fatty-acid composition of aortic plaques with serum (clear blood separated from blood clots) and human fat tissue samples from post-mortems. The blood and tissue samples reflected dietary intake. Their conclusions were as follows: "Positive associations were found between serum and plaque omega 6 (r = 0.75) and omega 3 (r = 0.93) polyunsaturated fatty acids, and monounsaturates (r = 0.70), and also between adipose tissue and plaque omega 6 polyunsaturated fatty acids (r = 0.89). No associations were found with saturated fatty acids. These findings imply a direct influence of dietary polyunsaturated fatty acids on aortic plaque formation and suggest that current trends favouring increased intake of polyunsaturated fatty acids should be reconsidered."

Ewa Stachowska et al writing in the *European Journal of Nutrition* in October 2004 obtained atheromatous plaques from 31 patients who underwent surgery due to atherosclerotic narrowing of the arteries.[237] Fatty acids were extracted and the conclusion was as follows: "We found spatial and positional isomers of sixteen- and eighteen-carbon fatty acids in plaques and adipose tissue, with elaidic acid (C18:1 trans-9) being the most abundant. Every plaque and adipose tissue sample contained linolelaidic acid (C18:2 trans-9 trans-12) which is derived exclusively from linoleic acid, as well as conjugated dienes of linoleic acid (CLA) produced during oxidative processes." In lay speak, this means – the most common fat we found in the plaques was elaidic acid – that's a trans fat. Every plaque sample contained linolelaidic acid – that's a trans polyunsaturated fat. No mention of saturated fat whatsoever.

Rats, fats and carbohydrate

We saw in Chapter Eight that Keys noted the significant correlation between the incidence of coronary heart disease and the average percentage of calories from sucrose in the diets – proof that he had been studying processed food (assuming that he had not been studying avocados). The logic analysis in this chapter proved that there was no way in which we could explain the observed incidence of high fat intake and high heart disease (USA), low fat intake and low heart disease (Japan), but also high fat intake and low heart disease (France) and low fat intake and high heart disease (Georgia). This could not be explained directly and it could not be explained through cholesterol *per se* or through cholesterol acting as a 'flip' switch in some way. However, if Keys had *not* confused saturated fat with processed food, there could be a consistent explanation for all of these observations.

The USA has probably the highest world intake of processed food; France and Japan have a very low intake of processed food. Georgia, although low in processed food, has carbohydrate consumption at the level you would expect for a low Gross Domestic Product (GDP) per capita nation. The two national dishes in Georgia are "Khachapuri" (cheese filled bread more like a cheese pie) and "khinkali" (spiced meat in a dumpling) "served in enormous quantities". The Georgian travel guide notes "Georgian men will down 15 huge dumplings like it's no big deal."[238] The presence of processed food/starchy carbohydrate in the USA and Georgia and the absence of such foods in the diets of France and Japan could, therefore, provide a consistent association for heart disease in all of these countries. 55% of Georgian men smoke,[239] so we should be cautious about causation.

Without knowing the national diets of the 14 countries involved in the two alternative Seven Country Studies done by Kendrick, we can note that the seven countries with the *highest* saturated fat intake and *lowest* levels of heart disease are all in the top 20 GPD countries per capita[240] – Switzerland highest at number four and Iceland the lowest at number 19. In contrast, the seven countries with the *lowest* saturated fat intake and the *highest* levels of heart disease were at an average (arithmetic mean) position of 101 in the world table – with Croatia the highest at 43 and Tajikistan the lowest at 149. The USA seems to be an exception, positioned nine in the world per capita GDP ranking, but making poor food choices. Japan is ranked 17 and has historically made good food choices, but is increasingly being infiltrated by western food and western girth.

The correlation with income is interesting *per se* (and could provide a plausible rationale for heart disease). However, I am sharing this to make the point that we have failed to separate macronutrients and it is not the presence of fat, but the presence, or absence, of carbohydrate, which can provide far more insight into epidemiological differences. The tragedy is then that avoidance of fat increases consumption of carbohydrate, as a proportion of the diet, and the desire of one man to prove what he set out to prove has resulted in hundreds of millions of people worldwide eating the exact opposite of what they should be eating.

You would think that we had moved on, from limiting our search for the suspect in heart disease to fat, as Keys was working in the 1950's. You would think that we had made the connection between the extraordinary and unprecedented amount of processed food and carbohydrate that we are eating (not least because we are following the advice and doing what we are told). You would think that we would *not* do another experiment without looking at both the absence and presence of fat and carbohydrate, or, better still the absence and presence of real and processed foods.

Sadly we have done no such thing. In August 2009 UK newspapers covered the story "Junk Food Dummies: How bingeing on burgers and chips can drain your brain power."[241] This was the media interpretation of a British Heart

Foundation funded study led by Andrew Murray at the University of Oxford.[242] Murray et al did some invasive tests on 42 rats. They were all fed a standard rat chow for up to two months. This had a composition of 7.5% "oil"; 17.5% protein and 75% carbohydrate and was 3.3 calories per gram. For nine days 21 rats were continued on this feed and the other 21 were put on a "high-fat" chow with a composition of 55% "oil"; 29% protein and 16% carbohydrate and was 5.1 calories per gram. The ratio of the first oil was 19 saturated: 18 monounsaturated: 62 polyunsaturated. The ratio of the second oil was 27 saturated: 48 monounsaturated: 25 polyunsaturated.

The conclusion was "Our study demonstrates clear detrimental effects of a high-fat diet on both endurance exercise performance and cognitive function in rats over just 9 d of feeding." But four things changed:

1) The diet – the first group of rats had no 'shock to the system' with a complete change in food intake;
2) The calorie intake – the article acknowledged that "the daily calorie intake of the high-fat-fed rats was 51% greater than their chow-fed counterparts";
3) The macronutrient composition changed dramatically; and
4) The type of fat changed dramatically. If I ate 51% more than I usually do for nine days (this is called the 'festive season' in real life) I would feel dreadful and substantially less capable of doing normal mental or physical activity. The average human being falls asleep after a 'Sunday lunch', let alone a nine day binge.

This was not a control experiment. The diet should have been varied as little as possible, but for the factor to be reviewed. Calories should have been held constant. If total fat were to be the thing measured then the type of fat should have been held constant and only total fat varied (and carbohydrate or protein kept constant). This would then facilitate observation of the impact of a swap of one macronutrient for another and the reduction of one as well as the increase of the other would need to be analysed. (By the way, the sedentary rats on the high-fat chow beat the sedentary ones on the normal chow on the cognitive test for completion time, so not even the conclusions were universal).

At a conference organised by the Association for the Study of Obesity in Cardiff, on 8 June 2010, called *Physical Activity, Obesity and Health*, Dr. Jason Gill gave a very interesting presentation on "Exercise, obesity and postprandial metabolism". While talking about fat in food, the pictures on the slide behind were of cola, burgers and fries – processed food and primarily carbohydrates. Gill referred to a study in The *Journal of the American Heart Association* where Merrill et al allegedly tested lipids after a high-fat meal.[243] The study subjects were fed "a high-fat breakfast purchased from McDonald's restaurant consisting of approximately two sausage McMuffins with eggs, one order of hash brown potatoes, and a glass of ice water." As soon as you know the food consumed, the conclusions are meaningless. This might tell us something about McDonald's food, it might tell us something about processed food, it might tell us something about hash browns and McMuffins, but it tells us nothing about real fat or real saturated fat.

The assumption that processed food, primarily carbohydrate, is a euphemism for saturated fat has been endemic for decades and our governments continue to perpetuate this fundamental error today.

How governments have confused fat and carbohydrate

The following table contains a full list of what the UK Food Standards Agency and the UK National Health Service list as sources of saturated fat. (I have changed the order to align items on the two lists. I have not changed the words).

Table 17: The UK Food Standards Agency and National Health Service lists of sources of saturated fats.[244]

	FSA	NHS
A	Fatty cuts of meat and meat products such as sausages and pies	Fatty meats and meat products, such as sausages and pies
B	Butter, ghee and lard	Butter, lard and ghee (oil made from butter)
C	Cream, soured cream, crème fraîche and ice cream	Cream, soured cream, crème fraîche and ice cream; full fat milk[xxxvi]
D	Cheese, particularly hard cheese	Cheese, particularly hard cheese
E	Pastries, cakes and biscuits	Biscuits, cakes and pastries
F	Some savoury snacks	Some savoury snacks, such as crisps
G	Some sweet snacks and chocolate	Sweets and chocolate
H	Coconut oil, coconut cream and palm oil	Coconut oil, coconut cream and palm oil

The *Dietary Guidelines for Americans* 2005 list: ice cream; sherbet; frozen yogurt; cakes; cookies; quick breads; doughnuts; margarine; sausages; potato chips; corn chips; popcorn and yeast bread as major sources of saturated fats. The Australian Government "Measure Up campaign" lists fatty processed meats and baked cereal based foods such as cakes, pastries and biscuits as sources of saturated fat, so this is not only a UK error.

[xxxvi] There is only one difference between the two lists – full fat milk is on the NHS list, but not the FSA list. Such language is misleading – "full fat" milk is still only 3.5% fat.

To determine the composition of example foods from the FSA and NHS lists of sources of saturated fat, I bought some products, which I would not normally touch, and analysed the ingredients and 'nutritional' information on the labels. For the nutritional information about real food I used the USDA database.[245] First, I will list the ingredients, then summarise the macronutrient composition of all products in a table and finally draw some conclusions. All ingredients are listed in descending order by weight:

A) Meat and meat products

I have included three products in this category. The products and ingredients are as follows:

- A sample pork chop: pork.
- A sample pork pie (branded): wheat flour, pork (24%), pork lard, water, pork fat, rusk (wheat flour, salt), salt, potato starch, pork gelatine, wheat starch, pepper, milk protein, yeast extract, sugar, dextrose, egg.
- A sample sausage & onion lattice (own label): pork (31%), wheat flour, vegetable oil, water, onion (5%), pork fat, potato starch, salt, yeast extract, sage, milk proteins, yeast, pepper, colour (plain caramel), glucose syrup, sage extract, black pepper extract, mace extract, nutmeg extract.

B) Butter, Ghee and Lard

As ghee is made from butter (and is very rarely used), I have included just butter and lard in this category. Butter contains butter and lard contains lard (pig fat in essence). Both are real foods and therefore contain no processed ingredients in their natural form.

C) Cream products and ice cream

I have included two products in this category: a sample carton of (own label) cream (fluid, heavy, whipping cream) and (own label) ice cream. The cream has the single ingredient cream. The ingredients for the sample vanilla ice cream are as follows: water, reconstituted dried skimmed milk, sugar, vegetable fat, buttermilk powder, dextrose, emulsifier (mono and di-glycerides of fatty acids), stabilisers (guar gum, sodium alginate), colour (annatto), natural flavouring, vanilla pods.

D) Cheese

I analysed two hard cheeses in this category, as these are the cheeses that we are particularly advised, by the FSA and NHS, to avoid: a sample own label ementaal contains cheese made from unpasteurised milk. A sample branded mature cheddar contains cheese.

E) Pastries, cakes and biscuits

I have included two products in this category: a (own label) pastry/cake and a (branded) biscuit. The ingredients are as follows:

- A sample chocolate éclair (own label) contains: stabilised whipped cream – whipping cream, dextrose, stabiliser (sodium alginate); choux pastry Éclair case – egg, wheat flour, vegetable oil, salt; chocolate fondant – sugar, milk chocolate (sugar, cocoa butter, milk solids, cocoa mass, whey powder, emulsifier (soya lethicins), flavouring), plain chocolate (coca mass, sugar, cocoa butter, cocoa powder, emulsifier (soya lethicins), flavouring), water, dried glucose syrup, vegetable oil).
- A sample packet of milk chocolate digestives (branded) contains: wheat flour (39%), milk chocolate (29%) [sugar, cocoa butter, cocoa mass, dried skimmed milk, dried whey, butter oil, vegetable fat, emulsifiers, (soya lethicin, E476), natural vanilla flavouring], vegetable oil, wholemeal (9%), sugar, glucose-fructose syrup, raising agents (sodium bicarbonate, tartaric acid, malic acid), salt.

F) Savoury snacks

I have included two products in this category: a (branded) crisp and a (own label) savoury snack. The ingredients are as follows:

- A sample tube of salt & vinegar crisps (branded) contains: dehydrated potatoes, vegetable oil, corn flour; salt and vinegar flavour (barley malt vinegar flavouring, lactose, acidity regulators, sodium diacetate, tridsodium citrate, malic acid), wheat starch, maltodextrin; emulsifier: E471, salt, rice flour, dextrose.
- A sample packet of cheese savouries (own label) contains: wheat flour, vegetable oil, cheese powder (10%), sunflower oil, yeast autolysate, sugar, glucose syrup, malted barley extract, raising agents (ammonium bicarbonate sodium bicarbonate), salt, whey powder, lactic acid, natural flavouring, pepper, cayenne pepper. Our governments advise us to favour carbohydrate and unsaturated fat. Presumably this product would meet approval, containing 50% carbohydrate and nearly 20% unsaturated fat (Table 19).

G) Sweet snacks and chocolate

I have included two products in this category: a (own label) snack bar and a (branded) milk chocolate bar. The ingredients are as follows:

- A sample chocolate chip chewy & crisp bar (own label) contains: glucose syrup, oat flakes, crisped rice (which contains rice flour, wheat flour, sugar, malted wheat flour, malted barley flour, vegetable oil, emulsifier – soya lethicins, anti-caking agent – calcium carbonate), peanuts, dark chocolate (7%) (which contains cocoa mass, sugar, emulsifier – soya lethicins, cocoa butter), vegetable oil, cornflakes (which contain maize, sugar, salt, barley malt extract, emulsifier – mono and di-glycerides of fatty acids), sweetened condensed skimmed milk (which contains skimmed milk, sugar), sugar, dextrose (which is another sugar), peanut paste, dark couverture chocolate (which contains cocoa mass, sugar, fat reduced cocoa powder, emulsifier – soya lethicins), glycerol, caramelised milk powder (which contains whey, butter, maltodextrin, sugar, skimmed milk) and anhydrous milk fat. (Pause for a moment to wonder just how so much rubbish can go into a 122 calorie snack bar).

- A sample milk chocolate (branded) contains: sugar, cocoa ingredients (cocoa butter, cocoa mass), skimmed milk powder, milk fat, lactose, whey powder, vegetable fat, emulsifiers (soy lethicin, E442), natural vanilla extract.

H) Coconut oil

Coconuts and their oils hardly deserve a mention in a table of food intake for the UK, or indeed the USA. World per capita consumption of coconuts is approximately 0.6 pound per person per year.[246] The average coconut weighs about five pounds, so that's about 12% of one coconut per person per year. Given that the people of Sri Lanka consume an average of 120 coconuts per person per year, one country is hugely distorting the figures by consuming 1,000 times the average. UK consumption of coconuts is negligible. You will rarely even find them in supermarkets. The coconut is interesting as a food because it has the highest saturated fat content of any product on the planet. Even more interesting is the fact that in Sri Lanka, the country with the highest consumption of the product with the highest saturated fat content, one or two deaths per 1,000 are attributed to heart disease, as compared to the one in two or three deaths in the UK and USA.[247]

The following tables provide a summary of the products detailed above. They have been separated into a table containing real food and one containing processed food. All data is based on 100 grams of product and all amounts for each macronutrient are in grams. The main macronutrient in each product is in bold. The main fat (saturated or unsaturated) is in bold.[xxxvii]

[xxxvii] Where the macronutrients – protein, fat and carbohydrate – do not add up to 100 grams, the remainder is water.

Table 18: Macronutrient composition of the *real* foods:

Product	Protein	Carb	Fat	Saturated	Unsaturated
A) Pork	**21**	0	3.8	1.5	**2.3**
B) Butter	Trace	0	**75**	**51**	24
B) Lard	0	0	**100**	40	**60**
C) Cream	2	3	**37**	**23**	14
D) Ementaal	**29**	0	**29**	**20.5**	8.5
D) Cheddar	25.4	0.1	**32.2**	**21.7**	10.5
H) Coconut oil	0	0	**100**	92	8

Table 19: Macronutrient composition of the *processed* foods:

Product	Protein	Carb	Fat	Saturated	Unsaturated
A) Pork pie	8.8	24.6	**30.6**	12.5	**18.1**
A) Sausage & onion lattice	8.7	20.3	**27.7**	12.3	**15.4**
C) Ice cream	3	**22.9**	10.1	**8.4**	1.7
E) Éclairs	6.7	**31.2**	28.1	13.4	**14.7**
E) Biscuits	6.7	**62.7**	23.4	**12.1**	11.3
F) Crisps	3.9	**50.0**	34.0	10.0	**24.0**
F) Savoury snacks	11.1	**49.8**	30.8	12.0	**18.8**
G) Chewy bars	7.0	**65.0**	18.4	7.7	**10.7**
G) Chocolate	6.6	**56.3**	32.5	**19.3**	13.2

My observations are as follows:

- There is a single ingredient in each real food – pork, butter, lard, cream, cheese, coconut oil. The list of ingredients in the processed foods is, frankly, horrific.
- I agree 100% that people should avoid every product in the processed food table. I disagree 100% that people should avoid any product in the real food table.
- Looking just at the processed foods listed by the FSA and NHS, other than the processed meat products, which do have fat as the main macronutrient,

all the other products are *not* primarily fat – they are carbohydrate. The real foods, in contrast, are either zero carbohydrate or virtually carbohydrate-free.
- The primary fat in the products in the table (real or processed) is *unsaturated* fat (mainly monounsaturated, some polyunsaturated), as often as it is saturated fat.

I suggested in Chapter Eight that we may have the makings of a heated agreement. May I suggest the following?

1) Public health advisors tell us to limit consumption of the following items and I would say cut out these processed foods all together:

A) Meat products, such as sausages and pies;
C) Ice cream;
E) Pastries, cakes and biscuits;
F) Some savoury snacks (I would advise all);
G) Some sweet snacks and chocolate (I would advise all, other than 85-100% cocoa content chocolate).

What we must do, however, is to stop calling these products saturated fats. The main macronutrient in the meat products analysed above is fat (primarily unsaturated fat), followed by carbohydrate and with protein a long way behind. Ice cream and the entire categories E, F and G are all primarily carbohydrates. The main fat in foods in categories E, F and G is invariably unsaturated fat. We can agree that they should be avoided/cut out altogether, but we need to advise this for the right reason. If there is any real meat, real egg, real milk etc in any of the above products, it will be the healthiest part of the product by some margin.

For hundreds of thousands of years we have eaten only real food with a single ingredient and probably only one or two foods at a time. With modern processed foods, we are hitting our bodies with multiples of unnatural ingredients at a time and this cannot be good for our health or biochemistry.

2) Surely we can agree that we need to stop calling real meat saturated fat. It is primarily water. Of the bit (approximately 25%) that it is not water, the protein and fat content varies between different types of meat (there is no carbohydrate content). The USDA composition for a cut of lamb (domestic, leg, sirloin half, separable lean and fat, trimmed to 1/4" fat, choice, raw), for example, is 27% protein and 73% fat, of which 53% is *unsaturated*. Meat is mainly unsaturated fat, not saturated fat – not that one type of real fat is better or worse than another. There is no justification whatsoever for our continued onslaught on meat. Meat is an excellent source of vitamins and minerals and human beings are unnecessarily missing out on the most nutritious food group on earth, as a result of misleading advice from our governments.

3) Consumption of coconuts and coconut oil in the overweight 'developed' world is so insignificant that it ridicules the FSA and NHS lists by being

included. If UK consumption of coconuts even reaches the 0.6 pounds per capita per year a) I would be surprised and b) this would be swamped by the 83 pounds of sugar that the average UK citizen consumes each year – or the staggering 124 pounds consumed by the average Australian.[248]

4) This leaves real dairy products as the only area for debate. Lard should be grouped with meat (it is pig fat), not with butter and ghee in category B.

In category C, real cream, soured cream and crème fraîche need to be separated from ice cream and any processed versions of cream and crème fraîche. The latter are processed foods – to be avoided for that reason. Cream and their variants (crème fraîche etc) and ice cream do contain more saturated fat than unsaturated fat, but the ratio is substantially higher with the processed food. Ice cream has five times the saturated fat to unsaturated fat ratio whereas cream has a ratio of less than two to one. Again, this is not to say that either saturated or unsaturated fat are better or worse than the other, but rather to make the point that nature puts different fats in foods in the 'right' balance. Food manufacturers have artificially decided what the ratio should be – more likely determined by cost, taste, look and feel and so on.

Real cheese in category D should similarly be distinguished from manufactured cheese (especially common in children's food – stringy cheese sticks for example).

I do *not* consider it reasonable for public health bodies to dictate that people should avoid whole dairy foods and/or advise people to eat low-fat dairy foods, without issuing an accompanying warning of what the consumer stands to lose by doing this. Dairy products are highly nutritious and they are excellent sources of protein and the fat soluble vitamins, A and D particularly, and this means they need to be delivered in fat to be absorbed by the body. How sensible of nature to put fat soluble vitamins in fat and how stupid of humans to remove the fat and thereby the delivery mechanism. Hard cheese is also a particularly good source of calcium, which can be a difficult mineral to consume in sufficient quantities in our diet.

Public health advice favouring manufactured spreads over nature's butter also makes no sense. Margarine is an unnatural product to which we have had little time, in evolutionary terms, to adapt to. Margarine was in fact banned in Canada until 1948. Legislation was introduced in 1940 to mandate the fortification of margarine to make it 'comparable' in nutrition to the butter that was rationed during the war. The addition of vitamins A and D to margarine remains mandatory in the UK, Belgium and Sweden. Fortification is voluntary in the Netherlands and voluntary for spreads in the UK.[249] Butter needs no such nutritional legislation. Butter's inherent stability (all the carbon links being naturally saturated with hydrogen), also makes it safer for cooking.

The National Food survey tells us that UK citizens eat 40 grams of butter, on average, per person per week.[250] This compares with 1,423 grams of flour[251] and 731 grams of sugar.[252] I think that we should worry far more about the empty sugar and nutritionally lacking flour calories that we consume, than we do our tiny butter consumption. I said as much to a biochemist whose help I was seeking to understand lipid metabolism. Unfortunately he was so believing of the 'fat is bad' hypothesis that, his response to this butter statistic was "it only takes a drop of arsenic to kill you." Butter and arsenic in the same sentence – there have been many days when I have wondered if I have any chance of trying to overcome sixty years of propaganda.

The ultimate irony is that an entire industry, worth five billion dollars in the USA (2008) alone,[255] has been built on destroying the reputation of butter and then trying to reproduce the substance. Butter is mostly saturated fat, naturally solid at room temperature and it has a natural colour. The first part of the imitation process is to take liquid oils, usually cheap and low quality vegetable oils, and then turn them into solid fats in some way. Hydrogenation is one way, increasingly less acceptable nowadays but still done. In this process the oils are heated and pressurised and hydrogen gas is added, along with a catalyst, like nickel, to produce the chemical reaction. This helps the oils to 'accept' the hydrogen atoms that they have been 'longing for'. Of course, the hydrogen atoms don't end up exactly where they 'should'. Some end up on the wrong side of the structure and you end up not with a saturated fat, but with a completely new fat completely alien to the body. (Do I think that putting alien chemicals into the human body can cause heart disease, cancer and all sorts of harm? I think that I would be naive *not* to think this).

The substance at the end of this process is grey, smelly and lumpy, so it is bleached, deodorised and emulsifiers are added to smooth things over. The mandatory vitamins are added in at this stage because none could have survived that process. Finally, the stuff needs some colour to make it look edible, so, of course, the preferred colour is butter colour. (Canada retained the strongest legislative position on *not* allowing butter colour to be used. As recently as July 2008 Quebec became the last Canadian province to repeal its law that margarine should be colourless).[254]

The processed spread is much cheaper, despite all the industrial operations needed. Real butter needs to come from a real animal and the best butter is hand churned. Checking my on line grocery store today, the cheapest butter that I can buy is nearly three times the price of the cheapest spread. The butter is sold in 250 gram packets. The spreads are sold in 500 gram, or one kilogram, tubs.

To conclude the 'how to imitate butter' process, you need a health claim, a name and a marketing campaign. The health claim can be two fold: a) this is *not* a bad saturated fat (tell them what you are not – don't tell them what you are); and b) some spreads add plant stanol esters and then 'sell' cholesterol lowering 'benefit'.[xxxviii] The name and the marketing campaign go hand in hand. While welcoming any attack on saturated fat generally, and butter particularly, the spread companies launch products called "Utterly Butterly", "Butter me up",

---

[xxxviii] If you don't have familial hypercholesterolemia and, for some reason I know not, want to lower your cholesterol, you can buy tablets containing plant stanol esters – you don't need to consume spreads.

"Butterlicious", "You'll Mutter It's Butter", "Don't Flutter with Butter", "You'd Butter Believe", "You'll Never Believe It, Believe It or Not", all spawned from the original "I can't believe it's not butter."[255]

You just couldn't make this up.

Chapter Thirteen

"Base your meals on starchy foods"

What are carbohydrates?

Carbohydrates are organic molecules in which carbon, hydrogen and oxygen are bonded together in the ratio $C_x(H_2O)_y$, where x and y are whole numbers that differ for different carbohydrates. The body will break down carbohydrates into their simplest form, which is carbon, hydrogen and oxygen in the ratio of 1:2:1 respectively. Carbohydrates are broken down during the process of metabolism to release energy. Carbohydrates are divided into three categories: monosaccharides; disaccharides and polysaccharides (saccharide derives from a Greek word meaning sugar).

1) Monosaccharides are also known as simple sugars and they contain one molecule (hence the pre-fix 'mono'). They include:

- Glucose (found naturally in fruit and grains);
- Fructose (found naturally in fruit);
- Galactose (found naturally in milk).

   The chemical formula for each of these is $C_6H_{12}O_6$.

2) Disaccharides are composed of two monosaccharides i.e. two simple sugar molecules (hence the pre-fix 'di'). Examples include:

- Sucrose (one molecule of glucose and one of fructose) – what we know as table sugar;
- Lactose (one molecule of glucose and one of galactose) – what we know as milk sugar;
- Maltose (two molecules of glucose) – less familiarly known as malt sugar.

   The chemical formula for each of these is $C_{12}H_{22}O_{11}$.

3) Polysaccharides are composed of many molecules, as the pre-fix 'poly' suggests. These include digestible forms of carbohydrate:

- Glycogen – is the form in which animals (including humans) store energy – in the liver and muscles in the body;
- Starch – is the form in which plants store energy – as in grains, pulses, potatoes and root vegetables.

   The chemical formula for each of these is $(C_6H_{10}O_5)_n$ – i.e. multiples of 6 carbon, 10 hydrogen and 5 oxygen combinations bonded together.

The indigestible forms of polysaccharides are collectively called fibre. Fibre contains sugars linked by bonds, which cannot be broken down by human enzymes, and are therefore deemed indigestible. There are two forms of fibre:

1) Insoluble fibre (which does not dissolve in water). This contains cellulose, hemicellulose and lignin. Cellulose can be found in whole-wheat flour, bran, and vegetables. Hemicellulose can be found in bran and whole grains. Lignin is a woody fibre found in wheat bran and the seeds of fruits and vegetables;

2) Soluble fibre (which dissolves, or swells, in water). This contains pectins, mucilages, and gums. They are not broken down by human enzymes, but instead can be fermented by bacteria in the large intestine. Pectin can be found in apples, strawberries and carrots. (Because it absorbs water and forms a gel, it is often used in jams and jellies). Mucilages and gums are similar in structure. Sources of gums include oats, legumes (beans, peas), guar and barley.

Since fibre is not digestible, it is not considered to provide energy (calories) to the body. This was the founding concept for the F-Plan diet, by Audrey Eyton. It was considered that, if calories were 'unavailable' to the body then people would lose weight. If you believe that energy in does equal energy out and that less energy in does not lead to less energy out, this may seem like a bright idea. But, if you know the correct definition of the first law of thermodynamics and the need to apply the second law correctly, this will more sensibly seem like a recipe for spending time in the bathroom.

What role does carbohydrate play in the human body?

In any definition of carbohydrate, the most common word seen is "energy". Carbohydrate provides readily available energy for the human body. Yet, surely in the midst of an obesity epidemic, the last thing that (overweight) humans need is easily available energy. We can make energy from fat and will do so in the absence of carbohydrate (in fact the body will *only* do so in the absence of carbohydrate).

The nutritional debate, as to whether or not humans need carbohydrate, centres on vitamin C. All other vitamins and minerals are found in animal foods (and some, like vitamin B12, are found only in animal foods). At the risk of killing any debate with facts, the USDA database, to which I frequently refer for comprehensive nutritional information, lists many animal sources of vitamin C – and in good quantities (veal thymus, for example, has 49 milligrams per 100 grams; chicken liver 28 milligrams per 100 grams of product and mollusc clams 22 milligrams). There are also substantial quantities of vitamin C in nuts, especially chestnuts. I have three points to make on the vitamin C debate:

1) Our ancestors lived for 1,200 generations through the ice age, and in many areas of the earth, with no consistent access to carbohydrate, if any at all. There are populations today that live solely on animal foods. Examples include: the Saami of northern Europe, living on fish and reindeer; some remote Siberians living on reindeer; Marsh Arabs living on buffalo milk,

buffalo, wild boar, water fowl and fish; the African Maasai and Samburu, living on meat (goats and sheep), milk and blood from cattle; and the Inuit of Greenland and Canada living on whale, seal, polar bears and even arctic fox. The latter is the most interesting population to note, as this was the culture studied in the 1920's by the anthropologist Vilhjalmur Stefansson. Stefansson lived with the Inuit for a decade and his study focused on the fact that the virtually zero-carbohydrate diet of the Inuit had no adverse effects on their health, nor indeed, on Stefansson's own health.[256] Stefansson (*Not by bread alone* 1946) also observed that the Inuit were able to get the necessary vitamins they needed in the winter diet, when even the limited plant matter found in summer was not available. Stefansson found that vitamin C could be obtained from raw meat (such as seal liver and whale skin). While there was considerable scepticism when Stefansson first reported these findings, they have been confirmed in recent studies.[257] It is likely that meat needs to be raw to provide vitamin C, as vitamin C is destroyed in cooking (the same applies in cooking vegetables and/or fruit, however, and this is not noted in our 'five-a-day' mantra).

2) Sugar, as the most refined carbohydrate of all, requires vitamins, such as B and C, and minerals for its digestion and metabolism and yet provides none in return. It follows that our need for vitamin C would be reduced if we avoided these substances and therefore, ironically, our need for carbohydrate (if there is any need for carbohydrate for vitamin C) would be reduced if we ate less (refined) carbohydrate.

3) We can say with confidence that, even if we need a few berries to provide vitamin C in our diets, especially in the absence of food like raw whale meat, we absolutely do not need refined carbohydrates at all and we do not need even 'good' carbohydrates in anything like the quantities advised by our governments and dietitians.

In conclusion, therefore, although we have a fundamental need for fat and protein, we either don't need, or need very little, of the one macronutrient that we are currently advised to ensure forms the vast majority of our diet – carbohydrate.

Getting energy from carbohydrates

Disaccharides and polysaccharides break down into monosaccharides, as the body breaks down carbohydrates into their simplest form. This is done in the presence of water (H_2O).

With disaccharides, $C_{12}H_{22}O_{11}$ gains two more H's and one more O (from H_2O) and becomes $C_{12}H_{24}O_{12}$, which is the same as two monosaccharides i.e. two lots of $C_6H_{12}O_6$.

With polysaccharides, any multiple of $C_6H_{10}O_5$ combined with the same multiple of water, adds two H's and one O making $C_6H_{12}O_6$, which is the chemical formula for monosaccharides. (Please don't be put off by the maths –

just add the H's together and the O's together and it is stuff you can do on your fingers).

I am indebted to Barry Groves for introducing me to the following concept.[258] I never knew calorie counting could be so much fun:

The disaccharides (sucrose, lactose and maltose) have the formula $C_{12}H_{22}O_{11}$. This has a molecular mass (decimal places ignored) of 342 g/mol. (Don't worry about the units "g/mol" – you don't need to understand what they mean for this – we'll call them units very soon). To break these down into the simple sugars, which is the form in which the body needs carbohydrate, water (H_2O) in the body provides the extra H's and O and we therefore end up with $C_{12}H_{24}O_{12}$, or, in fact two lots of $C_6H_{12}O_6$. Sucrose, lactose and maltose break down into different simple sugars – but all the simple sugars have the same formula.

The molecular mass of H_2O is 18 g/mol.
The molecular mass of $C_6H_{12}O_6$ is 180 g/mol.[259]

We started off with 342 units of, let's say, maltose. We added 18 units of water from the body and we ended up with two units of glucose at 180 each – equals 360 units. So, our original 342 units of carbohydrate ended up as 360 units of carbohydrate after being broken down by the body. This added 5% in mass and, therefore, if we started with 100 grams of carbohydrate, we end up with 105 grams of carbohydrate. If we assume that carbohydrates have four calories per gram, we started off with 400 calories of carbohydrate (maltose) and ended up with 420 calories of carbohydrate (glucose).

Polysaccharides are even more helpful to the body and unhelpful for calorie counters. Glycogen and starch have the formula $C_6H_{10}O_5$. This has a molecular mass (decimal places ignored again) of 162 g/mol. The body adds 18 g/mol with water and ends up with $C_6H_{12}O_6$, which has a mass of 180 g/mol. This time we started off with 162 units of, say, starch and we ended up with 180 units of glucose and we therefore added 11% in mass. In this scenario, we started with 100 grams of starch and 400 calories and we ended up with 444 calories. Hopefully even the most ardent calorie counters are starting to doubt the wisdom of basing their meals on starchy foods and/or counting calories.

For those who are still calorie minded, a rule of thumb for the body's daily requirement for protein is one gram per one kilogram of body weight. I weigh 50 kilograms, so my daily protein requirement, as a guide, is 50 grams. I would get this amount in one 200 gram tuna steak.[260] The calorie estimate for this tuna example is 144 calories per 100 grams – so I would need to consume nearly 300 calories of tuna to deliver my daily protein requirement. (10 grams of this 200 gram portion of tuna would be fat – supplying approximately 90 calories – so the whole food provides the energy – not just the protein). Both the protein and the fat in the tuna represent calories with 'a job to do' within the body – not merely calories that supply energy, for which I may or may not have a requirement that day.

Carbohydrates do not have these additional and vital roles – they merely supply energy. It will be useful for what follows to have a basic understanding of how carbohydrates are turned into energy, so let us look at this next.

Carbohydrate digestion starts in the mouth. Salivary amylase is an enzyme[xxxix] found in human saliva (also known as ptyalin) and this mixes with the food as we chew and starts the process by which starchy foods are broken down into simpler saccharides. Starch breaks down into maltose with the amylase in our salivary glands and digestive enzymes produced by the pancreas. Maltose, as we saw above, is a disaccharide with two glucose molecules and therefore starch that we eat is broken down into glucose, just as if we had eaten glucose in the first place. For the purposes of digestion, the body does not know the difference between glucose as the result of, say, sucrose intake (which breaks down into one molecule of fructose and one of glucose) and glucose produced by starch digestion. (Please note that this is just about digestion – none of this is about nutrients for now). I hope already that you can see the conflict between the two so called 'healthy eating tips': "Base your meals on starchy foods" and "cut down on sugar" – starch turns into sugar in just the same way.

The UK Sugar Bureau, which has the purpose statement "Improving knowledge and understanding about the contributions of sugar and other carbohydrates to a healthy balanced diet", uses this principle to suggest "The sucrose that we add to tea and coffee is exactly the same as the sucrose found in fruit and vegetables, and is used by the body in exactly the same ways."[261]

Kellogg's have also adopted similar tactics in their defence to the Advertising Standards Authority's review of a complaint made by the Children's Food Campaign. The latter were outraged by Kellogg's placing posters in bus shelters and running a TV advert campaign suggesting "Ever thought of Coco Pops after school?" Part of Kellogg's defence was that Coco Pops had no more sugar than other foods – one example given on their web site is "A bowl of sweetened cereals contains around two teaspoons of sugar – less than a couple of slices of toast and jam, a piece of fruit and yoghurt or a cup of sweetened tea."[262] The sugar in cereal is virtually all sucrose – table sugar, as is the sugar in a cup of tea. Jam will have some sucrose and some fructose and the fruit and yoghurt will have glucose and fructose, as well as sucrose and protein, fibre, vitamins and minerals – the latter are all lacking in the sugar in cereal. Hence, the argument that the body turns different saccharides into the same form during the digestion process is used disingenuously by food manufacturers to say "sugar is sugar", as Rachel Fellows from Kellogg's stated in a Radio 5 Live interview following the April 2010 *Which?* report into the sugar content of cereals. Nutritionally there is a significant difference, as whole grains (starch), fruit (fructose) and milk (lactose) have accompanying nutrients, which sucrose doesn't. If Kellogg's genuinely think that sugar is sugar, I invite the executive team to consume nothing but sucrose for a few weeks (it comes in a huge

---

[xxxix] An Enzyme is a protein (or protein based molecule) that speeds up a chemical reaction in a living organism. It acts as a catalyst.

variety of forms, so they need not be bored) and see how their health responds to calories without nutrition.

In what follows, don't worry about all the chemical terms – the key things to take away are: a) the complexity of the process – if this doesn't make you think twice about what you put in your mouth, I don't know what will; b) the way in which energy is being transformed continually in the body – not least with 50,000 enzymes with roles to play; and c) watch out for the term Acetyl-CoA – as we saw in the closing notes on cholesterol, in Chapter Eight, this is the building block for cholesterol and we are in a chapter all about carbohydrates – not fats.

The end goal of the energy cycle is a substance called ATP. ATP stands for Adenosine Tri-Phosphate. It is an organic compound made up of adenosine (an adenine ring and a ribose sugar) and three phosphate groups, hence, the name. ATP contains a large amount of chemical energy stored in its high-energy phosphate bonds. It releases energy when it is broken down into ADP (Adenosine Di-Phosphate). The energy is used for many metabolic processes. Hence, ATP is considered as the universal energy currency for metabolism. Plants make ATP during photosynthesis. Humans make ATP by breaking down molecules such as glucose.

There are three stages of the energy transformation process to turn glucose into our energy currency, ATP:

1) Glycolysis – this takes place in the cytoplasm[xl] and the goal of glycolysis is to break glucose down into two pyruvates, also known as pyruvic acid;[xli]
2) The Krebs Cycle (which was discovered by Hans Adolf Krebs in 1937 and is also known as the citric acid cycle) – this takes place in the mitochondria[xlii] and has two goals a) to convert pyruvate into Acetyl CoA and b) to perform the full operation of the Krebs cycle – i.e. to produce 2ATP's, 8NADH's,[xliii] 2 FADH$_2$'s[xliv] and 6 CO$_2$ per glucose molecule;
3) Electronic Transport Phosphorylation (also known as chemiosmosis) – this takes place in the mitochondria and the goal of this end part of the process is to break down NADH and FADH$_2$, generating the major part of the ATP production in the whole three stage process.

[xl] The cytoplasm consists of all of the contents outside the nucleus, but within the membrane, of a cell.

[xli] Pyruvic Acid is a colourless, water-soluble, organic liquid produced by the breakdown of carbohydrates and sugars during glycolysis.

[xlii] The mitochondria are the main sites of energy production in a cell.

[xliii] NAD stands for Nicotinamide Adenine Dinucleotide and is a coenzyme found in all living cells.

[xliv] FAD stands for Flavin Adenine Dinucleotide and is a coenzyme involved in several important reactions in metabolism. The H at the end of both FADH$_2$ and NADH indicates that the NAD/FAD has been reduced by accepting two hydrogen atoms (a net gain of two electrons, which makes it higher in concentrated energy).

So, carbohydrate metabolism starts with glycolysis, a process which releases energy from glucose (or glycogen) to form two molecules of pyruvate. Pyruvate/pyruvic acid is the pivot between glycolysis and the Krebs cycle. If oxygen is not available (the body is in a state of anaerobic respiration), pyruvate is converted to ethanol or lactate and energy can be produced for a limited period of time with lactic acid being an unpleasant side effect. If oxygen is available, the two molecules of pyruvate enter the Krebs cycle. The first step in the process is the conversion of pyruvate into a form that can enter the citric acid cycle. For this to happen, pyruvate loses one carbon, as carbon dioxide, to form acetyl coenzyme A (Acetyl-CoA being the start of the cholesterol production process). Acetyl-CoA is effectively an activated form of acetic acid (vinegar). It is Acetyl-CoA that enters the citric acid cycle. This reaction is irreversible and requires B vitamins for the conversion process (vitamin B2 is needed for FAD(H) and vitamin B3 for NAD(H) conversion respectively).

Just to show the energy generated:

- During Glycolysis, 2 ATP's are used up and 4 are generated along with 2 NADH.
- During the Krebs cycle, 2 NADH are produced from pyruvate to Acetyl CoA, 6 NADH from the Krebs cycle, 2 $FADH_2$ and 2 ATP's.
- The NADH and $FADH_2$ then go on to the electron transport chain and ATP is produced as follows: 3 ATP are produced per NADH and $FADH_2$ results in the production of 2 ATP for each $FADH_2$.

Overall we have: 4 ATP from glycolysis and 4 ATP from NADH in glycolysis; 24 ATP from NADH; 4 ATP from 2 $FADH_2$ and 2 ATP from the rest of the process resulting in 38 ATP – net 36 ATP given the 2 ATP used in glycolysis.

The key things to note are:

- Carbohydrate consumption produces Acetyl-CoA in the 'bridging' stage between the first and second stages of the metabolism process (between Glycolysis and the Krebs cycle);
- The conversion from carbohydrates into ATP – energy usable by the body – is very efficient and a lot of ATP is made from one molecule of glucose as a result of all the enzyme processes along the way – our body's spark plugs in effect;
- The conversion from carbohydrates into ATP requires B vitamins. Hence the argument that sugar provides energy is not strictly true. The body needs B vitamins from elsewhere to enable sucrose to be converted into usable energy. This is why sugar/sucrose has been called an anti-nutrient, as it depletes the body of vitamins from other food sources in its metabolism.

'Simple' vs. 'complex' carbohydrates

It has been wrongly assumed for some time that monosaccharides and disaccharides are absorbed quickly and polysaccharides more slowly. Hence the references that can still be found to 'simple/fast release' and 'complex/slow release' carbohydrates. Even by 1987, when Montignac's *Dine out and lose Weight* was published,[263] this myth had been dispelled and it was known that the glycaemic index was the most important measure of the impact of carbohydrates on the body.

The glycaemic index was developed by Dr. P. A. Crapo in 1976 and was defined as the area under the blood glucose curve induced by the food tested. I.e. a food would be consumed and the rise in blood glucose would be measured by calculating the total area below the raised blood glucose line. This would include the peak in blood glucose and the time period over which the blood glucose was raised. Glucose was assigned a glycaemic index (GI) of 100 and then all foods were measured relative to this. This index renders the notion of fast and slow release carbohydrates redundant with simple examples such as:

-   Fructose has a GI score of 20 and yet is a 'simple sugar' (a monosaccharide) as is glucose, which has the defining GI of 100;
-   Sucrose has a GI score of 75 as a disaccharide. Disaccharides are supposed to be simple/fast release carbohydrates, like monosaccharides – but the latter have such different GI scores;
-   White bread and potatoes have a GI score of 95 and some pulses have a GI of approximately 30 – all examples of polysaccharides.

We also know from glycaemic index studies that cooking foods and processing foods increases their glycaemic index, so cooked carrots have a higher glycaemic index (33 to 85) than raw carrots (16 to 30). One of the problems with the glycaemic index as a tool in weight loss is the huge variation in scores that can be found. In the cooked carrots example just above, the score of 85 for cooked carrots comes from Montignac and the score of 33 was found for peeled and boiled carrots in "the home of the glycaemic index" (www.glycaemicindex.com). Had the carrots been peeled, diced and boiled, their GI would have been 49, according to the same source. This source also lists raw carrots as having a GI of 16 compared to the 30 listed for raw carrots on the Montignac web site.[264] Counting calories is daft enough. If I were going to count anything, I would want it to be substantially more accurate and consistent than the glycaemic index.

Fructose

Fructose deserves a special mention in our chapter on carbohydrates, as we are learning more about this monosaccharide every day. I attended a conference on 7 September 2009 in Birmingham called *Fructose – the Lipogenic Carbohydrate* i.e. the fattening carbohydrate.

As we sat down in the meeting room, a slide was on the screen showing a typical continental breakfast. As the introductions started, numbers appeared next to each item on the breakfast tray to indicate the amount of fructose it contained: 10.4 grams in the cereal; 8.4 grams in the sugar bowl; 6.7 grams in a glass of orange juice; 5.2 grams in a coffee with sugar; 3.9 grams in a small portion of grapes; 3.6 grams in the jam and 1.6 grams in the croissant. There were 40 grams of fructose in total.

It was a privilege to hear Dr. Richard Johnson open the conference. Dr. Johnson had started his medical career specialising in infectious diseases and has become a leading expert on fructose (and uric acid) and he declared his possible conflicts of interest up front, for which he is to be respected. Quoting from an article written with eight colleagues, for the *American Journal of Clinical Nutrition* (AJCN) (2007), Dr. Johnson shared some historical facts about sugar consumption:[265] The average sugar intake in England per capita was four pounds in 1700 and 18 pounds in 1800 – just over quadrupling in one century. Intake increased further still after Prime Minister, William Gladstone, repealed the sugar tax (1874), reaching 100 pounds per person in 1950. Sugar consumption doubled in the USA and UK between 1900 and 1967.[266]

The key event that occurred in the early 1970's was the introduction of a substance called high fructose corn syrup (HFCS), which had certain advantages over table sugar in relation to shelf life and cost. "The combination of table sugar and HFCS has resulted in an additional 30% increase in overall sweetener intake over the past 40 years, mostly in soft drinks" (from the AJCN article). The article noted that consumption of these sweeteners had reached almost 150 pounds per person per year, by 2007 – more than 500 empty calories per day. Isolating consumption of HFCS, Americans consumed less than half a pound of the substance per person in 1970. By 2000, consumption had risen to more than 42 pounds per person per year.[267] It is worth seeing a copy of this journal article (freely available at ajcn.org), if only for the diagram of sugar intake alongside obesity prevalence since 1700. The correlation is striking.

High fructose corn syrup is made in different proportions of fructose and glucose, but the most common mixture is 55% fructose and 45% glucose, compared to the 50:50 proportions of fructose and glucose in sucrose. The fructose content is stated in the variant name: HFCS-42 is 42% fructose, HFCS-45 is 45% fructose and there is even a HFCS-90, which is 90% fructose.

This combination of fructose and glucose is particularly interesting. The glycaemic index of fructose, as mentioned above, is 20 and glucose, of course, is 100. The GI of fructose is low because fructose can only be metabolised by the liver and so most of the fructose consumed goes straight from the small intestine to the liver.

The single biggest dietary change that human beings have endured during the past 100 years is not just the increase in sucrose, but, specifically the increase in fructose. Although availability of carbohydrate would have been severely limited during the generations of our ancestors, as Gowlett stated, our access to carbohydrates would have gradually increased over the past 5,000 years. However, early consumption of carbohydrate would have been in the form of starch, such as potatoes and spelt (an ancient form of wheat) and starch is broken down into glucose molecules. It is the modern ingestion of carbohydrate, in the form of sucrose and HFCS, which has so dramatically increased fructose intake, as this comprises fructose and glucose and not just glucose.

As fat consumption has been demonised, numerous low-fat products have been made available to consumers and, as fat removed invariably needs to be replaced by something, sugar and HFCS have provided the low cost, long shelf life alternatives. This has substantially increased our fructose consumption and in an unprecedented way.

Because fructose is the main sugar in fruit, it has a 'halo' effect and is perceived as a healthy saccharide. This reputation as a healthy carbohydrate has been further enhanced because of the low glycaemic index of fructose and its consequential perceived suitability for diabetics. When I challenged a dietitian at a National Obesity Forum conference in June 2009 about the 400 empty sugar calories that the average Briton consumes each day, her retort was "What's wrong with that?" followed by a 'justification' that sucrose is merely fructose and glucose and the implication – what could be healthier? The reason why fructose has a low GI and the concomitant metabolism of fructose in the liver had been overlooked.

The notion that fructose is the most fattening carbohydrate incredibly dates back to 1916 with an article by Harold Higgins.[268] Higgins refers to fructose as levulose, an uncommon name today and the article is generally old fashioned in language and yet so modern in relevance. Higgins measured the Respiratory Quotient[xlv] for alcohol and different sugars and used this ratio to inform us about the metabolism of these substances by the body. The Respiratory Quotient for carbohydrate is 1.0; the RQ for fat is 0.7 and various figures are given for protein between 0.8 and 0.9. If the Respiratory Quotient goes above 1.0, this indicates that anaerobic (without oxygen) respiration is taking place. Under anaerobic conditions the cell cannot operate the citric acid cycle and the subsequent electron transport chain because both of these processes depend on oxygen. In this circumstance ATP can be generated with lactic acid fermentation – hence the burn that anaerobic exercise can generate.

Higgins' observations were: "The rise in the respiratory quotient after levulose and sucrose is distinctly rapid, being very marked even as early as the fourth to the eighth minute. With glucose and maltose, the definite rise in quotient does not occur until the twentieth to the thirtieth minute after the sugar was taken, although there is a small rise with maltose a little earlier." Higgins noted that these findings for levulose (fructose) and glucose were in agreement with the findings of Togel, Bresina and Durig three years earlier.[269]

Glucose and maltose having such similar outcomes is understandable, as maltose is made up of two glucose molecules. Fructose and sucrose having such similar outcomes is interesting for two reasons a) because fructose is the common denominator and b) we know that it is not the glucose in sucrose

---

[xlv] The Respiratory Quotient is the ratio of the volume of carbon dioxide expired to the volume of oxygen consumed by an organism or cell in a given period of time.

determining the rise, because we have measured this separately, so we know fructose is the sugar driving the observed higher Respiratory Quotient.

The Respiratory Quotient for the human subjects, following the consumption of fructose or sucrose, was regularly above 1.0 during Higgins' experiments. This meant that the person had entered a state of anaerobic respiration (no exercise was being undertaken). The conclusion reached was that the body could not metabolise the fructose or sucrose quickly enough to use it as energy and therefore it was concluded that fructose/levulose is more easily converted to fat by reason of its respiratory quotient being so often above 1.0.

Over 50 years later, Yudkin noted, almost in passing, "There is reason to believe that it is the fructose part of sucrose that is responsible for many of the undesirable effects of sucrose in the body."[270]

Sadly, we lost another two decades before this idea was taken further. Taubes reports that research on fructose-induced lipogenesis" was led by: the Israeli diabetologist, Eleazar Shafrir, at Hebrew University-Hadassah Medical School in Jerusalem; Peter Mayes, a biochemist at King's College Medical School in London and by Sheldon Reiser and colleagues at the Carbohydrate Nutrition Laboratory in Maryland. This was taking place in the 1990's, ironically in parallel with the development of the five-a-day campaign, to which we will turn next.

Shafrir noted that fructose places a metabolic load on the liver, which responds by converting it into triglycerides (fat) and then dispatching this in lipoproteins out from the liver around the body.[271] The title of the conference that I attended, *Fructose – the lipogenic carbohydrate* derives from this fact. Glucose entering the blood stream has the chance of being used for energy before being turned into glycogen and stored in the liver. Fructose goes straight to the liver to be stored.

Peter Mayes did some outstanding work on fructose, culminating in a key journal article in 1993.[272] Mayes determined that the metabolic effects of fructose are due to its rapid utilisation by the liver and it by-passing a key step in glycolysis, leading to "far reaching consequences to carbohydrate and lipid metabolism". These consequences are as diverse as increased secretion of very low density lipoproteins (triglycerides) and diminished ATP synthesis. Mayes also detailed how the pattern of fructose metabolism worsens over time, leading to raised triglyceride levels, decreased glucose tolerance, and hyper insulin sensitivity.

Dr. Lustig is one of the world authorities on fructose, if not the current lead. His video on youtube.com *Sugar: The Bitter Truth* is a revelation and will hopefully also be revolutionary.[273] Anyone with the courage to say "Coca-Cola: that's the smoking gun" deserves respect.

The Lustig work concurs with Mayes that the key issue with fructose is the fact that it is metabolised in the liver. Lustig compares the hepatic (liver) handling of a 12 fluid ounce can of fizzy drink with a 12 fluid ounce can of beer. Both have 150 calories. All the calories in the soda come from sucrose – so that breaks down into 75 calories as glucose and 75 as fructose. 90 of the beer calories come from alcohol and 60 from maltose. Lustig explains that 20% of the glucose calories and all the fructose calories reach the liver, so that totals 90 calories for the soda. All *but* 10% of the alcohol calories reach the liver and maltose breaks down into glucose, so 20% of these calories also end up in the liver – making 92 in total. The point made is that you wouldn't give a child a can of beer but giving them a can of soda, metabolically, is virtually the same.

Lustig concludes that "fructose is a poison" and presents a compelling case for this, accusing fructose of causing metabolic syndrome (obesity, type 2 diabetes, lipid conditions, hypertension and cardiovascular disease). He also notes an interesting role played by fructose in obesity – that it does not suppress grehlin, the hunger hormone and it does not stimulate insulin, or leptin, the latter being the signal to the brain that something has been eaten.

The final point to make on why fructose is increasingly being called the fattening carbohydrate is that it is more efficiently converted into glycerol than is glucose. From Chapter One, we noted that glycerol provides the backbone to join three fatty acids together in the form of triglyceride – human fat tissue. The combined potency of sucrose/high fructose corn syrup is as follows – as the fructose proportion heads to the liver for its metabolism it has little impact on blood glucose levels. The glucose proportion performs this role and stimulates the pancreas to provide insulin. Hence we have triglycerides being formed, courtesy of the fructose, and they are able to be stored, thanks to the glucose causing insulin to be provided. Food manufacturers may like to argue that all sugar is equal – but, when it comes to enabling fat to be stored, the glucose/fructose combinations are more equal than others.

With hopefully at least some doubt as to the wisdom of our current high and unprecedented, fructose consumption, let us look at another piece of advice trying to raise our fructose consumption even further.

Five-a-day

The five-a-day campaign is actually a different number-a-day campaign across more than 25 countries. The UK swears by five-a-day. The USA proposes nine-a-day: two and a half cups of vegetables and two cups of fruit every day. Australia suggests five portions of vegetables and two of fruit, where a portion of vegetables counts as 75 grams of cooked vegetables, one cup of salad vegetables, or one small potato and a portion of fruit would be one medium piece (150 grams), one cup of diced fruit pieces or canned fruit, or one cup fruit juice.

The European advice varies as follows: Denmark says eat six-a-day. The Irish have a food pyramid, not a plate (more American) and they go for four(plus)-a-day. The Swiss have five-a-day and tell citizens to go for a variety of colour in their choices. The Belgians and Austrians also favour five-a-day. Italy just says eat more fruit and vegetables – very libertarian. The Spanish have a pyramid with two rows to eat occasionally – the foods on these rows look like (red) meat, sausages, cakes and sweets – and then they have four rows to consume daily – in order of smallest to largest intake recommended – other meat/fish; dairy; fruit and vegetables and then grains. Hence, the Spanish have a free hand in choosing their number-a-day and they also have advice for moderate intakes of wine and beer along the side of their pyramid. The Greek food pyramid is simply called "The Mediterranean Diet" and they quantify three servings of fruit and six servings of vegetables a day. Latvia goes for percentages – 30% of daily intake should be in the form of fruit and vegetables. Germany (spot a centre of engineering expertise) has a three dimensional food pyramid indicating qualitative and quantitative nutritional information. They also have a staircase picture elsewhere on a public health website with fruit and vegetables on the bottom step (the largest group to be consumed); meat, fish and dairy on the next step; German sausages and whole grains on the next step and then other grains and finally junk on the final two steps.[274] This is getting closer to reasonable advice. I also heard anecdotally, from an attendee of the 2009 Amsterdam obesity conference, that the German delegates were recommending 500 grams of vegetables per day while fruit was not quantified. The Hungarians haven't gone for a pyramid, or a plate – they have a house with no numbers apportioned. The French have five-a-day *or fewer* – interesting.[275]

So where did the pick-a-number-a-day all start? It started as the "National five-a-day for better health" program in 1991 as a public-private partnership between the National Cancer Institute (NCI) and the Produce for Better Health Foundation. The programme started in California, the sunshine state, and has become the world's largest public-private nutrition education initiative. All States in the USA have a five-a-day co-ordinator and, as we can see above, the programme has spread as far as Australia and Latvia. (Five-a-day has since been trademarked by the National Cancer Institute).

The National Cancer Institute was established in 1937 and is the USA government's principal agency for cancer research and training. The Produce for Better Health Foundation can be found at the web site "fruitsandveggiesmorematters.org" and their purpose is to get us to eat more fruit and vegetables. The conflict of interest chapter comes later, but we can't move on without listing some of the sponsors of the Produce for Better Health Foundation:

- Logistics firms: C.H. Robinson Worldwide, Inc.; Caito Foods, Inc.; Capital City Fruit; Coast Produce Company and J&J Distributing.
- Specialist producers: Driscoll's (berries); U.S. Highbush Blueberry Council (blueberries); Ocean Mist (artichokes and fresh vegetables); Giorgio (mushrooms); Columbine Vineyards (grapes); Nature sweet tomatoes; Potandon Produce (potatoes) and Paramount Farms (nuts and flavoured nut snacks).
- General fresh produce firms: W. Newell & Companies; Eurofresh Farms; Giumarra Companies; General Mills (Green Giant brand); Sun-Maid raisins and dried fruit; Kagome juices and Duda Farm Fresh Foods.
- Other: such as BASF (the world's leading chemical company, and a provider of fungicides, insecticides and herbicides); Glad Products Company

(containers, bags and ovenware); Nunhems USA (commercial vegetable seeds); The Kidney Cancer Association and McDonald's.

With the exception of The Kidney Cancer Association and, ironically, McDonald's, the above represents a list of organisations that stand to benefit if there were a dictat from government that citizens should strive to eat (at least) five portions of fruit and vegetables every single day. Although we may mind less about tomatoes and berries being sponsored, than sugar and white flour, this is still a conflict of interest.

Why five-a-day? Why not? It's a memorable number. It would have seemed achievable and it was the number of digits on one hand and, I would suggest, no more scientific than this. It was never the outcome of evidence based, thoroughly researched, scientific investigation. It was a marketing campaign – and the most successful nutrition marketing campaign that the world has seen.

Having been launched with no evidence whatsoever, there have been numerous attempts since to post-rationalise and to justify this worldwide campaign. It must be noted at the outset that this was never intended to be an obesity campaign. The involvement of the National Cancer Institute suggests that it was intended to be a programme to help with cancer in some non-quantified way. If it were designed as a general healthy eating campaign – to what end? It is difficult to know what this programme was intended to be, other than an excellent commercial venture for all the companies involved at conception. With no evidence at the time (or since), of any benefit from eating a certain number of fruits and vegetables each day, it is incredible to realise how far this marketing programme has gone. Now, as with so many other elements of our diet advice, we reiterate the slogan daily with no idea from whence it came.

The Colorado Department of Public Health reviewed the campaign and reported that, from the introduction of the five-a-day Day for Better Health Program in 1991 to 1998, the percentage of Americans who 'knew' that they should eat at least five servings of fruits and vegetables each day increased from 8% to 39% and the average consumption of fruits and vegetables increased from 3.9 to 4.6 daily servings per American.[276] Most conveniently, in terms of dates, there was an article in the *Journal of the American Medical Association* (JAMA) in 1999 called "The Spread of the Obesity Epidemic in the United States, 1991-1998". This reported that, during this period (when fruit and vegetable intake increased by nearly 20%), obesity increased by 50%, from 12.0% in 1991 to 17.9% in 1998.[277] I'm not saying that five-a-day caused this, but it certainly didn't help.

Let us turn to the evidence for the condition that five-a-day was intended to help – cancer. In April 2010 a study was published in the *Journal of the National Cancer Institute* written by Paolo Boffetta, as the lead of a large group of European researchers.[278] The study sought to quantify if cancer risk were inversely associated with intake of fruit and vegetables. The article analysed data from the EPIC (European Prospective Investigation into Cancer) study, involving 142,605 men and 335,873 women for the period 1992-2000. This review of almost half a million people found that eating five portions of fruit and vegetables a day had little effect on cancer risk and the very small difference observed could be explained by other factors. The study also grouped participants into five categories from the lowest intake of fruits and vegetables (0 to 226 grams a day) to the highest intake (more than 647 grams a day). Significantly, the cancer risk did not vary between the five groups. The overall conclusion of the study was that: "A very small inverse association between intake of total fruits and vegetables and cancer risk was observed in this study. Given the small magnitude of the observed associations, caution should be applied in their interpretation."

One of the key arguments presented as justification for the five-a-day campaign (upon which the UK Department of Health alone has spent £3.3 million over the past four years), is that fruit and vegetables are highly nutritious.[xlvi] We must stop making general and unsubstantiated claims like this. A worldwide instruction to citizens of tens of countries, across three continents, should be based on clear empirical evidence (and that evidence should have been tested and verified before any public health advice was issued). Aside from the fact that there is no such evidence for the health benefit of eating a particular number of a random selection of fruit and vegetables on any medical condition, let us analyse this 'nutritious' claim theoretically – starting with vitamins first:

We learned about the fat soluble vitamins, A, D, E and K, in Chapter Twelve. The pure form of vitamin A (retinol) and vitamin K2 are only found naturally in animal foods (meat, fish, eggs and dairy products) and we can proceed on the basis that vitamin D can only feasibly be consumed naturally in animal foods. Seeds, nuts and their oils are the best source of vitamin E. Even where fat soluble vitamins are found in plant sources, as the name suggests, they need a 'fat' delivery mechanism. K1 is found in green leafy vegetables and avocado is also a good source. Because of the absence of a 'fat delivery mechanism', the K1 in, say, spinach has a bio availability (availability to the body) of 4%, which increases to 13% if it is cooked in butter.[279]

Vegetables have negligible or zero fat content, so no natural fat delivery mechanism. Two fruits do have a fat content – avocados and olives. If we compare the best source for each of A, D, E and K from avocado or olives, we find that 100 grams of olives delivers the equivalent of 20 micrograms of retinol (assuming that the body is capable of converting carotenes to retinol). Lamb's liver delivers 7,392 micrograms of retinol per 100 grams. That means we would need to eat three kilograms of olives (4,350 calories) or eight grams of lamb's liver (11 calories) to meet the recommended dietary allowance of vitamin A. Assuming again that our carotene conversion is optimal, 70 grams of carrots could provide the retinol equivalent, but we would need to eat them with

---

[xlvi] Fruit is also widely promoted for its antioxidant properties: a) the antioxidant role in the body is best played by vitamin E and b) if we reduce our exposure to free radicals (processed food, pesticides, smoking, pollution etc), we need fewer antioxidants.

199

(ideally) butter for this to be absorbed. For vitamin D, avocado and olives score zero; 100 grams of herring provides 40.7 micrograms. Avocado beats olives for vitamin E content – with 100 grams providing a respectable 2.1 milligrams. Sunflower seeds, however, provide 36.3 milligrams per 100 grams and almonds 24.7 milligrams. Avocado contains 21 micrograms of vitamin K1 per 100 grams, which is valuable, but no fruit or vegetable can provide K2.

The water soluble vitamins include the eight B vitamins and vitamin C. The best sources of the B vitamins are meat (especially organ meat), fish, milk and eggs. Whole grains and dried yeast are also a good source of B vitamins, but fruits and vegetables do not appear on lists of top sources of B vitamins. B12, of course, is only found in animal products and therefore must be taken as a supplement by vegans (vegetarians can get B12 in milk and eggs).

So we are left with vitamin C and fruit and vegetables do win the top spots here. Guavas and peppers provide the highest single source of vitamin C from fruits and vegetables respectively – with 228 milligrams per 100 grams for guavas and 183 milligrams per 100 grams for raw yellow peppers. However, as noted earlier in this chapter, the USDA database records many animal and nut sources of vitamin C and in substantial quantities. The more commonly consumed fruits don't compare quite so favourably with, say, the 43 milligrams of vitamin C per 100 grams of chestnuts: apples have 4.6 milligrams per 100 grams and bananas 8.7 milligrams per 100 grams. So, we don't even need fruits and vegetables for vitamin C, although they can be good sources of this vitamin.

On to minerals – we listed the macro and trace minerals in full in the opening to Part Three. If we look at the minerals with which people are more likely familiar: the best sources of calcium are dairy products and tinned fish; egg yolks, beef, cheese and liver are the best source of chromium; iron is best provided by organ meats; iodine is found in abundance in fish and kelp (seaweed); magnesium and manganese are plentiful in nuts and whole grains; good sources of selenium are organ meats, fish and shellfish and zinc is found in oysters, liver, meat, cheese and fish generally. Potassium is the one mineral for which fruits and vegetables are the best sources. Potassium, however, can also be found in all of nature's foods, so we don't need fruits and vegetables to obtain this mineral. Dried fruits and dark green vegetables are good sources of iron, but the organ meats are much better sources.

In conclusion, the statement in the *Dietary Guidelines for Americans*: "fruits and vegetables are excellent sources of vitamins" is not evidence based. A more accurate statement would be "low/zero-fat fruits are a good source of vitamin C and not much else; fruits with a fat content (avocado and olives) are poorer on vitamin C and better on other vitamins, but still no where near 'excellent'; vegetables are often a better source of vitamin C than fruit and can also provide some useful fat soluble vitamins when eaten with fat." For a short and accurate statement, the guidelines should have said "animal products are unbeatable nutritionally".

Even if eating a certain number of portions of fruit and vegetables a day does nothing beneficial for cancer and even if the vitamin and mineral analysis does not bode well for fruit and vegetables being a major benefit to health generally, does the five-a-day campaign still have merit? As this book is about the obesity epidemic, I will answer from that perspective. I can only conclude that five-a-day has *not* been a worthwhile campaign and I present the following arguments as to why it has in fact been deleterious:

- There is an opportunity cost of having spent so much time and money embedding a message that has not helped obesity (to be fair it was never intended to) when the benefits of embedding an equally simple, but far more effective message, could have transformed the obesity epidemic. The single public health message, which could have made an immense difference, would have been "eat real food."
- If the message had been "swap five-a-day", rather than "eat five-a-day", this could have helped – provided that junk were swapped out and *not* meat, fish, eggs, dairy and nutritious foods. My personal experience, working exclusively in the field of obesity, is that people are trying to eat five-a-day *in addition* to everything else they are eating, not instead of. This can only worsen obesity and, of course, obesity has worsened dramatically since the launch of five-a-day.
- As if it is not bad enough that people are trying to get their five-a-day on top of everything else, the means by which they are doing this is disastrous for obesity. People are adding more processed food into their diet trying to get their five-a-day. If you review internet advice sites for 'how to get your five-a-day', adding sweet corn to (white flour) pizza is one suggestion, eat tinned (syrupy) fruit is another, fruit juices and fructose rich drinks are frequently recommended. We are eating even more processed food trying to get our five-a-day, which is to our overall detriment.
- Five-a-day is not helpful for the increasing number of people who are increasingly carbohydrate sensitive and for whom fruit and high-carbohydrate vegetables are best avoided.
- Finally, for anyone who is overweight (that's two thirds of the 'developed' world), unlimited (green) vegetables and salads should be encouraged, but fruit/fructose is best avoided.

The first lesson in nutrition sets out that the body needs macronutrients (fat, protein and carbohydrate – the need for the latter is debatable) and micronutrients (vitamins and minerals). The best providers of the essential macronutrients are animal foods – meat, fish, eggs and dairy. The best providers of vitamins and minerals are animal foods again, with seeds and a few non animal foods (kelp and peppers) being useful. The most nutritious foods on the planet, therefore, are animal foods.

Where is the logic for our governments and dietitians telling us to replace the most nutritious foods on the planet with the one macronutrient that we arguably don't even need, and certainly don't need in the quantities currently recommended? How can our dietitians be so enthusiastic about processed foods, so lacking in micronutrients that they are invariably fortified? How did we get to the situation that low calorie is more important than high nutrition?

The attack on real food occurs at the highest level. Here is an extract from the Chief Medical Officer's report for England 2009 (published April 2010): "Meat, butter, cream and cheese can play a part in a healthy balanced diet. In excess they can cause health problems. Their high level of saturated fat *finds its way* into our diet in biscuits, cakes and pastries, as well as in meat" (my emphasis). If any meat, butter, cream or cheese have 'found their way' into processed foods: a) this didn't happen by magic – food manufacturers put them there; b) they will be the most nutritious ingredients in the end product; and c) this means that we need to avoid the processed foods themselves and not any real foods that may happen to be within them. This is rather like saying that grade A students are bad, because they might find their way into crime.

After all this, is there a perfect five-a-day? I set about doing what should have been done before any of this started. I went back to the nutrition database and repeated the exercise in the opening to Part Three and tried to see if I could get the RDAs from just five foods. This can be achieved with 100 grams of liver, 200 grams of sardines, 200 grams of whole milk, 100 grams of sunflower seeds and 200 grams of broccoli (1,300 calories). There will be infinite combinations of real foods that can provide the RDAs, but I started from the ones known to be highly nutritious.

For interest, I repeated the experiment for a vegetarian diet and the biggest challenge became vitamin D. The RDAs could be met with five foods: 500 grams of whole milk, 450 grams of eggs (10 medium eggs), 300 grams of spinach, 250 grams of raw mushrooms grown in sunshine and 50 grams of sunflower seeds (1,360 calories). Dietary advisors applaud people for choosing a vegetarian diet, but then tell them to avoid eggs and to consume low-fat milk. It then becomes practically impossible for a vegetarian to meet even minimal nutritional requirements. I had returned to eating meat and fish before the research for this part of the book, but, this exercise gave me great concern about what lasting damage I may have done to my health during years of not eating meat and fish. Gwyneth Paltrow may also be re-evaluating her diet after sharing her medical experience on her health website (June 2010). Paltrow's vitamin D levels were tested by doctors in New York, following a "pretty severe" bone fracture and they "turned out to be the lowest they had ever seen."[280]

Vegans can't get B12 naturally and they would need to eat 2.25 kilograms of (raw sunshine grown) mushrooms in a fat delivery mechanism (e.g. vegetable oil) to get the 'adequate intake' for vitamin D and an unusual food like oriental dried radishes to get their calcium – and to repeat this daily. For completeness, the five vegan foods would be 2.25 kilograms of mushrooms, 175 grams of porridge oats, 25 grams of sunflower seeds, 100 grams of oriental dried radishes and 300 grams of spinach (in more vegetable oil) and a vitamin B12 supplement. Without the calories in the vegetable oil, the vegan basket adds up to 1,644 calories – the highest of all three sample ways of getting our nutritional requirement.

The basket in the opening to Part Three would call for nine-a-day (liver, sardines, eggs, whole milk, sunflower seeds, oats, cocoa, spinach and broccoli). One of the problems of trying to pick just five foods is that we end up with many vitamins and minerals over, or under, represented in our diet. We should consume a wide variety of nature's food. This nine-a-day would be ideal, but the list of foods is not catchy enough for a marketing campaign, which, after all, is what this was. This 'perfect' basket also wouldn't lead to a large increase in fruit and vegetable consumption – which is what the 1991 meeting attendees were no doubt keen to achieve.

The biggest tragedy of five-a-day is that we missed the opportunity to deliver a message that could have made a difference to our health and weight. The drive to eat five fruits and vegetables a day would have been far better directed (and still could be) towards eating more of the most nutritious foods each day. Meat (ideally liver), fish (ideally oily), milk (whole), sunflower seeds and broccoli would be the optimal five-a-day. Mum and granny were right.

Chapter Fourteen

"Do more" – the role of exercise

Introduction

Can you imagine a caveman being transported to the present day in Doctor Who's Tardis, only to arrive at a step aerobics class? He would surely wonder why on earth people were deliberately expending invaluable energy (let alone in brightly coloured attire). He would ask why people were wasting fuel, which would take him days to hunt and gather. We would explain that these people are trying to burn calories because they are trying to lose weight or trying not to gain weight. In response to the incredulous look on the Neanderthal's face, we would have to explain – food is abundantly available nowadays, so we have created recreations for burning fuel. Surely his response would be: why do you eat the food in the first place?

The theoretical case

Gary Taubes shares an insightful anecdote in one of his videos on the internet.[281] He tells the story of how he came across George Cahill, Professor of Medicine, Emeritus, Harvard Medical School, during his research. Having realised that we best understood obesity before the Second World War and then that a couple of discoveries soon after were material, Taubes asked Cahill if anything discovered before 1965 had been overturned or found to be untrue. Cahill said that it had not been. When Taubes checked his specific understanding about the cause of obesity, Cahill replied: "That's true – carbohydrate is driving insulin is driving fat". Moments later he said "we're fat because we're sedentary. A calorie is a calorie."

Cahill returns to "a calorie is a calorie" because his belief that energy in equals energy out is so entrenched, it overrides even irrefutable evidence that he also holds to be true. John Taggart said, "We have implicit faith in the validity of the first law of thermodynamics. A calorie is a calorie. Calories in equal calories out and that's that," for the same reason. Dietitians regularly refer to the laws of physics or the laws of the universe (I don't know if they know to what they are referring). The misapplication is so widespread and common that perhaps we should expect nothing less.

The notion that the obesity epidemic has been caused by sedentary behaviour is just the converse of saying that the obesity epidemic has been caused by eating too much. They are equals and opposites of the same misapplication of thermodynamics and therefore we knock them down in the same way by clarifying:

- There is no law that says energy in equals energy out; the first law of thermodynamics is about conservation of energy;
- The conservation of energy law only applies to a closed system in equilibrium, so we cannot ignore the second law of thermodynamics, entropy;
- Even if you think that energy in precisely equals energy out *and* that we can ignore entropy *and* anything taking place endogenously in the human body, surely the corollary of energy in equals energy out would be that less energy in equals less energy out.

Those who believe that we are overweight because we are sedentary believe in "The General Principle". They believe that we are overweight because we have not expended enough energy. They believe that, if we increase energy out (do more) we will lose weight. Those who additionally believe in "The Calorie Formula" believe that, for every 3,500 calories worth of exercise we do, we will lose one pound.

Both beliefs above also rely on 'all other things being equal'. So exercise is no longer supposed to 'work up an appetite', it is supposed to use up 'love handles'. When we get hungry after exercise, as we undoubtedly will, we have to ignore that most basic of human drives – the urge to eat – and ensure that energy goes out, but not in. Both beliefs also rely on an assumption that we can ignore everything we know about biochemistry. Whether glucose or glycogen or fatty acids are available matters not – if we need energy, it is assumed that it comes from adipose tissue in the amount of one gram for every nine calories that we need.

Please note that most calorie theorists think that both energy in and energy out are responsible for the obesity epidemic. They think that we eat too much and do too little generally and that we eat too many lots of 3,500 calories and don't do enough 3,500 calories bouts of exercise more specifically. This chapter is only looking at exercise, but I didn't want you to think that I had put people in one camp or another.

The empirical case – UK

To prove the case that the obesity epidemic has been caused by sedentary behaviour, we need evidence to prove the following:

1) That sedentary behaviour is (solely or primarily) to blame for the obesity epidemic; *and*
2) That the increase in obesity can be accounted for, with reference to known changes in levels of activity; *and*
3) That the timing of the obesity epidemic can be explained by an equal and coincidental (literally coinciding with) change in activity. Figure 1, presented in the introduction, is invaluable for illustrating both the increase and the timing of the increase, which require explanation.

We also need to be able to explain how the emergence of obesity in babies (six months old) can be explained by sedentary behaviour, despite the fact that they have no means of controlling their energy out. We'll come back to that one.

Let us start with the UK evidence. Since the 1999 devolution of Wales, Scotland and Northern Ireland, the Department of Health has been responsible for the National Health Service in England alone. While the newly formed health services established their structures, the English publications continued to be issued and these are available and useful for research purposes.

In April 2004, the Department of Health published a document *At least five a week*, written by the Chief Medical Officer for England, Sir Liam Donaldson. The subtitle is "Evidence on the impact of physical activity and its relationship to health", so it is about the general health benefits of exercise and not specifically about obesity. However, it is clear that this document supports both the view that energy in equals energy out and the specific 3,500 calorie formula.

Early on in chapter two of the document, "The importance of physical activity for public health" (p17), we find the following statement: "Obesity levels in England are high and rising. Almost a quarter of adults and about 16% of 2-15 year olds are obese. These current levels of obesity are caused by an imbalance between energy expenditure and energy intake." There's "The General Principle."

Then, on p20, we have "This produced a difference of 66 miles walked per year between 1975-76 and 1999-2001. For a person weighing 65kg, this represents an annual reduction in energy expenditure equivalent to almost 1kg of fat." There's "The Calorie Formula" – at 4-5 miles per hour, a 65kg person walking 66 miles would use up approximately 6,000 calories, which, divided by 3,500 would be "almost 1kg of fat."[282]

As if it is not bad enough that we have the literal use of "The General Principle" and "The Calorie Formula", we also have an unjustifiable focus on energy out as the key factor in the assumed energy equation. Later on in the same chapter, we find the passage: "It is only recently in human evolution that energy expenditure (primarily searching for sustenance) has not been inextricably linked to energy intake. With the industrial revolution and more recently the emergence of technological advances, a serious mismatch has emerged between food availability and the energy required to access food – leading to a new pandemic of metabolic conditions such as obesity and type 2 diabetes." The focus again is on energy expenditure not being able to keep pace with energy intake.

Later still in the same chapter, this point is reinforced further: "What is known for certain is that people are insufficiently active to balance the energy (calories) they consume from food and drink, resulting in positive energy balance which translates in the longer term to increases in overweight and obesity". First, this is in no way known for certain. Had people consumed the same number of calories in the form of zero carbohydrate foods, they would have been unable to store fat and therefore would not have gained weight regardless of activity levels. Secondly, why hold food and drink constant and hold activity guilty for not having matched 'the positive energy balance'?

The chapter closes with the conclusion, "There is little doubt that physical inactivity is now a major public health issue. Obesity is the main visible sign of inactivity". The clearly implied direction of causation here is that inactivity causes obesity causes major public health issues.

The above clarifies the theoretical position of *At least five a week*. Let us now turn to the evidence presented. Given the emphasis apportioned to activity in the text, we should expect the evidence to be strong. There is a key summary table in this document, which lists the strength of the evidence available for the impact of exercise on a number of conditions and whether or not the benefits are preventative, therapeutic, or both. As this book is about obesity, I am content to accept the benefits proposed in the summary table, without going back to the original research for any or all of them to see how robust the evidence is. I have little doubt that I could find contrary evidence and/or critique the studies presented. However, I see nothing to be gained from such an exercise for what follows. We can proceed, therefore, on the basis that there is:

- A *high* level of evidence for strong *preventative* benefits of exercise on cardiovascular disease, type 2 diabetes, osteoporosis and colon cancer;
- A *high* level of evidence for moderate *therapeutic* benefit of exercise on lower back pain;
- A *medium* level of evidence for moderate *preventative* benefits of exercise on obesity and overall cancer;
- A *medium* level of evidence for moderate *therapeutic* benefit of exercise on cardiovascular disease, peripheral vascular disease, obesity, osteoarthritis, clinical depression and mental wellbeing;
- A *low* level of evidence and/or *weak* benefits for *prevention* of peripheral vascular disease and the whole category of psychological wellbeing and mental health; and
- A *low* level of evidence and/or *weak therapeutic* benefits for stroke and the category of psychological wellbeing and mental health (other than clinical depression and mental wellbeing, noted above as having medium evidence for moderate therapeutic benefit).

If we accept the evidence presented, following the report's comprehensive review of the benefits of exercise, we note at the outset that exercise is only claimed to have a medium level of evidence for moderate preventative and therapeutic benefits for obesity. Yet, in the same document, on p53, we have the following completely unsubstantiated assertion: "Low levels of physical activity in England are a significant factor in the dramatic increase in the prevalence of obesity."

I fortunately had the opportunity to clarify this contradiction. I attended a conference organised by the Association for the Study of Obesity in Cardiff, on 8 June 2010, called *Physical Activity, Obesity and Health*. The opening presentation was given by Professor Kenneth Fox, from the University of

Bristol, who was one of two senior scientific editors for *At least five a week*. Included in Professor Fox's presentation was the summary slide showing that there was medium evidence for moderate benefit of exercise on obesity. I asked in the question session if there were any evidence for sedentary behaviour being the cause of obesity and/or exercise being the cure and the reply was "it's still open".

At the same conference, Dr. Anton J.M Wagenmakers, a Professor in organic chemistry and biochemistry, gave a brilliant presentation on "Obesity induced impairments in muscle metabolism". Compelling evidence was presented for the muscle of sedentary obese individuals showing: low content of mitochondria; low capillary density; low fat oxidative capacity; low endurance; low muscle mass relative to body weight (that's an interesting point – obese people are less able to support their own weight, let alone move it). However, notice the control subjects – "sedentary obese" – and we immediately have a cause and effect issue. Central to the metabolic problems being observed was reduced glucose uptake and insulin resistance, but did a lack of exercise cause these or carbohydrate intake?

In the conference handout notes, Wagenmakers opened with "An inherent consequence of the adoption of a sedentary lifestyle, not compensated by a reduction in energy intake, is a gradual increase of adipose tissue mass." He then went on to say "The most striking change in skeletal muscle to a sedentary lifestyle is a reduction in the mitochondrial density..." So, we have an implicit assumption that the sedentary lifestyle is at fault. Not the energy intake (or, as I would clarify – *what* is consumed), but the notion that people were too lazy to compensate for their food consumption. I have no doubt that the metabolic consequences observed by Wagenmakers are relevant to sedentary obese people. I have little doubt that they would be observed in obese people alone. I have substantial doubt that they would be observed in the sedentary alone.

Interestingly, in his 2005 study on the potential role of mitochondrial dysfunction in insulin resistance, Wagenmakers demonstrated that metabolic consequences could be found without obesity or sedentary behaviour being implicated. He compared lean, non-smoking individuals with insulin resistance, with lean, non-smoking individuals without insulin resistance. The insulin resistant participants were offspring of parents with type 2 diabetes and the study concluded that insulin resistance could have a genetic causation connected to mitochondrial dysfunction.[283]

It seems far more plausible that carbohydrate consumption, especially processed carbohydrate, is a root cause of overweight *and* insulin resistance *and* other serious metabolic consequences, rather than sloth. Human beings have as naturally evolved to avoid expending energy as they have evolved to gathering energy. I do believe that inactivity plays a part in the vicious cycle, but not that it is the root cause. The 'but for' test for me comes down to modern processed food. This is the thing that has changed so dramatically during the time of the emergence of the obesity epidemic. Inactivity is a consequence of our current poor nutrition providing no useful energy for the mitochondria and a consequence of the overweight being less able to move and that's the downwards spiral.

No further evidence was presented throughout the day to even attempt to demonstrate that sloth has caused obesity or that activity will cure it. The conference proceeded on the basis that exercise is important for cardiovascular health and general wellbeing, but let's forget obesity and ignore the fact that this is an obesity conference.

So where does the claim that exercise is either the cause of, or shall be the cure for, the obesity epidemic come from? Not from this document, but that didn't stop the Department of Health building on *At least five a week* with the document: *Be active, be healthy: a plan for getting the nation moving,* which was launched by the Department of Health in February 2009. The 2009 annual report of the Chief Medical Officer (published April 2010) acknowledged the challenge: "Achieving this target will require more than central and local government commitment. Such rapid increases in activity have not been seen before in any country. What is needed is nothing less than a societal shift so that physical activity, rather than inactivity, becomes the norm in everyone's behaviour." This statement was in the chapter called "Moving to nature's cure" – sadly not a drive to eat real food, but a campaign for exercise.

The document *At least five a week* admits that the evidence for the benefits of exercise for preventing or treating obesity is not in abundance and not strong. *Be active, be healthy* almost accepts defeat at the outset by saying that the change in exercise levels 'required' has never been achieved. Despite this, exercise remains the only consistent message across three of the four UK government campaigns that I analysed in Chapter Ten. The FSA says "Get active and try to be a healthy weight." The National Health Service advice is "60 active minutes" and "Up and about" and the Department of Health advises we need to "Build activity into our lives".

As Ben Goldacre tweeted on 14 May 2010: "I hope all the people in government claiming the Olympics will improve the nations health have designed clear studies to assess this outcome." I also hope that, as we will see in the next chapter, 'all the people in government' have assessed whether the sponsors of the Olympic Games will have more impact on what is consumed than what is done.

The empirical case – USA

Turning now to the USA, it is one thing for me to say I can't find evidence to support a link between activity and obesity; it is more powerful when the American Heart Association and the American College of Sports Medicine say it themselves:

"Rapidly increasing rates of obesity reflect a lack of energy balance as large numbers of people are consistently expending fewer calories than they consume. Unfortunately, few reliable data are available on the relative contributions to this obesity epidemic by energy intake and energy expenditure, although both as well as individual variation are important. While more information is gathered on the varied causes of obesity, it seems vitally important for public health efforts to address both energy expenditure and energy intake.

"It is reasonable to assume that persons with relatively high daily energy expenditures would be less likely to gain weight over time, compared with those who have low energy expenditures. So far, data to support this hypothesis are not particularly compelling."[284]

There are three interesting points to note from this:

1) The emphasis on energy expenditure is similar in this American review to the UK documentation. The positioning is that people are expending too few calories, not that they are consuming too many;
2) There is a frank admission that there is not much data, it is not reliable and it is "not particularly compelling";
3) Despite admitting that there is no evidence to present a case for exercise, it is nonetheless recommended that people do more and eat less (note the order) while we gather more information.

The Franz systematic review of the efficacy of different diet and exercise programmes, presented in Chapter Seven, also rules out the idea that exercise can be a cure for the obesity epidemic. The four studies for exercise alone showed that this made barely one kilogram difference to starting weight over one year.

The obesity epidemic has been thirty years in the making. If we can't make a compelling case for the role of exercise by now, is it reasonable to suggest that is because there isn't one? If a comprehensive report, with 84 references, written by two organisations which, it would be fair to say, are likely to have a positive view of the benefits of exercise, can only find that the data "are not particularly compelling", perhaps it is time to look at the problem in a different way.

The second and third things that we need to prove, notwithstanding the fact that we could not prove the first, is that the increase in obesity can be accounted for with reference to known changes in levels of activity; and that the timing of the obesity epidemic can be explained by an equal and coincidental change in activity.

The Deakin study was the first to try to quantify the role played by energy expenditure vs. energy intake. It was led by Professor Boyd Swinburn, chair of population health and director of the World Health Organisation Collaborating Centre for Obesity Prevention at Deakin University in Australia. It was first presented at the European Congress on Obesity (Amsterdam) on 9 May 2009 and reported extensively in science journals and in newspapers worldwide in the same week.[285]

The experiment was solely focused on the USA and it was conducted with 1,399 adults and 963 children. The starting point was to establish the calorie requirement of each individual. From this, the research team calculated how much the adults needed to eat to maintain a stable weight and how much the children needed to eat to maintain a normal growth curve. Swinburn and colleagues then used the United States Department of Agriculture national food supply data (similar to the UK National Food Survey), to see how much Americans were actually eating, from the 1970's to the early 2000's. The researchers used the individual energy requirement and the USDA (per capita) energy intake to predict how much weight they would have expected Americans to have gained over the 30-year period, if food intake were the only determinant. The NHANES data was used to determine the actual weight gain of Americans between the 1970's and the early 2000's.

"If the actual weight increase was the same as what we predicted, that meant that food intake was virtually entirely responsible. If it wasn't, that meant changes in physical activity also played a role," Swinburn said. "If the actual weight gain was higher than predicted, that would suggest that a decrease in physical activity played a role."

The researchers found that the predicted and actual weight gain matched exactly in children, leading them to conclude that the increases in energy intake alone explained the weight increase during the period in question. "For adults, we predicted that they would be 10.8 kg heavier, but in fact they were 8.6 kg heavier. That suggests that excess food intake still explains the weight gain, but that there may have been *increases* in physical activity over the 30 years that have blunted what would otherwise have been a higher weight gain," Swinburn said.[xlvii] I emphasised the word increases – Swinburn has presented the case that exercise actually increased during the period studied and that the average weight gain would have been even higher, but for this. Swinburn thus argues that, far from sedentary behaviour being responsible for the obesity epidemic; increased activity levels have actually alleviated it.

Swinburn emphasised that physical activity should not be ignored as a contributor to reducing obesity and should continue to be promoted because of its many other benefits, but that expectations regarding what can be achieved with exercise need to be lowered and public health policy shifted more toward encouraging people to eat less. This conclusion was well received by the American Heart Association (AHA) and the American College of Cardiology (ACC). The AHA spokesperson, Dr. Gerald Fletcher said "This is a nice study. It reflects many of the things that we have predicted." The ACC spokesperson, Dr. Matthew Sorrentino concurred: "The main cause of the obesity epidemic in this country is the wide availability of high-caloric foods and the fact that we are eating way too many calories in the course of a day. Exercise has much less impact." Sorrentino's view was that about 90% of weight loss is achieved by cutting calories; only about 10% of weight loss is achieved by significantly increasing physical activity.[286]

Much as I like the conclusions of this study, it must be noted that this study relies on both "The General Principle" and "The Calorie Formula" and hence it is fundamentally flawed. Starting with a calculation of energy need, using USDA data for per capita energy intake and translating the difference into

---

[xlvii] Chapter 7 used the NHANES figure of a 20lb gain for the average American between 1974-1999. This is consistent with the 8.6kg in Swinburn's study.

pounds gained relies upon believing that any 'surplus' calories are directly converted to weight and that this conversion adheres to a formula. I have no reason to believe that anything other than the 3,500 calorie formula would have been used. We could dismiss this entire study, saying that it has been founded on wrong assumptions. However, there may be some validity in using current beliefs to undermine other current beliefs. In the absence of a contrary study, showing that inactivity can explain the timing and extent of the rise in obesity, Deakin provides a useful argument that food intake is the issue.

The final observation that we would need to be able to explain, if sedentary behaviour were the cause of obesity, is the emergence of obesity in babies (six months old). I was first introduced to this concept in the brilliant video *Sugar: The Bitter Truth*, by Dr. Robert Lustig.[xlviii] Lustig presented the composition of formula milk, using a can of Similac Isolmil as an example. The feeding guidelines on the Similac web site range from 1-2 weeks to 9-12 months, so this is clearly a product designed for babies. The can of baby formula, of the part that is not water, contained 43% corn syrup solids and 10.3% sucrose. "It's a baby milkshake," said a horrified Lustig. I wanted to analyse a product for myself, so I chose Similac Isomil Advance, Soy Formula and the composition of this was 50% corn syrup, 14.2% soy protein isolate, 10.4% high oleic safflower oil, 9.7% sucrose, 8.2% soy oil and 7.5% coconut oil.[287] If a baby is unfortunate enough not to be breastfed, the infant can be started on a diet of 60% sugar from the first moment something is put in its mouth.

Heinz is one of the best known brands of baby food in the UK. Their web site lists 61 product options for 4-6 month olds and provides nutritional information for these. The first four products on the list were breakfast options: three cereals and a yoghurt, ranging from 22-27% sugar content. Ingredients included maltodextrin, sugar and galacto-oligosaccharides. The latter is found naturally in breast milk, the first two clearly are not. Heinz Farley's Rusks are described as "a great way to gradually introduce your baby to solid foods". With the top two ingredients being wheat flour and sugar, we are indeed introducing baby early on to the two main ingredients it will consume for the rest of its 'plate or pyramid' life. The sugar content in Farley's Rusks is 29%, the same as in McVitie's milk chocolate digestive biscuits and more than in UK biscuit favourites such as Hobnobs (23.8%) and McVitie's plain digestive biscuits (16.6%). Heinz fed babies can also enjoy delights such as banana and chocolate dessert: "a taste sensation", "delicious tasty strawberry cheesecake" and even "scrumptious" mild sweet chilli with chicken sauce – all with added sugar. I've

---

[xlviii] There are a number of errors in this video, but this should not detract from its importance: 1) The countries in Keys' Seven Countries Study did not include Australia, Canada, England and Wales. The chart shown by Lustig is from the Keys presentation to Mount Sinai Hospital, 1953, not from the Seven Countries Study; 2) Lustig states that 150 'extra' soda calories a day will result in a 15.6 pound weight gain each year – they won't and 3) Lustig's Isomil comparison concludes that the baby food has 10.3% sucrose vs. 10.5% sucrose in cola, but this is not comparing like with like. The cola includes water and the Isomil data doesn't.

got my own view on the cause of obesity in six month old toddlers and it has nothing to do with sedentary behaviour.

The anecdotal case

The complete absence of evidence does not deter those who think that the obesity epidemic is the result of laziness, more politically correctly called sedentary behaviour. Where there is no evidence, anecdotal terminology is proffered: "kids watch TV all the time"; "we used to do more physical work"; "we have all these labour saving devices nowadays".

Let us take each of these in turn:

- "Kids watch TV all the time":

TV arrived in the 1960's, obesity took an upwards turn around 1980 (yes, when we changed our diet advice). A report in the British press in February 2010 noted that the average Briton was watching three hours and 45 minutes of television a day – adding up to a day a week – and that this was the highest level since 1992.[288] But that still means that we were watching the same number of hours of television in 1992 and yet obesity has gone up dramatically since this date. A 160 pound person (an average woman) will use up 272 calories watching television for three hours and 45 minutes.[289] Yes, it would be better for the woman's overall health if she were dancing or walking. However, if the woman went to the gym in the evening, instead of watching television, she may well get hungry with the increased demand for fuel. If Ms Average eats more than she has used up, especially in the form of carbohydrate, she could well end up fitter, but fatter. I suggest that it is not watching television *per se* that is a cause of obesity, but rather the snacks that we eat while watching television that cause obesity. Someone simply watching three to four hours of television in the evening and eating nothing during this time can only store as fat what they ate that day. Fat storage depends on carbohydrate and insulin. It cannot be caused by watching television.

Please note another fundamental error that is made with exercise and energy expenditure. Energy expenditure calculators work on the input of the weight of the person and the time a particular activity is undertaken or a particular distance travelled by a particular means. The calculator includes the basal metabolic rate in the estimated energy expenditure. Hence, if watching television requires 73 calories an hour (this is the calculation for our 160 pound person) and moderate walking (2.5 miles per hour) burns 218 calories an hour (for the same person), then going for a walk should really be viewed as the additional energy needed beyond doing nothing (i.e. 145 calories in this case). I understand that Weight Watchers allows people an additional four points if they jog for 20 minutes. Four points is approximately 200 calories and our same woman would use 169 calories jogging for 20 minutes, which would only be 145 more than if she were watching television. Jogging only needs twice as many calories as moderate housework and the latter can be sustained for much longer.

- "We used to do more physical work":

I searched for evidence for a dramatic reduction in activity levels coinciding with the obesity epidemic and found none. I did find evidence to the contrary. The report, "Physical activity and public health: updated recommendation for adults from the American College of Sports Medicine and the American Heart Association", (2007), notes: "Favorable trend data from 1990 to 2004 in the United States based on the CDC Behavioral Risk Factor Surveillance System indicate that over time fewer men and women reported no leisure-time physical activity" (CDC is Centers for Disease Control).[290] "The prevalence of leisure-time physical inactivity remained fairly constant through 1996, but more recently has declined in both genders. In 2005 23.7% of adults reported no leisure-time activity."[291] Figure 1 in the report showed a clear downwards trend from approximately 30% of adults *inactive* in 1990 to the 23.7% quoted for 2005.

Data is scarce for any quantification of physical activity (as opposed to inactivity), but there is an excellent document by Ross Brownson and Tegan Boehmer (2005) providing useful statistics on this topic.[292] This (American) paper notes: "The percent of the labor force in high activity occupations remained steady from 1950 to 1990 at around 16% to 17%." So, during the period when obesity increased from under 5% to over 20%, the proportion of people in high activity occupations remained steady.

The paper found the same evidence for improvements in leisure time activity, as was presented in the ACSM and AHA 2007 report above. The reference source used by Brownson and Boehmer was the National Health Interview Survey (NHIS) and they noted "Other data from the NHIS show stable rates of sedentary activity and slight improvements in recommended activity over the time period of 1985 to 1998."

This observation was corroborated by the *Time Magazine* article "Why exercise won't make you thin"[293]: "More than 45 million Americans now belong to a health club, up from 23 million in 1993. We spend some $19 billion a year on gym memberships. Of course, some people join and never go. Still, as one major study – the Minnesota Heart Survey – found, more of us at least say we exercise regularly. The survey ran from 1980, when only 47% of respondents said they engaged in regular exercise, to 2000, when the figure had grown to 57%. And yet obesity figures have risen dramatically in the same period."

Intuitively, we can summarise the activity trends, during the period in which obesity has dramatically increased, as follows: inspired by John Travolta, the Bee Gees, disco, Grease the movie and so on, we danced our way through the 1970's. The 1980's were the decade of lycra and aerobics, with Jane Fonda as global queen and the Green Goddess and Mr Motivator less well known in the UK. The 1990's, as Time Magazine noted, was the decade when gyms came to the fore and the 2000's have seen a notable dedication to running and cycling. Marathons, half marathons, 10 kilometre runs, six kilometre runs, 'Iron Men' contests, the London to Brighton bike ride – numerous challenges have been created as the thing to train for and to be sponsored for. The first New York

Marathon had 127 runners (1970). 43,660 finished the course in 2009.[294] Marathons around the world have seen similar growth in participation. Meanwhile, the gym and aerobics classes remain popular and dancing has enjoyed a resurgence thanks to the celebrity dance shows – *Dancing with the Stars* in the USA and Australia and *Strictly Come Dancing* in the UK.

The Brownson and Boehmer study did report some declines in activity levels. There was a downwards trend in walking and cycling, for transport purposes, with the car favoured instead. Daily activities were reviewed for the period 1965-1995 by gender. It was noted that, among women, there were slight increases for paid work and time spent in recreation. A slight decline was noted in time spent eating and a larger decline was observed for hours per week spent doing housework. For men, declines from 1965-1995 were observed for paid work and time spent eating and increases were noted for time spent watching television, doing household work and in recreation.[295]

Most importantly, Brownson and Boehmer considered the timescale argument (point 3 under our 'what must be proven' test above). They quantified the rise in obesity using data from the National Health Examination Survey, National Health and Nutrition Examination Survey (NHANES) I, and NHANES II, which showed "that the prevalence of obesity among adults aged 20 years or older was relatively constant from 1960 through 1980 (13-15%)". Subsequent data collected during NHANES III and the first 2 years of NHANES Continuous "showed an approximate 8% increase in obesity every 10 years (23.3% in 1988-1994 and 30.9% in 1999-2000)."[296]

The key passage in the journal is as follows: "The sharp increases in obesity over the past 25 years are difficult to explain based on available trend data. Based on available data, many structural changes in land use (e.g., suburbanization), travel behavior (e.g. more reliance on the automobile), and some types of physical activity (e.g. a lower prevalence of employment in active occupations) largely occurred several decades ago, most notably in the few decades post-WWII." Brownson and Boehmer ended by saying: "We may never have a full understanding of the causes for the rapid rise in obesity". I would add – but the notion that the rapid rise in obesity is due to sedentary behaviour has no evidence to support this.

- "We have all these labour saving devices nowadays":

Most labour saving devices were around by the 1950's – they have just become cheaper, better and more widely available since. The first automatic washing machine was developed by Bendix in 1937 and the first top loading washing machine was developed by General Electric in 1947. The first electronic vacuum cleaner was developed by Hoover in 1908 and 'hoovers' were in general use post World War II. The first electric mixer was launched in 1904 and the Sunbeam mixer was available by 1930. The labour saving device argument does not explain why obesity took off in 1976-1980 in the USA and a few years behind in the UK. This simply does not serve as an explanation for why American obesity rates have a pivot in them, at the point 1976-1980, as illustrated so well by Figure 1 in the introduction.

This argument, in fact all three of the anecdotal arguments, are also undermined by the connection between poverty and obesity. If having access to TV, *not* working manually and being able to afford labour saving devices were the cause of obesity, there would be a positive correlation between income/socio-economic group and obesity. The richer the person or family, the more inactive and obese they would be. In fact the exact opposite is true. There is a strong correlation between low income and high obesity.

One of the earliest articles to quantify the relationship between income and obesity was a study of a residential area in New York City, presented in the 1962 *Journal of the American Medical Association.*[297] Data was obtained from 1,660 people, selected as representative of 110,000 inhabitants of Manhattan. The results revealed a striking relationship between obesity and socioeconomic group. "The prevalence of obesity was 7 times higher among women reared in the lowest social class category as compared with those reared in the highest category." One of the three authors of the 1962 study, Albert Stunkard, wrote an article in *The New England Journal of Medicine,*[298] over 30 years later, noting "One of the most striking facts about obesity is the powerful inverse relation between obesity and socioeconomic status in the developed world, especially among women." The article went on to explore the three possibilities for direction of causation: that obesity influences socioeconomic status; that socioeconomic status influences obesity; or that a common factor or factors influence both obesity and socioeconomic status. The article concluded that all three played a part, but this need not concern us. We just need to establish that income and obesity being inversely correlated negates all three anecdotal arguments presented.

The document *At least five a week* concluded the same for England: "Obesity is related to social class in adults. Among those classified as 'professional' 16% of males and females are obese, while among those classified as 'unskilled manual' 23% of males and 29% of females are obese".[299]

Lower income individuals and families have less access to cars, more reliance upon public transport, fewer energy saving devices and they tend to be concentrated in manual labour occupations. The majority of roles in catering, cleaning and construction, as just three examples, are poorly paid and highly physically demanding. A coffee shop barista is on his or her feet all day long, for little more than minimum wage. Builders are the modern day equivalent of mine workers and the company owners tend to be the rich and inactive and the manual workers tend to be the poor and active. Builders are so notoriously overweight that cartoons and situation comedies feature 'the builder's bum' – the flesh on show where the trousers and top part with the strain of staying together. I have seen numerous overweight waiting staff and I suggest that the access to food in catering is the cause, not the lack of being active all day.

What does explain the correlation between poverty and obesity is food intake. Not the quantity (I haven't fallen for the energy in notion), but the type of food eaten. If you have any doubt whether McDonalds is more frequented by lower or higher income people a) by definition you are high income, because you haven't been in one and b) try to find an advert for McDonalds (or Wendy's, or Pizza Hut, or KFC, or any fast food outlet) that isn't based on price. Everything is "X for 99 pence or cents"; "buy this, get this free"; "get this whole bucket and fries to feed your entire family for ten bucks." Poor people eat poorly; it's a sad indictment of modern life.

The UK TV presenter Rebecca Wilcox did an experiment in the BBC Programme: *Who made me fat?*[300] She went into four of the leading supermarkets in the UK (ASDA, Morrison's, Sainsbury's and Tesco) and bought only the items on special offer. She left the shops with BOGOF's (Buy One Get One Free) in abundance for biscuits, crisps, fizzy drinks, cakes, sweets and so on. In one supermarket, she purchased a BOGOF offer on a 12 bag pack of crisps enabling her to get 24 bags of crisps for £1, likely the price of a small bag of salad in the same store. The more affluent shoppers are throwing cherries in the trolley without looking at the price. The lower income parents, with a family to feed, are trying to get the most food for the least money and this all too often ends up being manufactured, processed, nutritionally lacking 'junk'.

The Dr. Foster report (August 2008) noted that the five slimmest places in the UK were all in London and, after Shetland, the others in the top five most overweight places in the UK were all in Wales: Torfaen, Blaenau Gwent, Neath and Caerphilly.[301] The report presents a coloured map of the UK with the highest regions for obesity coloured red and the areas with the lowest incidence of obesity in green. West Wales and what we know in Wales as 'The Valleys', are a mass of red. The National Assembly for Wales report on GDP per head in European regions[302] stated that, "per capita GDP in West Wales and the Valleys represented 77.1% of the average for EU25 as a whole in 2004." (EU25 represents 25 European Union countries; Bulgaria and Romania have since joined to make the EU27).

If exercise were inversely correlated to weight, poorer people would be slimmer but, obesity is, in fact, positively correlated with poverty. The overweight unemployed are on the street corner; the slim executives are in the corner office.

Further observations

One of the most compelling arguments for me, against exercise being the key to the obesity epidemic, is the simple fact that we can eat in one minute enough fuel for one hour. The relative importance of *not* eating something vs. eating it and trying to use the fuel, is enormously weighted towards *not* eating something in the first place. This is not a new concept. Newburgh (1942) noted that a man can climb a flight of stairs or forego one quarter teaspoon of sugar.[303]

Those who think that sedentary behaviour is at the heart of the obesity epidemic think that, if only people did more, they would not be overweight. The UK government documentation reviewed earlier in this chapter placed so much more emphasis on what people do than what they eat. Childhood obesity particularly, has a worrying reliance placed on the idea that, if only we could get our younger people away from the screen and active in some way, all will be fine.

One of the best television programmes I have come across, as an obesity researcher, blew this theory apart with a simple and highly memorable experiment. The programme was called *30 Minutes* and it was about childhood obesity.[304] The presenter, Nick Cohen, took a boys football team from London, England, and split them into three groups. One third of the team were given an apple; another third a bag of crisps and the final group a confectionery bar. The teenagers were then asked to run around an athletics track continuously until they had burned off what they had eaten. They were invited to stop when they thought they had used up their energy intake and they did so after a couple of laps. They were asked to carry on until they had in fact used the energy equivalent of what they had consumed. The apple group needed to run for 13 minutes, the crisp group needed to run for 42 minutes and the confectionery group needed to run for one hour and five minutes to burn off their item. (The confectionery group was stopped long before the hour, as they were struggling to continue). Cohen explained that, if a child ate a bag of crisps, a confectionery bar, a burger and chips and had a fizzy drink, they would need to run continuously for five hours to burn that off.

As an additional point, if children are in the house and not able to access food, they cannot consume anything that could cause weight gain. If they are outside, possibly bored and have any money in their pocket, they can find a shop and buy calories. The biggest bang for the buck comes from the junk. I've watched children in newsagents (small stores for Americans) spend quite some time working out the most they can get for whatever coins they have on them.

In the *Larger than Life* TV programme, referred to in the introduction to Part Two and in Chapter Seven, Dr. Ian Campbell tried to analyse the weight that Lisa and Larry should have been gaining, according to the calorie formula. In the other two cases, Paul and Jacqui, he estimated how much exercise they would need to do to use up the calories they were consuming. With reference to Paul, Dr. Campbell said that "it is physically and physiologically impossible for Paul to burn off the calories he consumes." I.e., not withstanding the fact that Paul is bedridden, there is nothing he could physically do in one day that would match what he consumes in one day. The narrator added "To burn off what Jacqui eats in a day (15,880 calories) she'd have to walk briskly non-stop for almost two days."

This nicely illustrates a mathematical reality – a human can eat more in a defined period, than is physically possible to expend. We can, however, *always* adjust the intake to match the body's need. Why focus on the part of the equation that is the least malleable?

Michael Phelps (eight gold medals at the Beijing Olympics, 2008) arguably has the highest energy requirement in the world, with an estimated 12,000 calories needed to fuel his Olympic achievements.[305] Phelps doesn't swim an average 50 miles a week to compensate for his gluttony. His eating is driven by his activity. We should learn from this and prioritise food intake as the key determinant. We need to manage what people eat, not assume that activity can ever, let alone always, compensate for this.

Imagine that you and I had a competition. We each had to take one half of a number of pairs of twins and make sure that our group lost weight. Let us assume that one of us could pick the diet for both groups and the other could pick the exercise for both groups. Which option would you choose? I would opt for food and win every time. I would take my group off all processed food and put your group on unlimited (and only) processed food. You would no doubt schedule as much exercise as you could for your group and have my group totally inactive. My group would struggle to be inactive, as they would have so much natural nutrition and energy. Your group would struggle to be active, trying to live on non nutritious calories. If your group did manage to do more, I would expect them to eat more because the activity would make them hungry. With more processed food I am confident that your group would gain, while mine would lose.

The Department of Endocrinology and Metabolism at the Peninsula Medical School in Plymouth, UK, has made some very interesting findings as part of the "EarlyBird Diabetes Study."[306] The study identified a random sample of the 1995-96 birth cohort from Plymouth. 54 primary schools consented to take part. 307 children (137 girls, 170 boys, mean age 4.9), who started school between January 2000 and January 2001 were chosen for the study. The study was designed to try to understand why some children develop diabetes and others do not. However, it has also provided many invaluable insights into obesity and physical activity along the way.

The Peninsula research team have found consistent evidence for the concept of a 'set' activity level. The first study was presented in the *British Medical Journal* (2003).[307] The participants were 215 children (120 boys and 95 girls, aged 7-10.5, mean 9 years) from three schools with different sporting facilities and opportunity for physical education (PE) in the curriculum. School 1, a private school with some boarding pupils, had extensive facilities and 9 hours a week of physical education in the curriculum. School 2, a village school, offered 2.2 hours of timetabled physical education a week. School 3, an inner city school with limited sporting provision, offered 1.8 hours of physical education a week. The team said of the results: "Surprisingly, total physical activity between schools was similar because children in Schools 2 and 3 did correspondingly more activity out of school than children at School 1. Among the boys, total activity was higher in School 2 than in School 1 and School 3 with mean (standard deviation) units of activity a week of 39.1 (6.8), 34.7 (7.7), and 33.8 (7.8)."

The conclusion was: "The total amount of physical activity done by primary school children does not depend on how much physical education is timetabled at school because children compensate out of school."

The study was extended over a longer period of time and the researchers presented updated findings at the May 2009 European Congress on Obesity in

Amsterdam. The study group remained of similar size, 206 children, ages 7 to 11, from the same three schools in and around Plymouth. Over the longer study, the private school children had an average of 9.2 hours per week of scheduled activity, children at the two other schools got 2.4 hours and 1.7 hours of PE per week, respectively. Again, the study found that, no matter how much scheduled activity the children were given, they were similarly active overall. The children who had been doing organised PE were doing little outside school. The ones who had less scheduled exercise were more likely to head out on their bike, or play football, after school.

I have observed similar patterns with adults. Those who regularly go to the gym and participate in scheduled exercise classes, often have little energy and inclination to be active at other times. They report going to the gym on the way home from work and then "collapsing on the sofa" all evening. Those who don't have the time (or inclination) to go to the gym are more often active throughout the day, on their feet at work, running errands, cleaning, cooking and managing the household.

Conclusion

Theoretically, the idea that obesity is caused by sedentary behaviour and that exercise will be the cure, is fundamentally flawed as it relies upon both "The General Principle" and "The Calorie Formula".

Empirically, the 'sloth' argument has no substantiating evidence. We need to be able to prove that sedentary behaviour has caused obesity; that the increase in obesity can be precisely explained by an equally quantifiable decrease in activity and that the timing of the obesity epidemic can similarly be explained. On either side of the Atlantic, the evidence for even a general relationship is at best "moderate" and at worst "not compelling". For a specific correlation on amount and timing, the evidence is non existent. Anecdotal arguments can be equally easily undermined with evidence.

Working solely in the field of obesity, I have a number of final observations:

- I see no discernible difference between the size of people I see at the gym/pool and those I see in the high street. Look at the line up of the non athlete runners for a marathon or 'fun' run and they are a representative sample of that country's population.
- The two most difficult groups of people that I work with, from a weight loss perspective, are vegetarians and fitness enthusiasts. The vegetarians have cut out the only two zero carbohydrate food groups (although eggs are virtually carbohydrate-free) and therefore their food intake always impacts insulin and thereby facilitates fat storage. The fitness enthusiasts need carbohydrates to fuel their unnatural activities ('carb loading' being familiar terminology in fitness magazines). The human body can walk long distances and sprint short distances with little or no carbohydrate intake. The fitness fanatics, who cycle five hours up hill, as an example, report that they will faint/collapse if they don't have carbohydrate loaded meals and energy gels and bars. I believe them. If they want to lose weight, they need to cut both the

carbohydrate and the unnatural exercise and be more naturally active and nourished instead.

- The term "exercise addiction" was first used by Dr. William Glasser in 1976, who studied long distance runners. I see more incidence of exercise addiction than I do eating disorders and one often follows from the other. A person with an eating disorder can all too easily replace an obsession with food with an obsession with exercise (often not stopping the food obsession completely either). Withdrawal symptoms from not being able to exercise are well known and have been noted to appear within a week.[308]

I ask people who do 'unnatural' exercise why they do it and as many say that they enjoy it as those who readily admit that they don't. Probe the first group further and common elucidations are: a) that they like the effect more than the exercise itself;[xlix] b) that they don't enjoy it at the time, but do enjoy it coming to an end; and c) that they feel bad if they don't exercise. That's the withdrawal of addiction. It would be much better for overall health if these people did something more natural and something that they enjoyed. (The most extreme answer I received to that question is "you get to the point where you think you're going to die and then you get to the point where you wish you had.")

For those who don't enjoy exercise and also for many who think that they do, there is a pain/gain association. Sometimes exercisers will suffer pain in advance, so that they don't 'feel guilty' over consuming food or drink later on. Others have the gain first and can then be found in the gym 'working off' the indulgence as some kind of punishment. The phrase "no pain, no gain" is a favourite of fitness enthusiasts.

Just as we did with the five-a-day campaign, we should ask the question – even in the absence of evidence that sedentary behaviour has caused the obesity epidemic, or that exercise will cure it – is exercise a good thing to do?

If we follow the advice of pyramids and plates and base our meals on starchy foods, exercise is a vital thing to do. Carbohydrate can only be used for energy; it can't repair cells and perform the basal metabolic roles reserved for fat and protein. If we eat carbohydrate in the recommended quantity and *don't* 'get on our bike' we will store that carbohydrate as fat. If we more sensibly base our meals on foods such as meat, fish, eggs and vegetables, we don't have to make time for burning off carbohydrates. We can get on with our day and the body gets on with its planned maintenance.

My personal view on exercise is, just as I think that we should eat as we have evolved to eat, I advocate doing what we have evolved to do. I do not believe that there is anything natural about running marathons, pumping iron or spinning on stationary bikes. It is far more natural to walk, talk, dance, sing, cook, clean and tend the land. If there were a polite verb for sex, I would have included one. Human priorities have gone awry when 'grunting' is a solitary activity in the gymnasium, rather than a shared activity in the bedroom.

[xlix] This can be the during-exercise effect of the 'high', the 'burn', the endorphins being released or it can be the post-exercise effect on their body shape and structure.

Activity has a key role to play in childhood development. The damage done to our young people, by video and computer games, is multi dimensional. We have examples of repetitive strain injury in five year olds.[309] These 'games' are often horrifically violent and mentally disturbing. We have developed a teenage generation with an abnormal need for constant stimulus and with the concomitant attention span of toddlers. Perhaps worst of all, we have developed a self-reliant, less-social generation, more capable of interacting with a control pad and a screen than their fellow human beings.

Just as our mothers and grandmothers were right about food, so they were right about play. My brother and I would be encouraged out of the house after breakfast and discouraged from returning until the next meal time. We had no money in our pockets for sweets; snacks were simply not part of our vocabulary, so we developed a natural appetite for three good meals a day early on. We made friends; we explored; we invented things; we turned paving slabs into a hopscotch board; we resolved disputes; we appointed leaders; we agreed rules; we built things; we discovered wildlife. We had the most incredible social, emotional, mental and physical development – all through play. The tragedy of electronic entertainment is not that we sit on the sofa *per se*, but all that we have lost in so doing.

One of the obstacles to resuming the childhood that children should have is that parents fear harm coming to their young. The odds of a child in America being abducted are one in 347,000.[310] The odds of an American child being obese are one in five. Let the children play. The key thing is to let them play *without a snack.* As we will see in Chapter Sixteen the dangers are more likely in the sweets that we give children, than in the strangers from whom we try to protect them.

There are many good reasons to exercise, but to try to create a calorie deficit with the goal of trying to lose weight, is not one of them – not least because the body's natural response to this will be 'eat more/do less'. Our goal with activity should be the well established S's: stamina, suppleness and strength and all three of these can be achieved without running marathons. I would add another S – stress – as there is medium evidence for a moderate therapeutic effect of exercise on depression and mental wellbeing.[311] I suggest that alleviation of stress will especially require that the exercise is found to be enjoyable by the person. Dancing, yoga and/or walking a dog are all more likely to have benefits for mental wellbeing than 'going for the burn'.

As we will see in the final part of this book on "how can we stop the obesity epidemic", my recommended public health campaign message would be "eat naturally; move naturally". Walk, talk, dance, sing, cook, clean and tend the land, as captured above, is a fair summary of what we should do. Aerobics classes are not on the list, which takes us full circle to how we started this chapter.

Part Four

How can we stop The Obesity Epidemic?

Part Four

How can we stop The Obesity Epidemic?

One principle alone would be *sufficient* to stop the obesity epidemic. Whether it is *necessary* is the only matter for debate. That one principle would be a return to eating real food, as provided by nature and stopping the mass consumption of processed food, as provided by food manufacturers. The works of the explorer physicians at the turn of the twentieth century provide evidence for disease following 'civilisation' and the general absence of disease before 'civilisation'. Cancer was a key study area for many of these physicians. In parts of the world where there is still no processed food, and people are forced to live off the land, there is little or no obesity, heart disease, cancer, diabetes or other modern illness.[312] We say that we are the developed nations and condescendingly call such places 'under-developed', even primitive. If super morbid obesity is the pinnacle of developed societies, which really is the more advanced?

To achieve what sounds like a relatively simple goal will require some fundamental change in all of these 'developed' nations.

1) First, we must reverse the current advice. We must make a bold and clear announcement changing our advice back to what it was before we started the obesity epidemic. We must return to knowing that "Farinaceous and vegetable foods are fattening, and saccharine matters are especially so". This will mean a concomitant pardon for fat (as found in real food). The clear distinction needs to be made that it is *not* "fat is bad and carbohydrate is good", but "processed food is bad and real food is good".

2) We need an organisational design review, as would be done with major restructuring in the private sector, thus aligning strategy, shared values and all the processes necessary to achieve change. We need one body managing obesity, one goal, one message, not the many bodies with the multiple messages that we have now. This body needs to have the authority to intervene, with similar methods that we have adopted to tackle cigarette smoking and alcohol abuse. The clear target needs to be processed food and not any real food, as provided by nature. This will involve new incentives and retraining and all of these will be covered in detail in Chapter Sixteen.

3) We start Part Four with something that needs to happen immediately – no progress can be made until we end conflicts of interest. We cannot move away from processed food towards real food when our diet advice and agencies have been so comprehensively infiltrated by the food and drink industry. Surely it can't be that bad. Well, let us see...

Chapter Fifteen

Conflicts of interest

Fiction or fact?

Imagine you are a multi billion dollar food/drink company. Your stakeholders are essentially customers, employees and shareholders. The company needs to grow – growth means more returns for shareholders and employees may also benefit from higher returns. For real growth (beyond price inflation), you need any, or ideally all, of the following options: existing customers to buy more current products; existing customers to buy new products; new customers to buy current products and new customers to buy new products – and that is generally recognised to be the order of difficulty.

Unless a private company, you have to report quarterly to world markets and your financial position is affected every time you do this and hence you are under continuous pressure to meet, if not exceed, expectations (you have to manage expectations very carefully, however, as exceeding them establishes a new norm). You are also doing none of this in isolation – you have competitors who also want to grow. In fact they want to grow faster than you, so that they can get a better financial position from an influx of investors keen to benefit from their dividends.

The fact that real growth can never be sustained seems to have been overlooked by financial markets and investors. If the Top 10 listed companies in the USA were countries, with their revenue equating to GDP, they would fall into the range occupied by the Top 55 countries in the world.[313] America's largest company, Wal-Mart, was noted in the 2010 Fortune 500 list as having a revenue figure of \$408 billion. According to the International Monetary Fund list of companies by GDP, Wal-Mart would knock Sweden out of 22nd place on the world ranking. The compound interest calculation tells us that just 3.5% sales growth a year (a 'reasonable' shareholder expectation) would double the company revenue every 20 years.

So, expectations are unreasonable, you need growth and the last thing you want is anything that can threaten current revenue, let alone future developments. As a food/drink manufacturer you cannot afford to have any public health advice going against any of your products or planned developments. This would be disastrous. It would be really helpful in fact if public health advice could be promoting your products – this would be idyllic. PepsiCo, the top company on the food consumer products Fortune 500 list, would surely welcome universal low calorie advice to be reiterated. Pepsi Max, Diet Pepsi – you have many options to satisfy this want – even cherry flavour.

Kellogg's, sixth on the Food Consumer Products Fortune 500 list, would no doubt be thrilled to hear the public being told to eat breakfast. Even better that the public are actively told to avoid bacon and eggs and thus (sugary) cereal becomes the normal start to the day.

It would be really helpful for food/drink companies if the public received a consistent message (supporting your products). That USA food pyramid is just great for a cereal company – five to eight ounces of grains per day and three cups of milk – cereal is surely the easiest way to get those. The UK 'eatwell' plate even has a box of cornflakes on it – branded (Kellogg's) in some versions. "Base your meals on starchy foods". Even the confectionery and soft drink producers have nothing to complain about – the 'eatwell' plate has that great 8% segment (let's round it to 10% – that's a good 200-250 calories a day for us). The USA government 'allows' the same with the discretionary calories covered in Chapter Thirteen. This is terrific stuff.

But, irritatingly, there are rogue traders – nutritionists who tend to (quite outrageously) care about nutrition and the nutritional quality of things that we put in to our bodies. Many of them are telling people to avoid processed foods and sugar. Fitness instructors are telling people to avoid refined carbohydrates and to only eat whole grains, heaven forbid. Even chiropractors, for goodness sake, are advising people to avoid processed food, especially carbohydrates, to lose weight and ease the burden on joints and frames. This must stop.

Imagine then if you could contain dietary advice – particularly all access to public health advice – to one organisation. If only that one dietary organisation could have a monopoly on all dietary advice. Wouldn't it be great if laws were passed so that no nutritionists, chiropractors, or any other qualified therapists could provide advice or run a practice – that only the members of one dietary association could do this. How much easier things would be if food and drink companies could then sponsor just that one organisation and try to ensure that only the 'right' messages got out?

The plot for the next John Grisham novel? Sadly not. This is reality in 46 of the 50 States of America.

The American experience

The Commission on Dietetic Registration (CDR) is the credentialing agency for the American Dietetic Association (ADA).[314]

Their mission statement is "CDR protects the public through credentialing and assessment processes that assure the competence of registered dietitians and dietetic technicians, registered."[315]

The vision statement is "The nation recognizes seeks out and relies on competent CDR credentialed registered dietitians and dietetic technicians, registered, for food and nutrition expertise."

The CDR was formed in 1969. In 1976 the ADA constitution was amended to allow for registration separate from Association membership (this ensured that all dietitians would be part of the movement going forward, by virtue of being a dietitian rather than needing to be a paid up member of the ADA). In

1984 the first registration eligibility reciprocity agreement was signed with the Canadian Dietetic Association. In 1991 registration eligibility reciprocity was extended to foreign countries whose goals were comparable to CDR's. In 1992 the first such agreement was signed with the Dutch Association of Dietitians. In 1995 the CDR filed registration eligibility requirements and reciprocity agreements with the USA Trade Representative Office and World Trade Organization. By 2010, 79,411 dietitians were registered with the CDR.

At the time of writing this book, 46 out of the 50 States of America have passed laws to regulate who is able to provide nutritional advice through licensure, statutory certification or registration. The full list of which states have passed each level of restriction is published in Appendix 4.[316]

The most restrictive level is *Licensing* – where statutes include an explicitly defined scope of practice and performance of the profession is illegal without first obtaining a license from the state. Nonlicensed practitioners may be subject to prosecution for practicing without a license. 35 states have gone for this highest level of legislation. 25 of these 35 bills were standard ADA bills – the statute has clearly been submitted by the ADA to establish the monopoly position of their dietitian members. Of the 35 states that have passed bills for licensing regulations, 16 have stated that only dietitians can practise in the field of nutrition. Nutritionists may no longer do so. They must retrain as dietitians and become members of the ADA and be recognised by the CDR, or face prosecution. This is clear monopoly practice.

In nine states, nutritionists have been allowed to continue to do their jobs in accordance with their professional qualifications. However, the precise qualifications deemed acceptable have been narrowly defined by the state and many have added an additional requirement to complete 900 hours work under the supervision of a dietitian. This is insulting and restrictive.

A further 10 licensed states have also granted monopoly rights to dietitians, as their statutes use the terms dietitian and nutritionist, interchangeably, but to mean dietitian – defined as a dietitian, again, registered with the ADA and CDR. As an example of legislative clauses, here are some extracts from the Tennessee statute:

- "American Dietetic Association – When the acronym A.D.A. appears in these rules it is intended to mean American Dietetic Association".
- "Dietitian and Nutritionist – A licensed health care professional practicing dietetics/nutrition. 'Dietitian' or 'nutritionist' may be used interchangeably."
- "Registered Dietitian (R.D.) – A person who is currently registered by the Commission on Dietetic Registration of the American Dietetic Association."
- "It is unlawful for any person who is not licensed in the manner prescribed in T.C.A. §§ 63-25-101, et seq., to represent himself as a dietitian or a nutritionist or to hold himself out to the public as being licensed by means of using a title on signs, mailboxes, address plates, stationery, announcements, telephone listings, calling cards, or other instruments of professional identification or to use such titles as 'dietitian/nutritionist', 'licensed dietitian', 'licensed nutritionist' or such letters as 'L.D.N L.D.' or 'L.N.'"[317]

This makes the law very clear – these statutes serve to meet the requirements of the ADA i.e. thou shall be a dietitian registered by the CDR of the ADA, or thou shall be prosecuted.

The second level down is *Statutory certification* – which limits use of particular titles (e.g. dietitian or nutritionist) to persons meeting predetermined requirements, while persons not certified can still practice the occupation or profession. Ten states have opted for statutory certification.

One state, California, has opted for *Registration*, which is the least restrictive form of state regulation. As with certification, unregistered persons are permitted to practise the profession.

Four states, Arizona, Colorado, New Jersey and Wyoming have, thus far, refused to pass the ADA sponsored legislation.

Dietitians in America, therefore, enjoy a unique monopoly position and they have unfettered access to hospitals, schools, large institutions, prisons – all public health diet advice. When Michelle Obama launched her childhood obesity initiative, at the United States conference of mayors on 20 January 2010, she said that mayors were key to making the plan work. In subsequent speeches, no mention of mayors was made. Perhaps someone had explained to the First Lady that mayors were not allowed to help with dietary programmes. As a result of the legislation passed by previous government, that was the domain of dietitians. Thanks to the elimination of, or at least strict control over, nutritional practice, in over ninety percent of the States in America, dietitians also have sole access to private health advice. So, it is critical for us to know who is behind this monopolistic advice.

The *partners* of the American Dietetic Association (ADA) are as follows.[318] The 2008 or 2009 revenue figures, for each sponsor, are alongside:[319]

- Aramark (a 'dining away from home' company) – $12.3 billion;
- Coca-Cola – $31.4 billion;
- GlaxoSmithKline – $45.2 billion (not listed on the web site, but listed in the 2008 ADA annual report);
- National Dairy Council – The National Dairy Council is the nutrition research, education and communications arm of Dairy Management Incorporated. (All but one of the current spokespeople for the organisation is a registered dietitian);
- PepsiCo – $44.3 billion;
- Unilever (including spreads) – $55.8 billion (using a Euro dollar exchange of 1.4 for this Anglo Dutch company).

The *premium sponsors* of the American Dietetic Association (ADA) are as follows:

- Abbott Nutrition (infant formulas, nutrition bars etc) – parent company revenue was $30.8 billion;
- Corowise (including products designed to lower cholesterol) – parent company, Cargill, revenue was $116.6 billion;
- General Mills ("the world's sixth largest food company") – $14.9 billion;

- Kellogg's – $12.7 billion;
- Mars – $30 billion;
- McNeil Nutritionals (makers of Splenda sweeteners) – the revenue of the parent company, Johnson & Johnson, was $63.8 billion;
- SoyJoy (sugared cereal bars) – the revenue of the parent company, Otsuka Pharmaceuticals, was $9.2 billion (on the web site, but not in the 2008 annual report);
- Truvia (sweetener) – the parent company is Cargill, as above (on the ADA web site, but not in the 2008 annual report).

That adds up to $467 billion worth of revenue amongst a dozen organisations that sponsor the ADA.

There are also *event sponsors* listed in the 2008 annual report:

- American Beverage Association, formerly the National Soft Drink Association – this is the 'voice' of the soft drink industry – Coca-Cola and PepsiCo are members, as examples;
- ConAgra Foods – producers of an assortment of processed foods for stores, restaurant and food service establishments;
- Post Cereals – a cereal manufacturer;
- Safeway – grocery retailer.

There is also mention in the 2008 annual report of funding from the Grocery Manufacturers Association. Finally, the annual report thanks donors who made gifts of $10,000 or more to support research, education and public awareness initiatives: Abbott Nutrition; Almond Board of California; American Council for Fitness and Nutrition; Aramark; The Beef Checkoff, through the National Cattlemen's Beef Association; The Coca-Cola Company; Colgate Palmolive; Consultant Dietitians in Health Care Facilities DPG; Corowise brand; Dietitians in Nutrition Support DPG; Ecolab Inc.; Ensure; General Mills; GlaxoSmithKline Consumer Healthcare; Kellogg Company; Kraft Foods; Mars, Incorporated; McNeil Nutritionals, LLC; Mead Johnson Nutritionals; National Dairy Council; PepsiCo; Unilever and Washington State Dietetic Association.

For the year ending 31 May 2008, total revenue for the ADA was just short of $32 million. $2.7 million was noted as coming from sponsorship. I have no idea how much it costs to sponsor legislation in 46 states across America. More than a couple of millions I suspect. Lobbying may have been funded directly from partner/sponsor organisations, but this is not about a forensic exercise in multi billion dollar balance sheets. This is about two thoughts to put to you:

1) What do the American Dietetic Association and their partner/sponsor organisations from the food, drink and drug industries stand to gain from this legislation?
2) What does America and its 309 million citizens stand to lose?

National dietary associations

The sponsors of the Dietary Association of Australia (DAA) include Kellogg's, Nestle and Unilever.

The sponsors of the British Dietetic Association (BDA) are apparently confidential. I wrote to the BDA on 14 December 2009 asking for the details of their sponsors. I received no reply so I wrote to Pauline Douglas, the chair of the BDA, on 15 January 2010 and received a reply within a couple of hours from the partnerships and sponsorship officer at the BDA. The email said:

"The BDA does work with a wide variety of organisations – including commercial companies, business groups representing major commodities (e.g. flour, fish, sugar), not-for-profit associations and government departments.

"As you will be aware, the specific financial details relating to individual projects are confidential and we would not share this information outside the BDA.

"The BDA is proud of its partnerships and we have strict guidelines governing our collaborations to maintain an ethical and consistent approach."

I wrote back to say "I don't understand the secrecy, as other organisations openly share this kind of information on their web sites." (I then included the links to the American Dietetic Association, Dietitians Association of Australia, National Obesity Forum and The Association for the Study of Obesity, as examples). I continued...

"Please are you able to explain why the British Dietetic Association sponsors need to be confidential, when those of other organisations are not and please are you able to share any more about the links with sugar? I can't think why an organisation advising about healthy eating would want any association with such a product?"

I received the following reply: "There is no secrecy, we acknowledge the role of partners on each project as the collaboration is under way, it's just not currently compiled into a single list." And the email went on to say:"... we have been delighted to work with the Sugar Bureau..."

How can any dietary association be *delighted* to work with the Sugar Bureau? How can I "trust a dietitian to know about nutrition" (their little slogan) when they so joyfully partner with the least nutritious substance that we consume on a staggeringly regular basis? I expect that a number of dietitians are unaware of this and, hopefully, equally appalled.

I wrote to the Department of Health on 6 May 2010 informing them of the BDA non disclosure position: "As dietitians have a virtual monopoly on delivering Department of Health and NHS dietary advice – throughout the public sector and, more often than not, the private sector, I think that non disclosure is unreasonable. I respectfully request that the sponsors of the BDA, the body comprising the UK's dietitians, be disclosed." I received a reply on the 10 May 2010: "The BDA is independent from the Department of Health and is not accountable to it. I would therefore advise you to pursue the matter with the BDA directly."

I wrote back the same day: "But the British Dietetic Association has a virtual monopoly on nutrition and diet advice in all Department of Health institutions – hospitals, surgeries, clinics and they are the first point of contact for diet consultations. The Eatbadly Plate is on the walls of schools, clinics and hospitals nationwide with pictures of a box of cornflakes, white bread, white bagels, sugared baked beans, sugared tins of fruit, sugared yoghurts, sweets, cakes, Battenberg cake, cola drink etc. Surely you should know who their sponsors are? We have an obesity epidemic and our advice is compromised. The Department of Health cannot just turn a blind eye." I got the same reply two days later: "I can confirm that the BDA is independent from the Department; the Department is therefore unable to intervene in this matter."

The chief executive's foreword (Andy Burman) in the 2008-09 annual report of the BDA notes "We now have our first national partners with Danone and Abbott and we hope to announce new partners over the coming year or so." There is reference to a "Bird's Eye" education award, but no mention of other partners or sponsors. The accounts for 2009 showed a turnover of £2,359,013 with no details of the source for this revenue. The notes to the accounts, which could add detail to this number, are for the eyes of BDA members only.

A press release, dated 1 March 2007[320] entitled *Kellogg's: commitment to health and wellbeing*, informed me that Kellogg's had been the lead sponsor for the British Dietetic Association's annual obesity intervention campaign since 2002 (and may still be). The press release gave this as an example of Kellogg's commitment to a major programme of educational initiatives. The two other initiatives detailed were:

- Provision of "nutrition information to healthcare professionals – an example being sponsorship of the National Study of Obesity conferences"; (I'm not sure if Kellogg's meant the National Obesity Forum or the Association for the Study of Obesity – it may be difficult to keep track of one's involvement in the obesity world).
- "Since 1997 Kellogg's has invested more than £600k in the development of a network of Breakfast Clubs throughout the UK called *Breakfast Clubs Plus*... By April 2007 more than 1,000,000 breakfasts will be served at breakfast clubs supported by Kellogg's."

The opening of the press release reminds us that "Kellogg's offers a wide range of cereals (45 different products) to help consumers choose what's right for them."

Could the same happen in the UK as has happened already in the USA? I have little doubt that the BDA would like to have a monopoly position in much the same way as their American counterparts. The BDA is a trade union, after all, and such bodies are intended to act in the interests of their members.

Dietitians came up with a definition for themselves, which was accepted by 34 dietetic association members at the ICDA (International Confederation of Dietetic Associations) on 24 May 2004 in Chicago. "A dietitian is a person with qualifications in nutrition and dietetics recognised by national authority(s). The dietitian applies the science of nutrition to the feeding and education of groups of people and individuals in health and disease. The scope of dietetic practice is such that dietitians may work in a variety of settings and have a variety of work functions."

That's a harmless enough description, and not one that would lead me to worry that dietitians were determined to eliminate any competition around them. The BDA council (2007) defined a dietitian as follows:

"Registered Dietitians (RDs) are the only qualified health professionals that assess, diagnose and treat diet and nutrition problems at an individual and wider public health level. Uniquely, dietitians use the most up to date public health and scientific research on food, health and disease, which they translate into practical guidance to enable people to make appropriate lifestyle and food choices.

"Dietitians are the only nutrition professionals to be statutorily regulated, and governed by an ethical code, to ensure that they always work to the highest standard. Dietitians work in the NHS, private practice, industry, education, research, sport, media, public relations, publishing, NGOs and government. Their advice influences food and health policy across the spectrum from government, local communities and individuals." (NGOs are Non Government Organisations).

Dietitians do indeed have unique access to the NHS, private practice, industry, education, research, sport, media, public relations, publishing, NGO's and government and that is one of my key concerns given their conflicted relationships.

Just for completeness in this section, the sponsors of the UK National Obesity Forum include: Abbott Pharmaceuticals (makers of the diet drug Reductil, withdrawn from Europe in January 2010); Canderel (sweetener); GlaxoSmithKline (Alli); Lighter Life; Roche (Xenical); Safeway and Slim Fast.[321] To be fair, the National Obesity Forum also has some suitable partners – The Royal College of Paediatricians, All-Party Parliamentary Group on Obesity and The Department of Health. However, the introduction to the list of partners says "In pursuing our aims we have been assisted by, or worked jointly with the following organisations" and one suspects that the more suitable partners have been 'worked with' and the other companies more likely 'assisted by'.

The sponsors of the UK Association for the Study of Obesity include: The Cambridge Diet, Coca-Cola, GlaxoSmithKline, Kellogg's (again), Roche and Slim Fast and these are prominently featured and thanked in conference material and newsletters.

British Nutrition Foundation

The British Nutrition Foundation (BNF) was founded in 1967 and its web site says that this organisation "...exists to deliver authoritative, evidence-based information on food and nutrition in the context of health and lifestyle. Accurate interpretation of nutrition science is at the heart of all we do."

The BNF's "Sustaining members"[322] are: British Sugar PLC; Cadbury; Coca-Cola; Danone Waters and Dairies UK Ltd; J Sainsbury PLC; Kellogg's; Kraft Foods UK Ltd; Nestle UK Ltd; PepsiCo; Premier Foods (RHM Technology Limited); Tate & Lyle Sugar; Unilever PLC; WM Morrisons Supermarkets PLC. Presumably sustaining members are members that keep the organisation going?

The BNF's "members"[323] are: 3663 (the UK's leading food service company); AgroFresh; AHDB Meat Services Ltd; Ajinomoto/ Nutrasweet Switzerland AG; Arla Foods UK PLC; ASDA Stores Ltd; Associated British Foods PLC; Bernard Matthews PLC; Coca-Cola; Dairy Crest Ltd; GlaxoSmithKline; H J Heinz Ltd; Home Grown Cereals Authority; Innocent Drinks; J Sainsbury PLC; Kellogg's; Kerry Foods; Lighter Life; Marks & Spencer PLC; Mars UK Ltd; McCain Foods Ltd; McDonald's Restaurants Ltd; NcNeil Consumer Nutritionals (makers of Splenda and Benecol amongst other products); Müller Dairy; Nabim (the representative organisation for the UK flour milling industry); National Starch; Northern Foods PLC; PepsiCo UK Ltd; Pizza Express; Potato Council Ltd; Procter and Gamble Limited (Pringles); R Twinnings & Co (tea producers); Slimming World; The Co-Operative Group Ltd; The Jordans and Ryvita Company Ltd; United Biscuits (UK) Limited; Wagamama (restaurants and take outs); Waitrose Ltd; Weetabix Ltd; WM Morrisons Supermarkets PLC and Yoplait Dairy Crest.

The 2008-09 annual report shows that income for this financial year for the BNF was £1,581,298, of which 54% came from donations and subscriptions – presumably from the members; 40% came from projects – the report detailed examples of reports funded by the Food Standards Agency and the European Commission and 6% from publications, conferences and investments.[324]

The chairman of the board of trustees to the BNF is Paul Hebblethwaite. He has a stated affiliation with Cadbury Schweppes (having worked there for the majority of his career between 1984 and 2007).[325] Hebblethwaite has run his own consultancy since 2007, called *Sustained Advantage Ltd* which offers strategic advice to food and related industry partners in the areas of innovation, efficiency, quality, reputation and sustainability.

The honorary vice president listed in the 2008-09 annual report of the BNF is Mr IGT Ferguson, chief executive, Tate & Lyle Sugars. The honorary treasurer is Mr CJ Hart – formerly research and development manager, Weetabix Limited.

Professor Anne de Looy, professor of dietetics, University of Plymouth, is a scientific governor and a member of the board of trustees. A fellow researcher, Helena Wojtczak, sent me a publication endorsed by Professor de Looy, suggesting that there may be a P missing in her surname, as the brochure, called *Losing Weight & Keeping it Off* contained gems such as:

- "Puddings, cakes, biscuits, cereal bars and confectionery all contain carbohydrate, but choose those with a lower fat content. Some lower fat examples include: arctic roll, sorbets, fruit yoghurt, trifle, rice pudding, currant buns, fig rolls, jelly beans and mints." (I kid you not).

233

- "Have up to three snacks a day and choose fruit or low-fat types of biscuits, confectionery or buns such as iced buns, currant buns or scones."
- "I welcome this leaflet which contains sound, practical advice on long term weight loss. It reflects the current scientific consensus of the importance of a well-balanced, high carbohydrate diet in weight control". Anne de Looy, professor of dietetics, Centre for Nutrition and Food Research, Queen Margaret College, Edinburgh.

This booklet is available on the Sugar Bureau's web site.[326] Wojtczak was given her copy by Carisbrooke House, a general practice in St Leonards On Sea, east Sussex, UK and she has also seen them being given out by a local pharmacy on the King's Road in London.

Industrial governors of the British Nutrition Foundation include Ms J Batchelar, Sainsbury's director of brand; Mr R J Fletcher, director scientific affairs, Kellogg Europe (also a member of the board of trustees); Mr D Gregory, technical director Marks and Spencer PLC; Mr Hebblethwaite is noted as an industrial governor and a former science director of Cadbury Schweppes; Miss A Heughan, external affairs director Unilever Bestfoods UK (also a member of the board of trustees) and Mr J W Sutcliffe, chief executive grocery Associated British Foods PLC (also a member of the board of trustees).

As a member of the Association for the Study of Obesity, I received an email on 8 February 2010 inviting me to a conference on sweeteners being run by the British Nutrition Foundation. The one day conference was called *The Science of low calorie sweeteners – separating fact from fiction*. Speakers included Mary Quinlan, manager of sweetener technology development, Tate & Lyle and Dr. Colette Shortt, McNeil Nutritionals Ltd (makers of Splenda). I shared the audacity of the invitation on my Facebook page on 9 February 2010 saying: "Can you believe this? I've been invited by the Association for the Study of Obesity to a conference run by the British Nutrition Foundation on "Sweeteners". Speakers include Ms sweetener development from Tate & Lyle and Dr. someone from Splenda. Why are the ASO/BNF facilitating access for sweetener manufacturers to obesity professionals? Am I supposed to be converted into thinking I must go and munch some artificial chemicals?"

I was obviously not alone in spotting this conflict of interest. The Independent newspaper (Phil Chamberlain and Jeremy Lawrence) ran an excellent story on 22 March 2010 called: *Is the British Nutrition Foundation having its cake and eating it too?*[327]

In Chapter Ten we saw that government healthy eating messages are confusing and even the source of government messages is confusing. One common tip, however, is "Base your meals on starchy foods" (Food Standards Agency's top tip) and the eight government guidelines for healthy eating state "Eat plenty of foods rich in starch and fibre". Both the FSA and the BNF promote the 'eatwell' plate, which recommends 33% of intake in the form of starchy carbohydrate and 100% of intake can contain insulin stimulating carbohydrate. My number one tip is "eat real food" and I would advise restricting even 'good' carbohydrate for weight management. How many of the sponsors of the BNF would remain if these were the main pieces of advice from the organisation? I suspect no more than AHDB Meat Services Ltd and possibly Dairy Crest.

The BNF's 2008-09 annual report gives details of the education programme that it runs. *Energy Balance* is an interactive tool designed to help children aged 8 to 11 years old understand how to balance energy in and energy out. The annual report notes that there were 648,662 visitors to the site and 1,500,000 downloads. My heart sank when I read those statistics – that is a vast number of UK children growing up having been taught the misapplication of thermodynamics. I wonder what will happen to those who may study applied mathematics or physics later in education and whether this incorrect information will be corrected. The energy (calorie) obsession also plays into the hands of the many sponsor organisations who want UK PLC to continue eating processed food – so long as they can count the calorie content of this food.

Princess Anne, the Princess Royal, is patron of the British Nutrition Foundation and the Queen of England is the patron for the British Dietetic Association. I wonder if either of these members of the royal family knows that they are patrons of societies so intimately connected with the food industry.

And three more...

The International Life Sciences Institute (ILSI) "is a nonprofit, worldwide organization whose mission is to improve public health and well-being by engaging academic, government and industry scientists in a neutral forum to advance scientific understanding in the areas related to nutrition, food safety, risk assessment, and the environment. ILSI receives its funding from its industry members, governments, and foundations."[328] The board of trustees lists 31 members, including representatives from: Kraft foods; Sanofi-Aventis; The Coca-Cola company and Coca-Cola Europe; PepsiCo; Mars; Kellogg's Europe; Monsanto (agricultural company); Lotte Company (Korean food company); Kikkoman Corporation (soy sauce); Akzo Nobel (powder coatings); Danone; Nestle and General Mills.[329] The organisation arranges events such as the "Symposium on Saturated and Trans Fats: where do we stand?" (Sydney, Australia, 17 June 2010). The programme details open with "Saturated Fat, Trans Fats, and adverse Health Impact, are issues that we hear often in the press. As we know, the press can sensationalise and take key pieces of information out of context. So what are the facts?" With the board of trustees as is, we can probably guess where they stand and 'facts' can likely be found to support this position.

The British newspaper *The Guardian* reported "In the lead-up to the international conference on nutrition in 1992, where the first ever plan of action for world nutrition was to be devised, preparatory meetings turned into spats over whether sugar should be mentioned. The anti-sugar nutritionists found themselves at loggerheads with ILSI-sponsored scientists who claimed that there was no evidence to discredit sugar. Indeed, two ILSI delegates were senior executives at Mars and Coca-Cola – two of the world's biggest sugar users. The outcome was that the world's first plan of Action for nutrition does not provide any guidelines for sugar consumption."[330] The report does indeed *not* mention sugar once in its 50 pages.[331]

The Department of Health, Change4Life programme, managed by the UK National Health Service, has the logos of 75 partner organisations on their web site.[332] Kellogg's, PepsiCo and Unilever are the familiar names that stand out. The £75 million programme was criticised for the involvement of Business4Life partners from the outset. Marketing Week[333] noted that Richard Watts, co-ordinator of the Children's Food Campaign at lobby group Sustain, was concerned that allowing companies to use the Change4Life logo gave companies "tacit support". Unilever used the Change4Life logo along the Flora London Marathon route. Kellogg's have been sponsors of the Amateur Swimming Association's (ASA) awards scheme, with the "Kellogg's Swimtastic Awards" as a key annual event. In 2009, these awards featured a new logo: Swim4Life. Bruce Learner, corporate social responsibility manager at Kellogg's, said: "Our partnership with the ASA began in 1996, since then more than 15 million swimming awards have been presented to youngsters across the country."[334] The ASA annual report (2004)[335] said, under the heading "Another Grrreat Year", "It's been another financially successful year for the Kellogg's Frosties ASA Awards Scheme..." Under the heading "Swimtastic", the report continued: "The Annual Awards Gala Dinner, now known as Swimtastic, was held... Tony the Tiger was of course around to lend a helping paw of support to everyone."

Kellogg's were regularly featured in the British press during February, March and April 2010 following their campaign "Ever thought of Coco Pops after school?" Christine Haigh of the Children's Food Campaign noted that the cereal maker's advertising did not align with its role as a partner for Change4Life. "It's outrageous that Kellogg's, which is a partner of Change4Life, is encouraging children to eat more of their sugary products," she said. *The Guardian* reported in April that 26 people and organisations complained to the Advertising Standards Authority that the advert was irresponsible because it targeted schoolchildren, and encouraged them to eat a snack that was particularly high in sugar.[336] The ASA rejected the complaints, accepting the Kellogg's argument that although Coco Pops are approximately 35% sugar, there is no current UK or EU definition of "high" as far as sugar content is concerned.

I wrote to both Kellogg's and the Department of Health and received an email back from the Department of Health on 11 March 2010 saying "Whilst this work cited for Coco Pops is not activity to support Change4Life, we understand the concerns raised and are seeking a meeting with Kellogg to discuss the matter with them." Kellogg's sent me back a comprehensive defence of sugar,[337] essentially saying that Coco Pops were no worse than other products laden with sugar. Quite so – no worse, no better.

This, of course, is a brilliant growth strategy, backed by a strong marketing campaign. Kellogg's could double sales overnight if everyone who consumed a bowl of cereal for breakfast consumed another bowl during the same day. Special K has the two week challenge: "for 2 weeks, eat a bowl (up to 45g) of any of the 10 varieties of Special K cereal for breakfast. Then have another for lunch OR your evening meal." Kelloggnutrition.com suggests: "Cereal for Supper. What's cooler and quicker than a bowl of Kellogg's cereal with summer fruits and fat-free milk?" The Coco Pops campaign was just another strand of the 'double the sales' idea – if we can get kids to eat Coco Pops when they get in from school, as well as in the morning, mums will be buying twice as much cereal each week.

Last, but certainly by no means least, the Food Standards Agency. The Food Standards Agency was set up by an Act of Parliament, dated 11 November 1999. The agency came into being on 3 April 2000. The remit is set out in the Food Standards Act:[338]

1) "There shall be a body to be called the Food Standards Agency.
2) "The main objective of the Agency in carrying out its functions is to protect public health from risks which may arise in connection with the consumption of food (including risks caused by the way in which it is produced or supplied) and otherwise to protect the interests of consumers in relation to food.
3) "The functions of the Agency are performed on behalf of the Crown."

The summary of the overall purpose of the act is as follows: "An Act to establish the Food Standards Agency and make provision as to its functions; to amend the law relating to food safety and other interests of consumers in relation to food; to enable provision to be made in relation to the notification of tests for food-borne diseases; to enable provision to be made in relation to animal feeding stuffs; and for connected purposes."

You would read this act and envisage that this new agency would have far reaching powers to demand information and enforce standards in the area of food hygiene and safety. You would not read this act and imagine that, ten years later, the Food Standards Agency would be a) starting a consultation on their proposal for a tax on saturated fat; b) that they would have been involved in nutritional food labelling, let alone having caved in to the food industry on this; c) that they would be issuing press releases, on a regular basis, on anything from advertising to children to salt consumption; or d) that they would have developed the 'eatwell' plate and managed to get it posted in schools, hospitals and surgeries UK wide.

The 'eatwell' plate has also been adopted by the British Dietetic Association and concomitantly into local authorities and health boards UK wide. It has been adopted by Diabetes UK,[1] the British Heart Foundation, Cancer Research UK and the plate is even on netmums.[339] That's our gateway to health for the children of the future, and the gatekeepers for our major modern illnesses, signed up to promoting the consumption of unprecedented levels of (processed)

---

[1] Diabetes UK lists Kellogg's as one of their corporate sponsors.

carbohydrate, in complete contrast to how we have eaten for tens of thousands of years.

Even more worrying, the 'eatwell' plate is featured on web sites for numerous food and drink companies. I stopped looking after the first six companies that came to mind all endorsed the plate: Sainsbury's; Kellogg's; PepsiCo; Coca-Cola; Nestle and Premier Foods. The latter is "the UK's largest food producer" with brands including (best known for): Cadbury (confectionery); Mr Kipling (cakes); Rank Hovis (bread); Hartley's (jam); McDougall's (flour); Fray Bentos (pies and processed meat); Gateaux (cakes); Birds (custard); Batchelors (soups); Homepride (flour) and many more. When the food and drink industry are so actively embracing public health advice isn't it time to wonder just how healthy that advice can be.

The FSA appears to have carved out a role for itself, in telling the citizens of the UK what to eat, and my reading of the Food Standards Act sees this as overstepping their remit.

We also did not need the FSA straying into this arena. We have more than enough bodies falling over themselves telling us how to eat. In just the UK, we have the Department of Health, which is the policy body and the National Health Service, which is the operational part of the Department of Health. Both of these conduct studies, produce reports and issue advice, as we saw in Chapter Ten. The FSA is still a government agency, even though it reportedly "works at 'arm's length' from Government because it doesn't report to a specific minister and is free to publish any advice it issues". The British Nutrition Foundation is a registered charity. Why is a charity, with a sponsorship list like a who's who of the food and drink industry, telling us what to eat? We have the British Dietetic Association with their dietitians trained to promote the 'eatwell' plate UK wide. Doctors and nurses probably also have advice that they pass on to patients. We have special reports commissioned, such as the Foresight report, to give us more advice. In the 2009 Annual report, the Chief Medical Officer for England presented a full list of all the reports that he had commissioned during his tenure – they ran into pages. We do not need another agency giving us diet advice and we absolutely do not need one that can't tell the difference between processed food and saturated fat.

The details of the board of the FSA are openly available on their web site.[340] There are 13 board members and a headline summary of their areas of expertise are as follows: Jeff Rooker, chairman, a member of parliament for 27 years and then minister for food safety; Dr. Ian Reynolds, deputy chairman, healthcare and meat hygiene; Professor Graeme Millar, chair of the food advisory committee in Scotland, 20 years in the NHS in Scotland; John Spence, chair of the food advisory committee in Wales, career in environment, health, drugs and alcohol; Professor Maureen Edmondson, chair of the food advisory committee in Northern Ireland, food science, agriculture and bacteriology; Professor Sue Atkinson, public health management, hygiene and tropical medicine; Tim Bennett, farming and meat hygiene; Margaret Gilmore, writer and broadcaster in homeland security, environment and food safety; Clive Grundy, human resources, with corporate experience in a catering and food service company; Michael Parker, finance, an economist and accountant; Chris Pomfret, marketing, worked for Unilever frozen foods and ice cream since 1971; Nancy Robson, consumer policy, meat quality and catering standards; Dr. David Cameron, food manufacturing, now runs his own company offering training in food safety and hygiene. Far less by way of conflict of interest here, Unilever aside, but far more concern about relevant competence. This would be a strong board for the agency that was set out in the Food Standards Act – the one intended to deal with food safety, hygiene, meat standards and so on. This is not a board suited to managing dietary and weight loss advice for the UK, let alone when the UK is facing an obesity crisis.

The FSA board takes advice from the Scientific Advisory Committee on Nutrition (SACN). Hannah Sutter, in *Big Fat Lies*[341] highlighted the lack of expertise in the area of obesity on the SACN board, concluding "an impressive list of names, but only one is an expert in diabetes and only one has a specialist interest in obesity."

I noted in Chapter Eleven that the FSA had asked SACN to review "the evidence of carbohydrate on cardio-metabolic health". The SACN terms of reference for the carbohydrate working group state: "The Scientific Advisory Committee on Nutrition is requested by the Food Standards Agency and Department of Health to provide clarification of the relationship between dietary carbohydrate and health and make public health recommendations. To achieve this they need to review:

- "The evidence for a role of dietary carbohydrate in colorectal health in adults (including colorectal cancer, IBS, constipation) and in infancy and childhood"; (IBS = irritable bowel syndrome)
- "The evidence on dietary carbohydrate and cardio-metabolic health (including cardiovascular disease, insulin resistance, glycaemic response and obesity);
- "The evidence in respect to dietary carbohydrates and oral health;
- "The terminology, classification and definitions of types of carbohydrates in the diet."

This is the only working group, as far as I am aware, which has any remit close to reviewing the overall impact of carbohydrates on health. The remit should be simple and broad – to review the impact of 30 years worth of low fat/high carbohydrate dietary advice on human health and obesity.

There are seven members of this working group and the trial of carbohydrates is in their hands. The first member is a former advertising and marketing director for J Walter Thompson (Mrs Christina Gratus). Absolutely no offence is intended when I say this is a waste of a place on this important committee. Replace Gratus with Gary Taubes and you would add to the group an exceptional, independent scientist who has researched this topic full time for five years. Next we have Anne Anderson, Professor of food choice at University of Dundee. I do not know what she can contribute to the investigation. Dr.

David Mela, our third member, works for Unilever and has an interest in food choice and eating behaviour – no doubt – and he is conflicted and he has no place on this working group. Professor Alan Jackson is a nutritionist specialising in pregnancy and foetal development, and has declared interests in Nutricia (a specialised unit of Danone food company) and Baxter Healthcare. I would suggest that he does not bring enough relevant experience to the group to excuse the conflict (if one ever can). Professor Ian Johnson (head of human nutrition, Institute of Food Research), has a specialist interest in dietary fibre and I would assume, therefore, is positively disposed towards carbohydrate – as the only source of dietary fibre. The chair of the group is Professor Ian MacDonald (professor of physiology at Nottingham University), and his research interests include nutritional and metabolic aspects of obesity, diabetes and cardiovascular disease. That is more like it – relevant areas of expertise. However, the SACN 2008 annual report lists Professor MacDonald's declared interests as Mars Europe and Coca-Cola Europe. That should rule him out from the group, let alone the role of chair. Finally, we have Professor Timothy Key, an epidemiologist specialising in cancer, and the lead investigator from Oxford on the EPIC (cancer) study. Not exactly relevant areas of expertise, but could be a useful member? You would think so, until you see his declared interests. Professor Key is a member of the Vegetarian and Vegan Societies. He must be a fan of carbohydrates, or he would have starved to death by now.

On line and on screen

Kellogg's are at the forefront of being embedded with the world of obesity. Sponsors of the USA, Australian and British Dietetic Associations, sponsors of the Association for the Study of Obesity and the British Nutrition Foundation, it is not surprising that they are leading the way in on line messages to consumers.

The company's annual report is a good starting place to understand organisational priorities. The opening statement in the 2008 annual report for Kellogg's says: "At Kellogg Company, our goal is to drive sustainable and dependable growth by leveraging the talents of our people and the power of our brands, and by fulfilling the needs of our consumers, customers and communities." Sales in 2008 were nearly $13 billion, making Kellogg's the world's leading producer of cereal. More than 1,500 products were marketed in over 180 countries. Kellogg's "met or exceeded" all growth targets, even during the recession, and the opening statement from the chair and president ends with …"we remain committed to delivering sustainable and dependable growth into the future." The word "growth" appears 24 times in the brief opening statement. The word "obesity" appears once in the 98 page report: "Our innovation teams develop nutritious foods that take into account major public health issues, such as diabetes, heart disease and obesity." In the 2009 annual report, the word growth appears 85 times; the word obesity not once. Why would Kellogg's sponsor so many different dietary organisations when obesity does not appear to be a subject worthy of mention in the annual reports?

The opening statement admits: "We are aggressively embracing digital media, which affords an efficient, cost-effective way to target specific audiences, providing an excellent platform for developing our brands. We have already tapped the Internet to gain significant brand development traction for Special K, Frosted Flakes, Apple Jacks, Kashi, Rice Krispies, Morningstar Farms and Pop-Tarts. In addition, we are successfully building relationships with moms around the world through Kelloggs.com and KelloggNutrition.com. Our strength in brand building allows us to successfully drive new business opportunities that expand our portfolio and reach more consumers". (I wonder how 'moms' feel about being targeted in this way).

As Sally Fallon Morell said at the inaugural European Weston Price Foundation conference in London, March 2010, mothers are the gatekeepers of health. This view was strongly endorsed at the same conference by Natasha Campbell-McBride. The healthy mother, with the healthy digestive tract and optimal immune system has the best chance of giving birth to a healthy baby. The choices made by mums as (invariably) the purse keepers of the household are absolutely critical to the health of their child and, collectively, our entire future population. Real food fans such as Fallon Morell and Campbell-McBride want the gatekeepers of health to be eating real food, as provided by nature and not processed food as provided by food manufacturers. Food manufacturers want the converse.

Just as Kellogg's shared in its annual report – more and more companies are moving their advertising to on line mediums. I subscribe to a service called *Response Source*, which is like a dating agency for journalists wanting 'experts' and 'experts' wanting PR opportunities. I was intrigued to see a request from The National Magazine Company, on 3 January 2010, requesting prizes or special offers geared towards weight loss and healthy eating to feature on a new Natmags website: www.dietdiaries.co.uk. The website was being developed in partnership with GlaxoSmithKline. The website features diet diary blogs from women taking the drug, Alli, and other content from Natmags websites such as Cosmopolitan, Company, handbag.com, netdoctor and allaboutyou. Further requests for support for dietdiaries.co.uk followed on 21 January, 16 March, and 7 April and then I stopped taking note of them. I have subsequently seen the site and seen adverts for Alli and the dietdiaries site on other National Magazine web sites. This is likely a lucrative partnership for Natmags and GlaxoSmithKline. Do readers of National Magazine publications know that this partnership exists? Do people know that Natmags is behind netdoctor and allaboutyou?

If you think that you are not influenced by advertising while browsing on line, visit dailymail.co.uk and look at any article that attracts your attention. Then look at the Jan Moir article about the death of Stephen Gatley, which attracted such outrage that advertisers, including Marks & Spencer PLC, insisted that their adverts were removed from the page, to ensure no association with the article.[342] The page remains noticeably bare today.

I referred to the television programme *30 Minutes,* presented by Nick Cohen, in the chapter on exercise. Cohen opened with the stark financial reality "Far more money is spent researching how to make children eat than how to make them read." This was the voice over as nine year old Jake was walking around a grocery store wearing special glasses to show market researchers, for whom he was working, what was attracting his attention. Cohen noted that three and a half million adverts were on children's television in the UK in 2003. This will have increased dramatically with the expansion of digital TV and vastly more channels since then. (The USA has had hundreds of television channels for some time and may be surprised to know that the UK only added a fifth channel, *Channel 5,* in 1997).

Cohen noted "According to research we commissioned from Nielsen, 1,150 junk food ads were shown across children's television every day. McDonald's spent £32 million on TV advertising; nearly £13 million was spent by Coca-Cola and nearly £7 million by Pringles." All of this data was for 2003-04 for just the UK. Since 1991 no adverts, which set out to attract the attention of children under 12 years old, have been allowed on Swedish commercial TV stations. Tessa Jowell, the secretary of state for culture, media and sport at the time of the programme declared herself "sceptical" about such an intervention. Cohen said "the government pretends that children are savvy consumers who can't be manipulated; why they believe in Father Christmas, Ms Jowell never explains."

The programme was aired at the time that videos and other recording devices were becoming increasingly commonplace, such that consumers could skip adverts more easily. Needing to find alternative ways to reach young consumers, the programme noted that just under half of the schools in the UK had a permanent 'bill board' in the canteen – a Coca-Cola or PepsiCo vending machine. The government requirement for school capital projects to be privately funded had also led to branding in everything from exercise books to playing fields. "Eat football, sleep football, drink Coca-Cola" was the banner adorning the playing field at Bexley Heath School. It was accompanied by a large Kellogg's Frosties banner, behind the goal posts. In December 2008, the lobby group Sustain and the Children's Food Campaign published an excellent exposé of educational material produced by the food industry entitled "Through the Back Door."[343]

Magazines and newspapers

The print media provides regular examples of conflicts of interest. On 22 January 2010 there was a news story "Nine in ten food allergy cases 'are all in the mind'."[344] The headline was dangerously wrong at the outset. Food *allergy* is absolutely not in the mind. Food allergy is the life threatening condition where, for example, someone with a peanut allergy could suffer an anaphylactic shock after even coming close to a peanut, (and the person likely has problems with many, or all, nuts). My cousin discovered that her son had a nut allergy when he was a toddler and she kissed his cheek after a Chinese meal and a trace of nut oil, from a dish eaten hours earlier, almost killed him. A friend of mine has a life threatening allergy to kiwi fruit. This is not in his mind – it can kill him.

This article was about food *intolerance* – best defined as the 'too much/too often' problem where the body literally becomes intolerant to an over-consumed substance. It's the body's way of saying "I can't tolerate this substance any more". Wheat is the most likely food intolerance in the UK, USA and Australia. Why? Because we eat it several times every day: wheat toast or wheat cereal for breakfast; wheat muffins, wheat biscuits, wheat cereal bars etc for mid morning; wheat sandwiches or wheat pasta salad for lunch; more wheat snacks in the afternoon; wheat pasta, or wheat pizza or wheat pies or wheat pastry for dinner and then more wheat snacks in the evening. Indeed, the Flour Advisory Bureau statistics tell us that UK flour consumption per capita was 74 kilograms in 2008/09. That means *1.4 kilograms* of flour consumed per average person in the UK per week. I cannot find a single ingredient that we eat more of.

So, who stands to lose most by people in the UK (or the USA or Australia for that matter) believing that they have food intolerance? The Flour Advisory Bureau and food manufacturers reliant upon flour – cereal and bread manufacturers, biscuit and cake manufacturers and so on. Towards the end of the article you discover that the study that concluded that 'food allergy/intolerance is all in the mind', was funded by the Flour Advisory Bureau.

On 18 May 2010, Peta Bee reported in the UK *Daily Mail* "Giving up bread can make you fat: Gluten is good for you." The expert in this report was Dr. Emma Williams of the British Nutrition Foundation. Excellent job done there, keeping the many food industry sponsors of the BNF happy.

On 18 January 2010, the headline news was "Ban butter to save thousands of lives says heart surgeon." Shyam Kolvekar called for a ban on butter and said people should switch to 'a healthy spread'. Mr Kolvekar's comments were issued by KTB, a public relations company that works for Unilever, the makers of Flora margarine. The head of the London chapter of the Weston Price Foundation, Philip Ridley, spent the morning cycling around London delivering leaflets on the nutritional benefits of butter vs. the health concerns about hydrogenated vegetable oils. By lunchtime, the surgeon's hospital, University College London Hospital (UCLH), had distanced itself from the surgeon saying that his views were personal ones and did not necessarily represent those of the NHS trust. Felicity Lawrence, writing in *The Guardian*[345] on 23 January 2010 noted that the UCLH had received a fee from KTB for filming Kolvekar performing heart surgery, as part of Unilever's campaign to highlight the dangers of eating too much saturated fat.

Just to be fair, I'm a huge fan of eggs, but vested interest is just that – whether you like the product or not. On 9 March 2010, an unnamed *Daily Mail* reporter wrote the article "There's a cracking idea! Eggs are a superfood... and eating one a day could help you lose weight." Towards the end of the article we discovered that these latest findings were funded by the British Egg Industry Council.

On 22 May 2010 there was a press release by Weight Watchers "The 57 million Americans currently living with 'pre-diabetes' could benefit from a group weight loss program, like Weight Watchers, according to a new study published in this month's *American Journal of Lifestyle Medicine.*" We know that type 2 diabetes and weight are substantially correlated. We know that losing weight will help reduce the risk of type 2 diabetes, but this is a rather tenuous link to justify the headline in *Diabetes Health* "Attending Weight Watchers Meetings Helps Reduce the Risk for type 2 diabetes."[346]

On 26 May 2010 there was a press release: "Lack of exercise key to increased BMI in children – dietary sugars are not the driving factor behind rising BMI levels in children in Great Britain." The press release was made by the Ware Anthony Rust PR Agency on behalf of The Sugar Bureau.

The UK women's monthly magazine, *Glamour* and glamour.com announced a major new partnership with Kellogg's Special K in a press release on 26 February 2010.[347] Managed by Carat Sponsorship, "The biggest selling glossy women's monthly and its digital site will be working with Kellogg's on a fully integrated long term promotional campaign, bringing the Special K girl to life, and positioning Special K as the cereal of choice to manage readers' shapes." The arrangement was launched in the March issue of Glamour and is running as a three page promotion in every issue this year. Simon Kippin, publishing director for Glamour, was quoted as saying, "This long-term campaign recognises the strong reader relationship our magazine and website can offer a client, communicating with a large group of hard-to-reach consumers who see Glamour as a trusted source of advice. The commitment from Special K through the year allows a strong evolving message to develop and grow for maximum impact." From Laura Bryant's perspective, as brand manager for Kellogg's Special K, "This deal with Glamour is a fantastic opportunity for us to bring the Special K girl to life throughout the year and reach our target audience of shape watching women every month." So, Kellogg's get access to "hard-to-reach" consumers (over 500,000 of them) and *Glamour* 'sells' their readers.

I came across all of these examples easily, during the spring months of 2010, while finishing the manuscript for this book. We do not need to search for such stories – they are continually under our noses. We just need to be very tuned in to who is behind the messages we are receiving on a daily basis.

Sporting events

Detailing the full history of the relationship between sport and the food and drink industry could be a book in itself. The London 2012 Olympic Games can be used as one timely example and the finale to this conflict of interest chapter. This sporting event, par excellence, is sponsored by, amongst others, McDonald's, Coca-Cola and Cadbury.

McDonald's have been associated with the games since 1968. They are a TOP sponsor – which means "The Olympic Partners Programme". This gives

McDonald's: exclusive marketing rights in the restaurant and food service category; the rights to use the Olympic rings in global marketing activities; exclusive sponsorship opportunities with national Olympic teams around the world and status as the official restaurant partner of the Olympic Games through 2012. "McDonald's has been a proud Olympic partner for nearly three decades because we believe in the spirit and ideals of the Games," said Jim Cantalupo, McDonald's chairman and chief executive officer. "As a global brand serving 47 million customers every day, we share the same core principles of teamwork, excellence and being the best that make the Olympic Games a model of excellence for the world."[348] (Please note the focus on the company and not the product).

Michael Phelps won his eighth gold medal, at the Beijing Olympics, on 16 August 2008. Two days later he was at the McDonald's, just 20 minutes away from the Water Cube, for a photo shoot. Rebecca Adlington won two gold medals in the same Water Cube, also shattering world records. She was asked in her post win interview how she planned to celebrate. "'I'm going to go to McDonald's,' she told The Independent on Sunday with a sheepish grin.[li] 'After all this hard work, and watching what I eat, I just fancy a burger and some chips.'"[349]

The cola drink available in McDonald's is Coca-Cola and not Pepsi, which is just as well, because...

Coca-Cola is "proud to be the longest continuous corporate partner of the Olympic Games" – an involvement that dates back to the Amsterdam games of 1928 and has just been extended to 2020 "extending this extraordinary relationship to nearly a full century", in the company's own words. Coca-Cola's web page on the Olympics proudly states: "As an organization, The Coca-Cola Company shares the Olympic Values, which embody the discovery of one's abilities, the spirit of competition, the pursuit of excellence, a sense of fair play and the building of a better and more-peaceful world."[350] No mention of the "nearly 70 different beverage products". Strangely silent on the 140 calories, 39 grams of sugar and 34 milligrams of caffeine per 355 millilitres of Coca-Cola. No mention of the ingredients list, with the empty calories: carbonated water; high fructose corn syrup; caramel color; phosphoric acid; natural flavours and caffeine. The marketing people must know that they need to promote the company and not the product that it makes when the web site nutritional information needs to say what the product is *not*, rather than what it is: "*Not* a significant source of fat calories, saturated fat, trans fat, cholesterol, fiber, vitamin A, vitamin C, calcium and iron".

Cadbury is a relative newcomer, having sponsored the Sydney Olympics, in 2000, and the Commonwealth Games in Manchester, in 2002, and Melbourne, in 2006. Their announcement that they were going to sponsor the 2012 Olympics was criticised by the National Obesity Forum. Board member, Tam

---

[li] The Oxford English Dictionary defines "sheepish" as "embarrassed through shame". I hope that Adlington was sheepish.

Fry, was quoted as saying "I would be very concerned that it is encouraging children to eat chocolate because it is all part of the promotion of unhealthy food to children." Cadbury's response was the one that we commonly hear: "Treats can be consumed responsibly – the key is how to balance consumption of treats and physical activity."[351] I.e. processed food is part of a balanced healthy diet. Cadbury have the 'eatwell' plate on their side in this respect.

In the programme *Who made me Fat?*,[352] Rebecca Wilcox wrote to Lord Sebastian Coe, chair of the London Organising Committee of the Olympic and Paralympic Games, about the association of McDonald's, Coca-Cola and Cadbury with the 2012 games. Wilcox had two requests for interviews rejected, but she did receive a letter saying: "At the London 2012 games there will be a wide range of food and drink options available including McDonald's, Coca-Cola and Cadbury products. These companies have a great heritage in supporting the Olympic movement and in promoting balanced active lifestyles. We are proud to be working with them to deliver a successful Olympic Games... Put simply, without commercial partners, the Games would not happen."

A journalist asked me which part of researching for and writing this book had most shocked me and it is this chapter. Yes I was stunned that not one of seven UK government and obesity organisations could source, or provide evidence for, the calorie formula. Yes I was shocked to find that we have never even done the fat/heart study, let alone proven causation, but the depth of the involvement of the food industry in our dietary advice was way beyond anything I could have ever conceived. The legislative monopoly of dietitians, backed by the billions of dollars of the American food and drink industry, is nothing short of scandalous and I hope that highlighting what has happened in the USA can avoid the same happening in the UK, Australia and other obese nations. From our web pages to magazines, from industry sponsored health stories to the pinnacle of sporting prowess, the giants of the food and drink industry are omnipresent.

As we shared in the opening to this chapter, companies aim to grow. Kellogg's, McDonald's, PepsiCo, Coca-Cola, and others involved in various ways in the obesity industry, are no exception. If the numerous activities described in this chapter did *not* increase sales, organisations would not spend millions of pounds on them. Given that they do spend this money, *de facto*, it increases consumption. We know that the dietary advice 'avoid fat/eat carbohydrates' is far more favourable to food and drink organisations than the message 'avoid processed food/eat real food'. Such organisations will be only too happy that we have been calling processed carbohydrate saturated fat since Ancel Keys started the war on the wrong macronutrient. It is in the interests of these companies that the food pyramid and the 'eatwell' plate prevail. Sadly, it is not in the interests of those fighting the obesity crisis.

It is my absolute belief that growth in sales for the food and drink industry goes hand in hand with growth in obesity. To reverse this epidemic, sales of these organisations need to shrink, not grow. Our waistlines are not going to shrink otherwise.

As I write, the football teams have just boarded planes worldwide to attend the 2010 football world cup. A couple of sponsors are all too familiar – Coca-Cola and McDonald's. Another global sporting event, another opportunity to have one's brand associated with the implication of energy expended, with the intent of increasing energy consumed. The only words that come to mind to close this chapter are those of Scott Adam's character, Dilbert: "We are doomed."

Chapter Sixteen

The organisational design of obesity management

The role of government in the obesity epidemic

I believe that our governments caused the obesity epidemic. With the dietary advice change in America first, followed by the UK and then other 'developed' countries, the U-turn from "carbohydrates are fattening" to "base your meals on starchy foods" caused the obesity epidemic. I am somewhat torn, therefore, in terms of the role government should play in resolving the obesity epidemic.

On the one hand, I am naturally inclined towards Henry David Thoreau's view of government: "That government is best which governs least." On the other hand, there is an argument that government is going to be necessary to reverse the damage done over the past 25-30 years. Overriding both of these, I believe that the most likely resolution of the obesity epidemic will come from a 'bottom-up' revolution. Let us explore these further...

If government has serious intentions toward addressing obesity, I see two options for consideration. Option one would be to remove itself completely from the field of obesity, on the basis that the current repetition of the wrong messages is doing more harm than saying nothing at all. If government is *not* inclined to change current advice, the less it promotes the current messages the better. Much as I think that in principle we should interfere as little as possible in the lives of others, I think that this would fail. We would be left with the messages that we have now and these would continue to be reiterated by the food and drink industry and no improvement would be made. Option two, is therefore my preferred option. We need government to stand up and say we got it wrong in 1983 (1977 in the USA) – we were right the first time – and we need to return to what we believed throughout history up to those dates. We actually need strong and independent government more than ever to counterbalance the numerous messages that are being given to consumers every day from the food and drink manufacturers. Another compelling reason for calling upon government to act is that this would speed up the change process dramatically. While I do think that 'bottom up' renaissance will lead the way, 'top down' reform would be so much quicker and literally could save and improve lives from the moment of change. Surely that is within the remit and ethics of government?

So, how can we achieve the effective leadership that we need?

Organisational design – general principles

I worked as a human resources director/vice president, in global corporations, for a number of years and one of the topics that most interested me was organisational design. The Burke Litwin model is more sophisticated, but I particularly like the simplicity and effectiveness of the McKinsey 7-S model.[353] The 7-S model, in essence, is a framework for addressing all necessary aspects of the design of an organisation. The S's stand for structure, strategy and systems (called the 'hard S's', as these are the ones that are actively determined) and shared values, skills, staff and style (called the 'soft S's', as these are more subtle and style, for example, is an outcome rather than something that can be worked upon). I prefer to use the Mars Incorporated variation of the McKinsey 7-S model. The word "skills" in the McKinsey model refers to the competencies of the organisation – the things it does best. Mars changed this S to strengths of the organisation accordingly and took skills to mean all the value that people could bring, dropping potential confusion with staff.

Our governments could apply private corporation principles to great effect and I recommend a complete organisational design review of obesity (health generally could benefit from the same approach). When HR professionals are trained to lead management teams through organisational design and major restructuring, the starting points are strategy and style. These two define the end in mind in a 'hard' and 'soft' way. Our strategic end in mind should be nothing short of stopping the rise in obesity and reversing the trend, so that obesity levels start to fall. I will come back to the specific measures that I would recommend to underpin this strategy.

Style is an interesting part of organisational design. It is often interchangeably referred to as culture and the best definition of culture I found was "it is the way we do things round here." Sticking to the country that I know best, the way to address style in the UK would be to ask those involved in obesity – how do you want to be seen by stakeholders? The answer to that question is remarkably consistent – organisations want to be seen as efficient, effective, customer oriented, highly competent and, bottom line, they want to be seen as having made a difference. Then you ask stakeholders how they see the management of obesity and the reality would be 'confusing', 'conflicting', 'don't know who is responsible for what' and 'not working'. This defines the gap between where obesity management is now and where it needs to be.

You can start to see how the S's inter-relate, as you can't work directly on style. You can't just declare that you want to be seen as an innovative and revolutionary organisation – you *structure* the organisation to make this one of the cores *strengths* and recruit and reward the right *skills* and establish innovation as a core *shared value* and you are more likely to achieve your desired *style*. The same goes for government and obesity. The three S's that need the most attention for public health management of obesity are structure, systems and shared values. The strongest companies in the world have the strongest shared values. The Mafia, the Catholic Church – whatever you think of their shared values – they make for incredibly strong and endurable entities.

Our governments need to establish strong shared values to address this epidemic. True independence and zero tolerance of conflict of interest must be one such value. Courage and preparedness to make tough decisions should be another. Open mindedness and the ability to change views are going to be essential. Being evidence based and at the forefront of the latest research is also imperative. There will be more – but at the moment we are simply holding on to flawed research from a post war study and attempts to repeatedly post rationalise it since.

In terms of structure, speaking for the UK again (but with wider application), we need a fundamental review of the management of obesity. We need one and only one source of information on obesity. That body must be completely transparent, independent and protected from any lobbying and sponsorship from the food, drink or drug companies. We cannot have the Department of Health, the National Health Service, the Food Standards Agency, the British Nutrition Foundation, the British Dietetic Association, local GP practices, local health authorities and so on all issuing public 'healthy eating' advice. Creation of a single body would also ensure that we don't have the situation, described in Chapter Fifteen, where the Department of Health 'washed its hands' of the British Dietetic Association's conflicts of interest. To avoid any baggage, we would best be served with the establishment of a new body. The Department of Health would likely need to be the overseeing body, but only if true independence could be guaranteed.

From structure flows systems. This term is all encompassing and covers any process, formal or informal, which supports the strategy. Every action in an effective organisation contributes to the purpose of the organisation and no activity detracts from it. Systems stay true to shared values and processes exist to deliver what is important to the organisation. With just one body, the systems for conducting research, establishing evidence based positions, consulting with people, communicating to the public and so on would be much easier and more effective.

The key strength of this single body needs to be focus. The organisation needs to be the centre of excellence for obesity and not dilute this strength straying anywhere else. This is still a wide brief – from breastfeeding, through childhood obesity, to the impact of hormonal changes and medication on weight, to weight management in the elderly – there is an entire weight life cycle to manage. The people working in and for this body need to have the skills to be role models for the shared values, to achieve the strategy and to complement the strengths of the organisation.

We already have objective measures for establishing optimum nutrition. We know which macronutrients are most needed by the body. We know the foods that provide the most vitamins and minerals. This should determine uniform healthy eating advice. We should never again talk about "recommended dietary allowances", or worse, "adequate intake". We should be striving for optimal health, not a minimal level. This is the way forward to remedy obesity, heart disease, cancer, diabetes or any modern illness.

Obesity is what we call a root cause illness. If our 'one national organisation' sets guidelines for optimum nutrition, based on consumption of real food, this will be a healthy diet for human beings suffering other conditions *per se*. Other conditions will also be seen less often and will be greatly helped by a reduction in obesity levels.

Organisational design – specific recommendations

I will continue to use the UK as an example, but the messages for what needs to happen specifically are equally relevant, or at least can be adapted, for any obese nation. I have set out the framework for a complete review of the way we manage obesity at national levels. There are three of the S's that I want to go into in more detail: strategy, systems and skills.

Strategy

With the goal of stopping the rise in obesity and then reversing the trend, the key messages that I would propose to achieve this are as follows:

The first thing that must happen is that we make an honest and clear announcement that we got some things wrong and we need people to forget any messages that they may have picked up in the past and follow the advice from the one new body going forward. This is easier said than done, as it impacts trust. However, check internet sites today, whenever a new government food initiative is launched, and the current level of trust could barely be lower. We changed our position in 1983 (albeit before the rapid communications facilitated by the internet) and we need to do it again. The UK changed its position on cholesterol – only no one knows. The UK changed its position on eggs – only no one knows. The USA changed its position on total fat – only no one knows. We'll address looking stupid shortly. All promotional material, the most obvious one being the 'eatwell' plate posters and tool kits, need to be removed, as part of a complete change of strategy and message.

"Eat naturally; move naturally" could work as a slogan for the overall campaign. With the emphasis in this book placed on food vs. activity, it won't surprise you that the key messages I propose are related to *what* we eat, rather than how much we eat or what we do. I propose three, and only three, dietary tips. These should be reiterated by one and only one body until they are even better known, and far more useful, than five-a-day:

1) Eat real food; don't eat processed food;
2) Eat three meals a day; don't snack unless you are slim and active;
3) Manage carbohydrates if you need to manage your weight.

1) The first message can easily be explained and embedded. Simple examples can illustrate the difference between real and processed food: Oranges grow on trees, cartons of orange juice don't; baked potatoes come from the ground, crisps and chips don't; fish swim in the sea, fish fingers don't. Children need to be taught this as early as possible and retain this fundamental healthy eating message for life. We can replace plates and

pyramids with posters of real foods (with a tick/'green for go' colouring) and processed foods (with a cross/no entry sign/'red for stop' colouring). The detail can follow, but the message needs to be clear, simple and very different to what we have now.

2) We need to reverse messages about portion size to achieve this goal. (Sadly, so much of what we need to do to reverse the obesity epidemic involves removing current messages from people's minds and replacing them with invariably the opposites). People should be eating three substantial meals a day – with lots of meat, fish, eggs, dairy products, vegetables and salads – to ensure that they don't need to snack. Snack foods are invariably carbohydrates – whether 'good', like seasonal, local, fruit, or 'bad', like sugared cereal bars with multiple ingredients, they keep the body in fat storing mode, not fat using mode, and therefore perpetuate the obesity problem.

3) Message (1) can help people understand the difference between real (good) carbohydrates and processed (bad) carbohydrates. Message (3) will be about educating people that fat can only be stored when we eat any carbohydrates, so, to manage obesity (fat storage), we need to limit the number of meals that contain even good carbohydrates (brown rice, whole wheat pasta, 100% whole grain bread, baked potatoes, fruit etc). The fewer carbohydrate meals a person has, the more weight loss will be facilitated. Salads and vegetables (not potatoes) can be eaten freely at main meals by most people.

I can visualise a diagram with an outer wheel and an inner wheel: The inner wheel shows numerous examples of salads and vegetables – indicating that these are good to eat with any meal and then one part of the outer wheel (taking up at least two thirds of the ring) would have pictures of real meat, fish, eggs and dairy and the remainder would have pictures of fruit, baked potatoes and whole grains. No junk segment, no refined carbohydrates, no sugared fruit or yoghurt, no processed meat, no processed food at all would go on this picture. We will know that we have achieved our goal of establishing a healthy eating message when food and drink industry sponsors abandon any diagram that we develop.

The one message I would suggest regarding activity is "move naturally". We are designed to walk, talk, dance, sing, cook, clean and tend the land and that is what we should do.

There is a particular aspect of strategy, which needs to be prioritised, and that is prevention. The recent emphasis on the management of childhood obesity is absolutely right in principle, just tragically misguided in execution. Childhood obesity is critical to avoid *per se*, but also for two specific reasons:

1) We know that the risk of overweight children becoming overweight adults is significant: "80% of children who are obese at age 10–14 will become obese adults, particularly if one of their parents is also obese."[354] "Adjusting for parental obesity, the odds ratio of an obese 1-2-year-old being obese as an

adult is 1:3, i.e. 30% more likely than a non-obese child. While for a child obese at age 15-17 years, the odds ratio is 17 fold. Among very obese children aged 10-14, the unadjusted odds ratio is 44 fold. Clearly, the increasing prevalence of obesity in childhood[355] is very likely to translate into greatly increased levels of obesity among adults, rendering them more susceptible to chronic, life-threatening illness."[356]

2) Although it is difficult to increase the number of fat cells in adults (super morbid obesity aside) "a significant increase in the number of fat cells has been shown to occur at key stages in childhood development."[357] We know that fat cells can *not* be reduced in number, only in size, so, if a child does increase their number of fat cells before adulthood, this fat cell capacity is with them for life. These fat cells will continually demand to be fed, giving the individual a life long increased drive to eat and a life long propensity for obesity.

Ensuring that our children reach the age of 21 with a similar BMI should be a fundamental goal of government, dietary advisors, parents and young people alike. To this end, the 'education' that is being given to children and parents is catastrophic. Here are three examples by way of illustration:

Our current diet advice has created completely the wrong view of calories. Instead of calories being seen as energy for the human body, they have become things to be avoided – even feared. The British TV presenter, Fearne Cotton, made an excellent programme *The truth about online anorexia,* which aired in April 2009.[358] Cotton visited a school in west London, UK and talked to a class of 10 year olds about body image and calories. Kira said the following: "I don't like my body" and "I think I weigh too much." When asked about calories she knew the calorie content of a small Kit Kat and said "I don't really count them (calories), but they are bad 'cos you have to try and spend all your time exercising trying to burn them off." That's what a ten year old thinks about calories.

Panorama, BBC 1, 13 April 2010 was called *Spoilt Rotten* and was about a number of children presenting a number of preventable conditions to staff at Liverpool's Alder Hay Hospital. Leon was the child I was most interested in. Aged five he weighed 145 pounds (65.85 kilograms) – the weight of an average 17 year old. Leon's mother, Sharon, is convinced that her son has a genetic disorder. She follows him from school with a wheelchair, because, at some point during the 700 yard journey, he 'can't' walk any further and needs to be pushed home. His doctor, Dr. Mohammed Didi, was trying to encourage the family to give Leon as much exercise as possible. Dr. Didi was unaware of the wheelchair until the programme production team informed him about it.

Sharon said "I just wish someone would put a camera in the corner of the house and watch my son, then come back and tell me I'm doing something wrong, because I guarantee they won't find nothing (sic)". So the production team did exactly that. They filmed Leon eating a banana in the final part of the journey, as he was being pushed in the wheelchair to home. When he arrived home, he thought he had left a piece of birthday cake from a party at school and he became quite hysterical. (If anyone ever doubts whether or not sugar is addictive, they should have watched this programme). His grandmother 'fortunately' found the cake and Leon ate it and was transformed immediately into a 'normal' child once more. The cake was two (slim) slices of chocolate log. Within minutes of finishing this, Leon was offered another snack. He was actually preoccupied at the time and mum had to interrupt him to clarify did he want strawberries or banana on his Weetabix. "Both", was the reply. The camera team stayed at the house for just two hours – enough time to see Leon have his actual tea of fish, mashed potato and mushy peas. The portion size would have been ample for my six foot tall husband. Before the production crew left, Leon was filmed sat on the sofa eating an apple.

When the presenter challenged Sharon about the amount of food she had given Leon, her defence could only be described as aggressive. "Why is that a lot of food?" she retorted "when the Weetabix is fibre with fruit on and it was fish, mash potatoes and veg?" "Was it chips and pizza?" The presenter could barely say the word "no" before Sharon closed the conversation with "there you go then." Mum flatly refused to accept any responsibility for her son's obesity. In her defence, she had followed the 'eatwell' plate well.

I attended a meeting at the Aneurin Bevan Health Board in Pontypool, south Wales in April 2010. Arriving early, I looked at some drawings of 'healthy' lunch boxes, done by children from a local school, Llanyrafon Primary. The pictures featured sandwiches, spaghetti, chocolate, pizza, pasta and fruit juice. It is difficult to draw pasta, so one lunch box had a label saying "pasta – this is because it has carbohydrate in it" and another said "yogat (sic) has carbohydrates in it – that's why it's in there." I estimated the children's ages to be approximately seven. The teacher likely put the word carbohydrate on the board, for this to be spelled correctly and yoghurt incorrectly. It would appear that our primary school children know lots about carbohydrates, but not the most nutritious macronutrients: protein and fat. The 'eatwell' plate proponents would no doubt be thrilled to see such young children thinking that carbohydrates are the most important food to consume.

My heart literally sank thinking about the scale of the task we have, if we are to stop 90% of these children being overweight or obese by 2050. If they were finishing primary school convinced that eating food as delivered by nature was the most important thing that they could do for their health and weight, we would have done a good job. Instead, our under tens think that sandwiches, spaghetti, chocolate, pizza, pasta and fruit juice should form the basis of a healthy school lunch and dietitians would most likely agree with them.

Unsurprisingly, we are failing in our targets. In October 2007, the Public Sector Agreement (PSA12) in the UK set "a long-term national ambition by 2020 to reduce the proportion of overweight and obese children to 2000 levels."[359] This was trying to build on the 1996 target for childhood obesity to "halt the year-on-year rise in obesity among children aged under 11 by 2010, in the context of a broader strategy to tackle obesity in the population as a whole."[360] "There is, as yet, almost no evidence that these policies have changed the trajectory of obesity growth."[361]

As a final thought on children – if you slap your child, be prepared for any person who may witness this to verbally abuse you, or even to call the police. Give your child glucose syrup, sugar, gelatine (derived from the collagen inside animal skin and bones), dextrose, citric acid, flavourings, fruit and plant concentrates, colours (including carmine, which is made from crushed insects – usually red beetles), glazing agents (including beeswax), invert sugar syrup and fruit extract and no one will bat an eyelid. That's the ingredients list for (sing along) "Kids and Grown-ups love it so, the happy world of Haribo". And – the slap is supposed to be a punishment and the sweets are supposed to be a treat. What could such a concoction do to the body of a child? I believe that loving a child (indeed any human being) and giving them a cocktail of sugars bonded together with animal innards are mutually exclusive acts.

Systems

The constitution of the World Health Organisation[362] sets out eight founding principles on the opening page. The eighth is: "Governments have a responsibility for the health of their peoples which can be fulfilled only by the provision of adequate health and social measures."

There are a number of formal processes and measures (systems) that the proposed 'one national organisation' should consider to address the obesity epidemic:

1) The banning of certain substances;
2) Fiscal policy (taxation);
3) Any measure that makes it easier for people to eat real food.

Food and drink companies will be delighted that I am not an obesity tsar, as this is what I would do if tasked with reversing the obesity epidemic:

1) The banning of certain substances

Unsurprisingly, from all that I have said in this book, I would target processed foods to attack the obesity epidemic. I would not tinker with bans on advertising; I would ban the key ingredients that make up processed foods. In the unlikely event that we were bold enough to ban sugar, trans fats and sweeteners, this one step would be *sufficient* to reverse the obesity epidemic (whether such bans are *necessary* is a matter for debate). It is questionable whether a number of products in the food chain should ever have been considered fit for human consumption. The USA Food and Drink Administration is able to grant approval for new creations with a 'GRAS' classification. This means "Generally Regarded As Safe". A cynic may say that the FDA is protecting itself and that you would be wise to do the same. In July 2010, there were 347, largely unrecognisable, substances on the GRAS notice inventory. Most have elicited no queries from the FDA.[363]

- Sugar: Professor Yudkin called sugar *Pure White and Deadly* back in 1972 and page two of his work of the same name asserted "if only a small fraction of what is already known about the effects of sugar were to be revealed in relation to any other material used as a food additive, that material would promptly be banned."[364] In the 1920's, Otto Warburg started work on the concept that cancerous cells and healthy cells were 'feeding' in different ways. His conclusion was: "But, even for cancer, there is only one prime cause. The prime cause of cancer is the replacement of the respiration of oxygen (oxidation of sugar) in normal body cells by fermentation of sugar."[365]

- Trans fats: The National Heart Forum summed up their position on trans fats in the opening to their paper calling for a ban on these substances: "Industrially produced Trans fats (IPTFAs) are harmful to health, they have no nutritional benefits and there is no known safe level of consumption."[366]

- Sweeteners: Dr. Ralph Walton, Professor and chairman of the Department of Psychiatry Northeastern Ohio University Colleges of Medicine, undertook a comprehensive review of studies available for just one sweetener: aspartame. It was called "Survey of aspartame studies: correlation of outcome and funding sources." The summary of the report stated: "Of the 166 studies felt to have relevance for questions of human safety, 74 had Nutrasweet® industry related funding and 92 were independently funded. One hundred percent of the industry funded research attested to aspartame's safety, whereas 92% of the independently funded research identified a problem." Walton's overall conclusion was "We have also become much more sophisticated about the impact of a variety of toxins on psychological processes. I am convinced that one such toxin is aspartame."[367]

Let us add another definition to the one with which we opened Part Three:

Food (noun): "Substance taken into body to maintain life and growth; nutriment."

Poison (noun): "Substance that, when introduced into or absorbed by living organism causes harm."[368]

Which noun more accurately describes sugar, trans fats and sweeteners?

As Yudkin said of sugar,[369] "Cutting down *any* other food is bound to reduce nutrients as well as calories." If he were writing today, Yudkin would no doubt add trans fats and sweeteners to the list of foods we can do without, with no loss of nutritional value. Trans fats have been banned in Austria, Denmark, Switzerland and New York City. Alan Johnson, former British Health Secretary, has just talked about doing so.[370] We have no need for sweeteners: they have been shown to have a similar effect on blood glucose levels to sugar;[371] they perpetuate our taste for unnaturally sweet things and food manufacturers would simply replace sugar with sweeteners if we ban one and not the other. If we eat sugar and trans fats instead of other food, we lose nutrition. If we eat them on top of the nutrition we need, we gain weight. I consider these three nutritionally

256

void ingredients to be the foundation of the key products that obese nations must stop eating.

I said in the introduction, if this sounds extreme, how does "90% of today's children being overweight or obese by 2050" sound?[372] But why would this be considered extreme? I am merely suggesting that we return to eating what we used to eat before we got too obese to function as human beings.

2) Fiscal policy (taxation)

I cannot conceive of any government having the courage to ban sugar, trans fats and sweeteners. Hence, if we lack the leadership qualities to ban nutritionally void substances, the minimum that we need is a deterring and punitive tax on each of them. We need to be very specific about the targets. In May 2009 Dr. Tim Lobstein called for a 'fat tax',[373] while talking about junk food and pizza. The reiteration of the notion that 'fat is bad' is incessant. We must stop this forthwith. The target of fiscal measures needs to be processed foods and no real food should ever be demonised again. Again, although this step may not be necessary, it would be sufficient and we are almost expecting the impossible from our populations to tell them to avoid processed food while the food manufacturers are simultaneously promoting BOGOF's (Buy One, Get One Free) on biscuits, cakes, confectionery and all the things that we need help to resist. David Kessler's book, *The end of overeating,* gives full details of what humans are up against in terms of food industry tactics.[374]

Taxation would merely be a return to previous public policy, albeit from centuries ago. Adam's Smith's The Wealth of Nations (1776) noted "Sugar, rum, and tobacco are commodities which are nowhere necessaries of life, which are become objects of almost universal consumption, and which are therefore extremely proper subjects of taxation." Just under one hundred years later, the sugar tax was repealed. If sugar is not banned, the tax needs to be reinstated.

I am most encouraged by not being the first to call for such taxes to be reinstated. In April 2009, Kelly Brownell and Thomas Frieden[375] called for the imposition of taxes on sugared drinks arguing that "Sugar-sweetened beverages (soda sweetened with sugar, corn syrup, or other caloric sweeteners and other carbonated and uncarbonated drinks, such as sports and energy drinks) may be the single largest driver of the obesity epidemic". Writing in 2009, they noted that "in the past decade per capita intake of calories from sugar-sweetened beverages has increased by nearly 30%;[376] beverages now account for 10 to 15% of the calories consumed by children and adolescents." Brownell and Frieden call for a penny-per-ounce excise tax, which would raise an estimated $1.2 billion in New York State alone.

The objective of such taxation should primarily be to reduce consumption, but any revenue generated can have an added benefit of subsidising real food and/or the health services that are impacted by such consumption. I would go substantially further than Brownell and Frieden propose. Using sugar as an example, I would put a minimum 100% (double the price of the product) tax on any product containing non naturally occurring sugar (any added 'ose').[lii] This would immediately discourage food manufacturers from adding sugar, completely unnecessarily, to ham, cottage cheese, tins of chick peas, kidney beans and other healthy products. I would put at least a 200% tax on any product where all sugars added together are the majority of the composition of the product. For any product (e.g. children's sweets) where the entire product is essentially sugars (with a bit of crushed animal innards, gelatine, for bonding), we should multiply the current price by four or five fold. The proceeds from taxes on sugar, trans fats and sweeteners should subsidise real food for people who are currently least able to afford it. We cannot hope to solve an obesity epidemic when we can buy ten doughnuts *or* one cucumber for the same price.

Other fiscal measures should be considered. Corporation tax can be raised on companies that make processed food and lowered, or eliminated, on companies that provide completely unadulterated natural food. The local butcher must become the provider of choice for meat, not McDonald's. Today, I can buy one pound (454 grams) of grass fed steak for the same price as a regular cheeseburger *and* medium fries *and* mayo chicken *and* a McFlurry original *and* a medium drink *and* a double cheeseburger.[377] This is not conducive to healthy eating – particularly in the sections of our population who can least afford, and most need, real food. Kessler details some of the most contemptuous examples of fast food: "One of the signature hamburgers at Hardee's is called the Monster Thickburger, which famously contains 1,420 calories and 108 grams of fat." "Yet even that pales in comparison to a slice of Claim Jumper's Chocolate Motherlode Cake ... 2,150 calories a slice". (Note the use of the word 'mother' to imply approval). Such inhumanity to man should be met with an "Inhumanity Tax". It's not far away from manslaughter, if you are familiar with the legal definition.

There would be additional benefits from such fiscal measures. The less processed food we eat, the less packaging is needed and the less drain on the world's scarce resources and the less rubbish created and the less need for land fill sites and so on. The 2010 report *What's Littering Britain?* by Tim Barnes, noted that 34% of Britain's litter comes from drink cans and bottles, 16% from confectionery wrappers and 13% from fast food. The most littered brand was Coca-Cola, followed by Walkers (crisps), McDonald's, Cadbury and Red Bull.

3) Any measure that makes it easier for people to eat real food

The 'one national organisation' should be creative in thinking of any other measures that can encourage healthy eating. The Children's Food Campaign is actively working to have drinking water available in all parks in the UK. Their July – September 2009 survey in parks across the UK[378] revealed that only 11% of the parks surveyed had water fountains and only one third of these were

---

[lii] As an example, fructose in a whole apple is fine, as this is the form in which nature intended us to eat fructose. Fructose added to sweeten other products is not necessary.

working. This is such a simple and good idea – we want children in our parks and we want them satiating thirst with easily available water, not leaving the park to find a fizzy drink.

Local produce providers could be helped to attend local bingo night. The household providers could have a fun night out and pick up the meat, fish, eggs, vegetables and dairy products at the same time. There will be many more ways to make healthy eating as easy as possible – we need to introduce any measure that could make a difference.

I have not proposed bariatric surgery as a solution, because a fundamental premise of this book is that we need to remember why we eat. Not only must we eat, we need to be able to digest what we eat. Campbell-McBride calls the gut the second brain of the body. Do we have full and certain knowledge of what will happen long term by surgically altering our digestive tract in such drastic ways? I sat next to someone at an obesity conference whose stomach had been stapled.[liii] He was unable to eat the lamb, as he knew he would not be able to digest it. He was, however, able to eat the bread, potatoes and the pastry based dessert. He was regaining weight at a steady pace. Bariatric surgeons are keen to stress that the expensive surgery 'pays for itself' in reduced cost to healthcare systems within two to four years.[379] There is nothing else that will work, they say, and the obesity journal evidence on low calorie diets lends support to this view. However, the one thing that we have *not* tried is eating the way we used to, before we got so obese and addicted. Would we really rather wire someone's jaw, or remove half their stomach, before doing everything we can to feed them real food? As Julian Hamilton Shield quipped at an obesity conference "if you attach your oesophagus to your anus, of course you will lose weight."[380] What are we doing to our fellow human beings?

Skills – training

I want to address two things under the skills sub heading – training and incentives.

To reverse the current advice and deliver new and consistent messages, we need to retrain people working in the field of obesity. We need to ensure that never again does a dietitian, nutritionist or dietary advisor glibly say "energy in equals energy out" (it doesn't) or "you can't change the laws of the universe" (but you can misapply them) or "you will lose two pounds of fat a week if you cut 1,000 calories a day" (you won't).

The British Dietetic Association (BDA) curriculum framework for the pre-registration, education and training of dietitians (2008)[381] is a 58 page document giving full details of all the training and education necessary for someone to qualify as a dietitian. The elements of the knowledge base (as the curriculum calls them) are: biochemistry; physiology; genetics; immunology; microbiology; clinical medicine; pharmacology; nutrition; sociology and social policy;

[liii] The Roux-en-Y procedure had been performed, which bypasses part of the small intestine. The small intestine is where almost all nutrients are absorbed.

psychology; communication and educational methods; food; food science and food systems management; dietetics; public health; research and evaluation; professional issues and organisations and management.

Nutrition and dietetics are arguably the two most relevant parts of a dietitian's training to any matters related to obesity. The indicative content in the nutrition part of the course includes "factors that determine food choice in achieving current dietary guidelines." The indicative content in the dietetics part of the course includes "the rational for modification of energy and nutrient intake." These seemed worthy of note, as the first aims to reinforce current dietary guidelines and the second seeks to justify the position taken on energy and nutrient intake.

We noted the BDA council (2007) definition of a dietitian in Chapter Fifteen. The relevant words here are "Uniquely, dietitians use the most up to date public health and scientific research on food, health and disease..." There is nothing in the curriculum (which came out a year after the dietitians defined themselves as above) to support this assertion. I regularly attend obesity conferences where I am a lone and unwelcome voice in amongst an overwhelming majority of dietitians. I have yet to find a dietitian who has come across the Minnesota experiment, let alone the most up to date public health and scientific research. None seem to be aware of the current and significant debate taking place about fructose. None can provide a reference for any allegations they repeatedly make about fat, cholesterol and heart disease. I say this not to criticise any individual dietitian, but to implore them to see that they are not being best served by their professional body and that they will need to do independent research for themselves, reading widely and discerningly, if they are to make a difference to their patients.

When I set out to study nutrition more formally, I investigated training as a dietitian. I rejected the prospect very quickly on two grounds a) my passion is obesity and with 1.1 billion overweight people in the world this is more than a big enough arena in which to specialise. I have no interest in food hygiene, food management systems, education or even in the nutritional aspects of any ailment outside obesity (unless obesity related) and therefore have no time to 'waste' on such topics when I could be spending that time reading obesity journals. b) Upon investigation of the weight management part of the course, I discovered that the first lesson is the calorie formula. I would be told that energy in equalled energy out and that to lose one pound of fat a deficit of 3,500 calories must be created. Thus the one part of the course that I would be interested in, would be of no use to me. Presumably I would need to reproduce answers that I know not to be true to pass, or fail as a result of giving my honest answer. A quick analysis of the 58 page curriculum document confirms that I made the right decision: the word weight does not appear once; the word obesity does not appear once; the word calorie does not appear once and the word diet only appears six times and in a very general context of the word diet e.g. UK diet or diet and lifestyle.

Some specialist obesity qualifications are being developed. The UK Weight Management Centre has a level 4 obesity management certificate. The curriculum reveals that, despite being a new course, this shows no sign of new thinking and energy in equals energy out remains at the heart of the programme. The part of the course on weight management features: "*Basic concepts of human energetics, Energy – Intake & Expenditure, Regulating Energy Expenditure, Control of Food intake*," i.e. energy in and out and how can we regulate energy in and out.

I believe that dietitians chose their vocation because they genuinely want to make a difference to the health and lives of others. I believe that they have the best of intentions, but have received the worst of advice during training. (I am only commenting on healthy eating and weight loss advice here. The rest of their training – food safety, food systems management and so on – may have been good). I implore dietitians, who really do want to improve the health of their nations, to challenge the training and education that they have been given. If you are studying at the moment – now is the perfect time to challenge. If you don't believe my questioning and research – please do your own. You must have seen by now many of the conclusions in this book for yourself, with your patients. I have met many dietitians at obesity conferences who already question the advice given and are very anti-sugar and concerned that they are being asked to recommend processed margarines, for example, above natural fats like butter and olive oil. We need you to play a key part in resolving this epidemic, but you will need to embrace nature's offerings if you haven't already done so.

The British Dietetic Association should ideally lead the way and it would be particularly valuable if the Dietitians in Obesity Management could play a key role in revised training for dietitians working in obesity management. I don't know what to advise for the USA. There is a mountain to climb to overcome the way in which the food and drink industry have been legally embedded to influence dietary advice. That's where the First Lady's focus should be.

Skills – incentives

The quality and outcomes framework (QOF) was introduced in April 2004 for the UK National Health Service (NHS), covering England, Wales and Scotland. It was introduced as part of the general medical services contract to replace other fee arrangements for general practices that were in existence at the time. The original arrangements allowed practices to earn up to 1,050 QOF Points across 146 different indicators. The general medical services contract was revised in April 2006 and the number of key clinical areas was increased. The total number of points available was reduced to 1,000 and 138 points were reassigned.

I used to run a manufacturing department for Mars Electronics (making coin mechanisms) and I soon learned that you get what you measure. When I joined the department our on time customer delivery performance was very poor. A quick review of the key performance indicators (KPI's) for the four shift managers revealed that they were rewarded on safety, housekeeping, quality, output and costs. The output target was based on the number of units built per shift. Hence, the production managers would make as many of the easiest to make coin mechanisms as possible, regardless of whether or not they met the customer order requirements. Trying to get the production managers to make what was needed was impossible for as long as their KPI's incentivised something else. All we needed to do was to change the output KPI to conform with customer requirements and we had four entire shifts of 120 people all making what the customer wanted.

I share this anecdote because analysis of the QOF will tell us exactly what UK general practitioners (GP's) and their practices will be trying to deliver. The clinical areas designated by the QOF are: asthma (4 indicators); atrial fibrillation (3); cancer (2); chronic kidney disease (4); chronic obstructive pulmonary disease (5); coronary heart disease (10); dementia (2); depression (2); diabetes (16); epilepsy (4); heart failure (3); hypertension (3); hypothyroidism (2); learning disabilities (1); mental health (6); obesity (1); palliative care (2); smoking (2) and strokes (8).

There are 650 of the 1000 points available in the clinical areas as follows: asthma (45 points); atrial fibrillation (30); cancer (11); chronic kidney disease (27); chronic obstructive pulmonary disease (28); coronary heart disease (89); dementia (20); depression (33); diabetes (93); epilepsy (15); heart failure (20); hypertension (83); hypothyroidism (7); learning disabilities (4); mental health (39); obesity (8); palliative care (6); smoking (68) and strokes (24). Organisational performance can earn 167.5 points; patient experience accounts for 146.5 and additional service can earn 36 points.

Each point is currently worth £120 to the GP and/or practice so that's £120,000 available for meeting these KPI's. My neighbour works as a GP practice manager and her job, essentially, is to get 1,000 points because points mean prizes. Given that the first requirement in each of the 19 clinical areas is to have a record of the patients with that condition, the practice can earn 27% of the points and money on offer by having one database recording all conditions for all registered patients.

Obesity earns eight points (out of the 1,000 available). That says something about NHS priorities in itself. To earn the eight points, the practice must be able to produce a register of patients aged 16 and over with a BMI greater than or equal to 30 in the last 15 months. The practice doesn't have to do anything about it – just record it. For recording this, and doing nothing more, the practice gets £960.

As a comparison, 89 points are available for coronary heart disease (CHD) targets. That equates to £10,680 in monetary terms. Examples of the 10 KPI's in this category include: the practice can produce a register of patients with coronary heart disease; the notes of these patients have a blood pressure reading in the past 15 months; the notes show that a cholesterol test has been done in the past 15 months. Each of these three measures can earn the practice nine points – more than the single category of obesity. These three simple recording measures together are worth over £3,000. Even more alarming is the reward that GP's can get for treating patients with CHD: another nine points if the patients are taking aspirin; another nine if they have a cholesterol level lower than the number 5mmol/l picked out of the air (this might be achieved artificially with statins); another nine if they are taking a beta blocker (please note the weight gain associated with these in Chapter Three); another nine if they are taking medication for hypertension (please note the weight gain associated with these in Chapter Three) and another nine if they had a flu jab.

The heart patient is quite likely to be a diabetes patient as well. The same boxes can be ticked if the diabetes patients have had a blood pressure test and a cholesterol test. One of the diabetes measures is simply having the BMI recorded. Again, if cholesterol is lowered to 5mmol/l or less, if the flu jab has been administered and if the patient is on medication for hypertension – more points and more money. We are literally paying doctors to multi-medicate our citizens. What was that Hippocratic Oath? First do no harm.

Just to prove that you get what you measure in the health service, just as you do in private sector manufacturing, in 2008/09 the average practice in England achieved 95.4% of the overall 1,000 points and £120,000 available. The average practice also achieved 97.8% of the clinical targets.[382]

I have much respect for our generalist medical staff – doctors and nurses. Patient A has depression, ten to fifteen minutes later and you are dealing with a possible broken bone; patient C has detected a lump in their breast and then the next person presents themselves as TATT (tired all the time). All of this can happen on a typical day before the morning coffee break. Nurses too are playing increasingly important roles in front line response in surgeries and hospitals. There is no way that doctors or nurses can know about any one condition to the level of a specialist and yet they know about all of them to an impressively high degree.

I sincerely hope that this book inspires doctors and nurses to change the lives of their patients. Please take down every copy of the pyramids and plates that you see. Please remove literature in your surgeries that speaks of 'good' and 'bad' cholesterol – this is insulting to you and your patients' intelligence. Please work only with dietitians and dietary advisors who recommend real food. Please don't refer patients to those who want to hang on to the advice that has led to the average UK citizen eating 1,536 calories of processed food each day.

People power

I hope desperately that this book has a significant impact on our public dietary advice and that we return to eating real food to the benefit of all modern illness, not just obesity. Hope is no where near a strong enough word – lives literally depend upon us doing this – not just saving lives, but the *quality* of lives that people are leading today. Many of our citizens are 'existing', rather than living, and this is a tragedy in a supposedly advanced species.

Hope is one thing – what I think will happen is another. I think that individuals will be the primary catalysts for change. There is inspiring evidence across the world that there is a growing momentum of people expressing similar views: a drive to eat for health, not to maximise the profits of the food industry; anger at the marketing of processed junk to our children; despair at the bad advice being given by our governments; disbelief at the absurdity of the idea that somehow real food is bad and processed food is good.

Every single one of us, as individuals, can stop this obesity epidemic. Let food and drink companies advertise to us all they like – we can commit to eating Mother Nature's food from this day forward. We can lobby government until they do help us. We have a forum now – it's called the World Wide Web and we can meet globally in a way we never could before. We can join organisations like the Children's Food Campaign and the Weston A. Price Foundation and unite together until we *can* get ten cucumbers for the price of one doughnut, or at least not the other way round. If we don't buy or consume processed food and drink – the food and drink industry will respond. Let their vast funds start going into how to help us eat nature's food in a convenient way.

Government should lead the way, I pray that it does, but I'm not relying upon it. We individuals can change the way every one of us eats and the government can play catch up at some embarrassing juncture. What has leadership come to when the people I follow on Twitter are more likely to change the world than our elected politicians?

What might stop us?

I have given a great deal of thought to what blocks progress. I think that the number one reason, for which we find ourselves in the current crisis situation, is ignorance. I did not know that we changed our diet advice in 1977-1983. I did not know how fundamental that change was. I did not make the connection with the obesity epidemic until I started researching this topic full time. One of the key aims of this book is to present facts and evidence, so that we can no longer plead ignorance.

There are of course those who will have read this far and do not believe any of this. You may still believe that the first law of thermodynamics says that energy in equals energy out, that we can ignore the second law and that the body is a cash machine for fat. You may believe that medication and hormones are just excuses – fat people are greedy and lazy, full stop. You may still be convinced that every person will lose 104 pounds in fat alone every year that they create a deficit of 1,000 calories a day. You may think that our change of advice had nothing to do with the obesity epidemic – the timing was just a coincidence. You may consider food pyramids and 'eatwell' plates to be role models of healthy eating. You may think that manufactured substances, chemically altered and fortified to emulate butter, are better than the real thing. You may still think that five-a-day does have some scientific basis. You may still think that fat is bad, not processed food, despite the fact that we've confused the two all along. You may not worry about the food and drink industry being integrally embedded with our 'healthy eating' advice. You may think that they have our best interests at heart.

I'm going to be blunt here: if you think that continuing to do what we have been doing for the past 30 years is going to solve the obesity epidemic, you are, by definition, mad. If you think that nature is out to get us, by putting killer substances in the same food that has all the nutrients, you are, by definition, paranoid. Please don't be offended if I move on and leave you behind from this point onwards.

I do think that the cholesterol propaganda has been so effective that I am not expecting this book to have convinced everyone by any means on this critical topic. I do hope that I have at least shared some interesting things that you didn't know, which I also didn't know before setting out on this journey. I hope that you are more thoughtful about the importance of cholesterol and more concerned about drugs that stop the body making it. I also hope that our foray into cholesterol and saturated fat has at least left you content that human beings can, and indeed should, eat nature's food. If you need convincing further, please read Kendrick's *The Great Cholesterol Con* with an open mind and see where you end up.

If this book has proved enlightening, there are three thoughts that are likely to come to mind:

1) "How can I help?"
2) "I don't want to look stupid."
3) "I've got too much to lose."

The first group are the ones who will lead the way. I salute you and the more of you there are the more chance we have of solving the obesity epidemic.

The second group are significant and critical for progress. I think that many of our health charities could be in this category. Surely organisations like the British Heart Foundation and the American Cancer Society are more interested in the *health* of their nations than the *wealth* of their nations' leading companies. Are these bodies really accepting dietary advice without question? Do they honestly think that sugary cereal is the optimal way for already sick people to start the day? I find it inconceivable that Charles Clark is the only diabetologist who has worked out that it is wrong to advise diabetic patients to base their meals on starchy foods.[383] My personal view is – telling diabetics to base their meals on the one macronutrient that they cannot handle is tantamount to medical malpractice. Diabetes UK must have worked this out. Being conflicted by having Kellogg's as a sponsor is not helpful. However, the leadership of this organisation needs to stand up and say "we got it wrong". There are 171 million diabetes sufferers worldwide and the World Health Organisation estimate is that this will rise to 366 million by 2030.[384] Surely that is worth a moment of "we were wrong"? According to the World Health Organisation *World Health Report* of 2003, 16.7 million people die of heart disease each year. Surely that's 16.7 million reasons, and growing, to contemplate that modern food may be responsible for modern illness and to suggest a return to real food?

Dietary organisations, public health advisors, doctors and dietitians may also think "I'll look stupid" if I say something this week and I said the opposite last week. I have three comments here: First, I bet Columbus looked a bit stupid to start with, but he soon had the last laugh. Secondly, if someone's ego is more important than the health of their patients, they're in the wrong job. Third, it is completely wrong to think that changing tack is in any way a sign of weakness. As Alexander Pope said, "A man should never be ashamed to own that he has been in the wrong, which is but saying in other words that he is wiser today than he was yesterday."[385]

The third group we need to neutralise. The food and drink industry has the most to lose, if people return to eating real food. Companies making things as diverse as plus size clothing to indigestion tablets also stand to lose if we go back to 'the good old days'. If you can think of a reason why the profits and returns to shareholders of these organisations are more important than global health, please let me know. Meanwhile, I will proceed on the basis that the consumption of processed food needs to be dramatically curtailed, not continually grown. Dietary organisations, not least in the USA, may also have something to lose, as they currently benefit from the financial sponsorship of the food and drink industry and they enjoy a legislation endorsed monopoly position. The food and drink industry is a huge group to be up against in the battle against obesity. Please let there be no other people in this group (doctors, individual dietary advisors, politicians etc), so that we have a decent chance of counterbalancing the enormity of this economic force.

The only question now is – which group will you be a part of?

Summary

The Obesity Epidemic

Summary

The Obesity Epidemic

Our dietary advice was right the first time and we need to go back to the certainty that "farinaceous foods are fattening and saccharine matters are especially so."[386]

We changed our advice for the wrong reason. We changed it to the wrong advice.

In the 1970's, the fact that (fewer than six) people (in one thousand) were dying from heart disease was of great concern to America. American public health advisors wanted a solution. Ancel Keys had spent the 1950's trying to prove that cholesterol consumption was the cause of heart disease. He failed and he acknowledged this. He then tried to prove that saturated fat consumption causes heart disease, despite this having no logic, not least because saturated fat and cholesterol (and unsaturated fat) are found in the same foods. At the time that Senator McGovern was looking for the first *Dietary Goals for the United States*, the Keys theory was *not* the only idea available for consideration, but it was the best promoted. The rest, as they say, is history.

The USA changed its dietary advice in 1977 and the UK followed in 1983. We told people that fat was bad and carbohydrate was good not because we *knew* either fat to be bad or carbohydrate to be good. At the time we changed our advice, the only 'evidence' for fat being bad was a feeble suggestion that, in seven hand picked countries, heart disease tended to be related to cholesterol levels, which tended to be related to saturated fat intake and so (that must mean) heart disease tended to be related to saturated fat, (although cholesterol intake was not directly related *per se)*. Association was never proven and causation was never alleged. We had no evidence that carbohydrate was good – just the admission that, if we tell people not to eat fat they must eat something and "it was advised that starchy carbohydrates should replace the reduction in fat as an energy source."[387]

We have not looked for proof since:

- "There has been no controlled clinical trial of the effect of decreasing dietary intake of saturated fatty acids on the incidence of coronary heart disease nor is it likely that such a trial will be undertaken." (COMA, 1984).[388]
- "It has been accepted by experienced coronary disease researchers that the perfect controlled dietary trial for prevention of coronary heart disease has not yet been done and we are unlikely ever to see it done." (Truswell, 1994).[389]
- "The ideal controlled dietary trial for prevention of heart disease has not yet been done and it is unlikely ever to be done." (FSA, 2009).[390]

Without doing the definitive study, we have nonetheless tried to post rationalise the U-turn in dietary advice. We claim that saturated fat causes heart disease directly; we claim that saturated fat causes heart disease through cholesterol; we claim that saturated fat is trying to kill us and unsaturated fat is trying to save us; we claim that a magic ratio of polyunsaturated fat to saturated fat, (unachievable with a natural diet) will save us; we claim that there is such a thing as bad and good cholesterol and that the former is trying to kill us and the latter is trying to save us; we claim that food we have been eating for thousands of years will kill us and modern-man-made-spreads will save us. We have claimed some quite extraordinary things since the Seven Countries Study and we have no more evidence now than we had then. We still have no consistent association; let alone got anywhere near proven causation. As for the possible benefit of carbohydrate – we have not even bothered to post rationalise this.[liv] To do so would be pointless – fat is bad, so we must eat carbohydrate, so it could only be unhelpful to find anything wrong with carbohydrate.[lv]

The ultimate irony is that if Keys did show anything, he likely showed a relationship between the 100% carbohydrate, sucrose, and heart disease: "The fact that the incidence of coronary heart disease was significantly correlated with the average percentage of calories from sucrose in the diets is explained by the inter correlation of sucrose with saturated fat."[391] Decades later we have not corrected this fundamental mistake and we still list biscuits, cakes and pastries – carbohydrates first and invariably *unsaturated* fat second – as saturated fats. The Chief Medical Officer for England blames the real foods meat, butter, cream and cheese for "finding their way into our diet in biscuits, cakes and pastries."[392] So, we changed our advice to try to alleviate heart disease and, as a result of this catastrophic confusion over macronutrients, our citizens are consuming more of the foods that should have been clearly identified as the culprits in the first place.

We have forgotten that we eat for nourishment. We have a vital need for nutrition and we have lost this basic value in our current dietary advice. If we had stayed true to the principle of why we eat, the most nutritious foods would be evidential in any analysis of fat, protein, vitamins and minerals. They are the liver, sardines, milk, eggs and greens favoured by our elders and not the fortified cereals and margarines favoured by conglomerates and, reprehensibly, far too many dietary advisors alongside.

An industry originated marketing campaign, five-a-day, has become the leading public health message in tens of countries across three continents and it is spoken of as if there is overwhelming evidence behind it, when the reality is that there is none. Worse, if the proponents of pick-a-number-a-day knew what

---

[liv] Other than to extol its calorie content compared to fat. We don't, however, promote protein in the same way, which has the same approximate calorific value as carbohydrate.

[lv] We have inadvertently found much 'wrong' with carbohydrate along the way – not least the fact that, at the level of carbohydrate intake recommended in dietary guidelines, VLDL and thereby cholesterol levels will rise.

Johnson and Lustig know, they would surely revise their opinion of fructose and never mention fruit juice again.

We have slandered and libelled the most nutritious macronutrient – fat and we have promoted and praised the least nutritious macronutrient – carbohydrate. We don't need to look far to understand why. The most nutritious foods on the planet are those provided by nature. The most profitable foods on the planet are those provided by food manufacturers.

As the demonisation of real food has gathered pace, fledgling and long standing food and drink companies have become multi-billion dollar empires. "The world's largest convenient food and beverage company", PepsiCo, is bigger than 60% of the countries in the world.[393] An immense and profitable industry has grown on the back of the low fat, high carbohydrate advice that we invented. Human beings have become high fat and low health in parallel.

When people talk about "the obesogenic environment", they do so as if this were some inexplicable phenomenon that crept up on the world and made everyone fat. *We created* this obesogenic environment; it did not happen to us. We told people to avoid real food and to eat processed food. We passed legislation to introduce trans fats and sweeteners into our food chain. We allowed our children to be given toys, cartoon characters and junk food by 'strangers'.[394] We have facilitated the comprehensive infiltration of the food and drink industry into our dietary advice – no where more so than in the fattest nation on earth, where we have gone as far as legislating the relationship. We put cakes, cola and sweets on government posters, pyramids and plates of role model healthy eating. We welcomed food and drink industry funds turning global sporting events into advertising arenas for their products. We continue to revere sports and pop stars, who are paid millions of dollars to endorse products that they likely don't consume themselves. We care more about the profitability of Kellogg's and McDonald's than we do the health of our citizens. Prove me wrong governments and take decisive and immediate action. Just don't act like this environment is nothing to do with you.

Had we changed our advice for the wrong reasons and to the wrong advice without consequence, we would have been fortunate. We have not been fortunate. We have paid an enormous price for this change; with a ten fold increase in obesity. Furthermore, more people are continuing to become obese and the obese are continuing to become more obese and we have not yet had the first generation born to our most obese generation. It is not unreasonable to say that on the back of one man's study, first adopted by one American Governor and then the world, we have an obesity epidemic.

Kessler tells a wonderful anecdote about Katherine Flegal, a researcher at the Centers for Disease Control and Prevention. The story goes that, when Flegal first reviewed the 1988-1991 USA obesity survey, she was convinced that the data must be wrong. Double, triple, checks later, colleagues confirmed that the data was right – one third of the population was now overweight. "In fewer than a dozen years, about 20 million Americans had joined the ranks of the overweight."[395] (Subtract fewer than a dozen years, say 11, from 1988-1991, to find the dates of the change in USA dietary advice). This epidemic took off so suddenly and it has taken hold like wild fire and we have barely had time to take stock to make the connection between the timing of the change in our advice and what happened since.

As obesity doubled for UK adults between 1972 and 1982 and then almost doubled again by 1989 and then almost another time by 1999, the urgency and desperation to lose weight was palpable. The advice that people were given was the same as the advice that made them overweight in the first place: eat less fat – eat more carbohydrate; eat less real food – eat more processed food.

Eat less/do more became such a common mantra that anyone who didn't 'get this' was declared stupid on the world wide web. What these critics didn't know is that we had evidence going back to 1917 that eat less/do more did not work. The level of failure was quantified in 1959 by Stunkard and McLaren-Hume at 98%. Another irony could be that we ignored the brilliant and unbiased study done by Ancel Keys and favoured instead the one where he set out to prove an already held view. Keys did the definitive study to show exactly what happens when we manage to restrict calorie intake and that even this can only be achieved 'in captivity', due to the hunger that ensues. We know from this Minnesota experiment and from Leibel et al that calorie restriction results in a disproportionate reduction in energy expenditure and metabolic activity and that the 'circular reference' will defeat the dieter in weeks.

As we tried to fix a crisis, without making the connection that we started it, we compounded the challenge by proceeding on the basis of flawed assumptions – theoretical and empirical.

The theoretical error we made was to simplify the application of the laws of the universe to the world of dieting – we got the first law wrong and ignored the second law. If we had considered both properly, we would have realised that obesity is not a simplistic outcome of energy in (overweight people eat too much) and/or energy out (overweight people are too sedentary). We would have realised that energy in can only equal energy out if the body makes no internal adjustment whatsoever. Not only is this biochemically impossible, the internal adjustment made by the body, in response to changes in energy intake and/or energy requirements, is likely far greater than any change in fat reserves that the body can or will make.

Empirically, we got hold of a calorie formula, we know not from where, which we hold to be true and continually prove to be untrue. Justin Stoneman was the first journalist I met to grasp the enormity of the lie that is the calorie formula. He made the analogy that, if we carried on teaching children that London is the capital of America, when we knew this to be wrong, there would be uproar. Quite so; yet when the hopes of 1.1 billion overweight people depend upon an equally wrong, but vastly more serious, untruth, we continue to lie.

We know that any answer to the obesity epidemic must explain what has *changed* since circa 1980. The answer, therefore, can *not* be found in something we have been eating for over one hundred thousand years (real food – especially fat). The answer can *not* be found in anything we have been eating *less* of during the past thirty years (real food – especially fat). The answer *can* be found in anything we have *not* been eating for over one hundred thousand years (processed food – especially carbohydrate). The answer *can* be found in anything we have been eating *more* of during the past thirty years (processed food – especially carbohydrate).

The answer similarly can *not* be found in the other half of the energy in equals energy out oversimplification. Sedentary behaviour did not cause the obesity epidemic. Exercise will not cure it. The conclusion of the one study that tried to quantify the contribution played by energy intake vs. energy expenditure (Swinburn) was that Americans had been expending more energy during the period in which the average person gained 20 pounds.[396]

When we put together the following...

1) Obesity is not a simplistic imbalance of energy in and energy out but a far more complex matter of how, biochemically, the body can store or utilise fat. Carbohydrate is the unique macronutrient that facilitates fat storage and prevents fat utilisation.
2) Fat/protein calories have jobs to do within the body – they contribute to the 'up to' 85% of energy requirement determined by metabolic rate. Carbohydrate doesn't; this needs to be burned as fuel or it will be stored as fat.
3) Insulin has been called the fattening hormone for good reason and only carbohydrate calories stimulate the release of insulin; fat/protein calories have no impact on insulin.
4) A calorie is not a calorie – if it were the second law of thermodynamics would be violated. Fat/protein calories have substantial metabolic advantage over carbohydrate calories. A low carbohydrate diet can thus simulate a low calorie diet, as if a 25% reduction in calorie intake had been made, but without the accompanying desire to eat more and do less.
5) Isolcaloric studies, back as far as 1956, have shown low calorie diets to be far less effective than low carbohydrate diets (even if the reviewers did not do the correlation analysis to conclude this).

... all routes lead to carbohydrates as being uniquely suited to weight gain and uniquely unsuited to weight loss. The macronutrient that we have been advising people to eat more of is the very macronutrient that enables fat to be stored and disables fat from being utilised. Carbohydrates, not calories, are the critical determinant of obesity and the epidemic thereof.

We opened this book with Colleen Rand's brilliant study of how much people would rather be something else than obese. The precise numbers were that 100% of those researched would rather be deaf, 89% would rather be blind and 91% would rather have a leg amputated – than be obese. Proposed solutions are that we wire the jaws, or staple the stomachs, of our fellow humans. The suggestion that we might return to eating the way that we did, before we needed to invent such drastic procedures, is instead seen as radical.

The decision made by humans to move away from the diet that we have evolved to eat has led to two thirds of the 'evolved' world being overweight and a number wishing that they were literally anything else, rather than obese.

As Barry Groves observed: "Man is the only chronically sick animal on the planet."[397]

Man is the only species clever enough to make his own food and the only one stupid enough to eat it.

How many more obese humans do we plan to produce before we stop feeding them man-made food? Will the man-made obese ever forgive us for what we have already done? Will we ever forgive ourselves if we make any more? Is it really so preposterous to suggest that we simply return to eating the real food that our planet provides for us? The real food that we used to eat, before we got so fat we'd rather be blind.

The End

The Obesity Epidemic

Glossary of Terms

ATP: stands for Adenosine Tri-Phosphate. It is an organic compound made up of adenosine (an adenine ring and a ribose sugar) and three phosphate groups, hence, the name. ATP contains a large amount of chemical energy stored in its high-energy phosphate bonds. It releases energy when it is broken down into ADP (Adenosine Di-Phosphate). ATP is considered as the universal energy currency for metabolism. Plants make ATP during photosynthesis. Humans make ATP by breaking down molecules such as glucose.

Body Mass Index: a measure of weight in relation to height. It is calculated by measuring weight in kilograms divided by height in metres squared. It should be viewed more as a useful guide than a precise science. A BMI of less than 18.5 is considered underweight; a BMI of 18.5-24.9 is considered normal; a BMI of 25-29.9 is considered overweight and a BMI of 30 or more is considered obese.

Basal Metabolic Rate: the energy (calorie) requirement of a person in a resting state.

Calorie: a gram calorie is "The amount of energy required to raise the temperature of 1 gram of water from 14.5°C to 15.5°C, at standard atmospheric pressure." A "kilogram calorie" is the amount of energy required to raise the temperature of one kilogram of water by one degree Celsius. The Kilogram calorie is also known as: the large calorie; a food calorie and/or Calorie with a capital C.

Cholesterol: ($C_{27}H_{46}O$): a waxy lipid found in all body cells and critical for the working of the body.

Cholesterol measurement comparators: The USA favours mg/dl for cholesterol measurement, Europe and Australia favour mmol/L. To convert mmol/L to mg/dl, multiply by 38.67. To convert mg/dl to mmol/L, divide by 38.67.

Chylomicrons: are the largest lipoproteins. Chylomicrons are formed in the intestine, as a result of digestion, and chylomicrons are the transport mechanism for taking dietary fat (and cholesterol) from the digestive system into the blood stream and from there to the different parts of the body.

Coenzyme Q10 (CoQ10): a naturally occurring compound found in every cell in the body. It is also called ubiquinone, from the word ubiquitous, which means "found everywhere. It plays a key role in energy production in the body and has been called the energy spark plug for the body.

Cohort: This is a term used frequently in epidemiological studies. It means a different demographic group of people. A cohort is typically a discrete group, which does not overlap with another group being studied. In the Seven Countries Study, as an example, the cohorts were defined as the different regions/towns studies within each of the seven countries.

Corticosteroids: are steroid hormones that are produced in the adrenal cortex, (specifically and interestingly, they are synthesised from cholesterol within the adrenal cortex). There are subsets of corticosteroids – two key ones being glucocorticoids and mineral corticoids – listed elsewhere in this glossary.

Cytoplasm: The cytoplasm consists of all of the contents outside the nucleus, but within the membrane, of a cell.

Diabetes: Type 1 tends to develop in children, adolescents or young adults and tends to have genetic origins, although type 1 has recently been observed to develop in older people and not necessarily with a hereditary connection. With type 1, no insulin is produced by the pancreas. Type 2 has tended to develop in older people and is commonly described as a state of insulin resistance – the pancreas does produce insulin but the cells have become resistant to insulin. Type 2 diabetes is also now being seen in children, which is extremely worrying in that it can be seen as analogous to an 'overworked' pancreas – no longer able to cope with continual (refined) carbohydrate consumption.

Enzyme: a protein (or protein based molecule) that speeds up a chemical reaction in a living organism. It acts as a catalyst. There are three types of enzymes in the human body: metabolic enzymes, which run our bodies; digestive enzymes, which digest our food; and food enzymes from raw foods, which start food digestion. There are approximately 50,000 enzymes in the human body.

The Endocrine system: one of the nine systems in the human body. This system is made up of the endocrine glands that secrete hormones. There are eight such glands: the pineal; pituitary; thyroid; thymus; adrenals; pancreas; ovaries (females) and testes (males).

Epidemiology: the study of how often and in what circumstances different illnesses occur in different populations/groups of people.

Glucagon: a hormone released by the pancreas which stimulates the liver to convert stored glycogen into glucose when blood glucose levels fall too low.

Glucocorticoids: The adrenal cortex produces corticosteroids (steroid hormones). Three of these (cortisol, cortisone and corticosterone) are collectively known as glucocorticoids. Glucocorticoids play a key role in the utilisation of carbohydrate and regulation of blood sugar levels especially and fat and protein to a lesser extent.

Glycerol: has the chemical compound $C_3H_5(OH)_3$. Glycerol is a sugar alcohol and it has many other names – glycerine, glycerine, 1, 2, 3-trihydroxypropane etc. The 1,2,3 reference indicates that glycerol has three hydrogen/oxygen groups that can bond with the COOH group at the end of fats.

Glycogen: the storage form of glucose in the body. The body can store approximately 100 grams of glycogen in the liver and 250-400 grams in the muscles. The glycogen in the muscles can only be used by the muscles, but the glycogen in the liver can be used wherever energy is needed by the body.

Hypothalamus: a part of the brain (at the base), which contains cells that perform a number of functions such as the regulation of hunger, respiration, body temperature and it acts as the control centre for the endocrine (hormone) system.

Insulin: a hormone produced by the pancreas which acts to regulate blood glucose levels. Insulin does this by turning glucose into glycogen, which can subsequently be stored as fat. Insulin also facilitates the movement of glucose from the blood stream into body cells, including fat cells. It has been called the fattening hormone, as a result of these roles.

Isocaloric: where calories are kept the same and the composition of carbohydrate, fat and protein are varied. This enables the impact of what is eaten, rather than how much, to be assessed.

Lipase: the enzyme that breaks down triglycerides into fatty acids and glycerol.

Lipolysis: the hydrolysis (breaking down) of lipids (fats). Metabolically it is the breakdown of triglycerides into free fatty acids within cells.

Lipoproteins: are microscopic bodies found in our blood stream. We can think of lipoproteins as tiny 'taxi cabs' travelling round the blood stream acting as transporters. They are needed because the vital substances fat and cholesterol are not water soluble, so they cannot exist freely in blood. The lipoproteins, therefore, carry fat and cholesterol around the body to perform their critical tasks.

Macro minerals: minerals present in the body and used by the body in amounts greater than 100 milligrams per day: calcium; chloride; magnesium; phosphorus; potassium; sodium and sulphur.

Macronutrient: the collective term for carbohydrate, fat and protein –the three macronutrients that we consume in large quantities – hence the pre-fix macro. Rarely is a food solely one macronutrient – far more commonly foods are fat/proteins (meat, fish, eggs, dairy etc) or carbohydrate/proteins (vegetables, fruit, pulses, grains etc). Sugar is one of the rare foods that is 100% carbohydrate (no fat or protein). Oil generally and olive oil, as an example, is 100% fat (no carbohydrate or protein).

Melatonin: a hormone secreted by the pineal gland during the hours of darkness, which regulates the pituitary gland and is associated with the biological clock. Melatonin is derived from serotonin, with which it works to regulate the sleep cycle.

Mineral corticoids: regulate minerals and therefore water balance in the body, through the regulation of potassium and sodium. The mineral corticoid, aldosterone, has a key role to play in the regulation of salt and water balance.

Mitochondria: the main sites of energy production in a cell. They contain a number of pathways, including the pathway for oxidising fat for fuel.

Pancreas: is a gland organ playing dual roles in the digestive and endocrine systems of the body. It is both an endocrine gland, producing several important hormones, including insulin and glucagon, as well as an exocrine gland, releasing pancreatic juice containing digestive enzymes that pass to the small intestine. These enzymes help to further breakdown carbohydrate (pancreatic amylase), protein (protease) and fat (lipase).

Pancreatic amylase: the enzyme that breaks down polysaccharides into simple sugars.

Poly cystic ovary syndrome (PCOS): a syndrome of ovarian dysfunction. It can be observed with an ultrasound, or it can be diagnosed by noticing an over production of androgens (hormones) and/or infrequent/irregular or absence of ovulation.

Protease: the enzyme that breaks down protein into amino acids. It is produced by the stomach, small intestine and pancreas.

Pyruvic acid: (also called pyruvate) a colourless, water-soluble, organic liquid produced by the breakdown of carbohydrates and sugars during glycolysis.

Serotonin: a neurotransmitter that is primarily found in the pineal gland, digestive tract and central nervous system. It is synthesised from the amino acid tryptophan. It plays a key role in mood and appetite and is crucial in maintaining a sense of well-being. Serotonin is sometimes called the 'feel good' hormone.

Trace minerals: minerals present in the body and used by the body in amounts smaller than 100 milligrams per day: chromium; copper; fluoride; iodine; iron; manganese; molybdenum; selenium and zinc.

Triglyceride: (also called TAG, Triacylglycerol, Triacylglyceride) is the structure formed by three fatty acids bonded together with glycerol. It is the form in which human fat tissue is stored.

Abbreviations

As a board member of two organisations, I see too many TLA's (Three Letter Abbreviations) and I invariably spell these out in full, so as not to trouble my reader. In the unlikely event that I have not used the full version recently before a TLA, here are the abbreviations used in this book (these are global terms, unless indicated otherwise):

ACC: American College of Cardiology (USA).

ACSM: American College of Sports Medicine (USA).

ACTH: Adrenocorticotrophic Hormone.

ADA: American Dietetic Association (USA).

ADH: Anti-Diuretic Hormone.

AHA: American Heart Association (USA).

AI: Adequate Intake – nutrition guideline in the absence of an RDA (USA).

ASO: The Association for the Study of Obesity (UK).

ATP: Adenosine TriPhosphate.

BBC: British Broadcasting Corporation – the British media channel (UK).

BDA: British Dietetic Association or the British Diabetic Association (spelled out in full, when first used in a new passage, for clarity) (UK).

BMI: Body Mass Index.

BMR: Basal Metabolic Rate.

BNF: British Nutrition Foundation (UK).

BUPA: British United Provident Association (global health care company).

BOGH: Balance of Good Health – the plate preceding the 'eatwell' plate (UK).

CDR: Commission for Dietetic Registration (USA).

CHD: Coronary Heart Disease.

COMA: Committee of Medical Aspects of Food and Nutrition Policy (UK).

CVD: Cardio Vascular Disease.

DCCT: Diabetes Control and Complications Trial (UK).

DEFRA: The Department for Environment, Food and Rural Affairs (UK).

DETR: the Department of the Environment, Transport and the Regions (UK).

DoH: Department of Health (UK).

DOM: Dietitians in Obesity Management (UK).

FDA: Food and Drug Administration (USA).

FSA: Food Standards Agency (UK).

FSH: Follicle Stimulating Hormone.

GDP: Gross Domestic Product.

GRAS: Generally Regarded As Safe (USA).

HDL: High Density Lipoprotein.

HFCS: High Fructose Corn Syrup.

HGH: Human Growth Hormone.

HHS: Department of Health and Human Services (USA).

ICSH: Interstitial Cell Stimulating Hormone.

IDL: Intermediate Density Lipoprotein.

LCD: Low Calorie Diet.

LDL: Low Density Lipoprotein.

LH: Luteinizing Hormone.

MAFF: Ministry of Agriculture Fisheries and Food (UK).

MONICA: A World Health Organisation study "Monitoring Trends In Cardiovascular disease."

NACNE: National Advisory Committee on Nutrition Education (UK).

NCEP: National Cholesterol Education Programme (USA).

NHANES: The National Health and Nutrition Examination Survey (USA).

NHS: National Health Service (UK).

NICE: National Institute for Clinical Excellence (UK).

NOF: National Obesity Forum (UK).

ONS: Office of National Statistics (UK).

PCOS: Poly Cystic Ovary Syndrome.

RDA: Recommended Dietary Allowance (USA).

SACN: Scientific Advisory Committee on Nutrition (UK).

TSH: Thyroid Stimulating Hormone.

UKPDS: United Kingdom Prospective Diabetes Study (UK).

USDA: United States Department of Agriculture.

VLCD: Very Low Calorie Diet.

VLDL: Very Low Density Lipoprotein.

WHO: World Health Organisation.

Appendix 1

"Popular Diets: A Scientific Review"[398]

	Authors & publication	# of people	Duration	Carb grams/ day	Kcal/ day	grams lost/ day
1	Rickman, JAMA (1974)	12	7 days	7	1,325	-442
2	Benoit et al, Ann Intern Med (1965)	7	10 days	10	1,000	-660
3	Yudkin & Carey, Lancet (1960)	6	14 days	43	1,383	-200
4	Fletcher, Br J Nutr (1961)	6	14 days	36	800	-223
5	Lewis et al, Am J Clin Nutr (1977)	10	14 days	27	1,115	-371
6	Kasper et al, Am J Clin Nutr (1973)	16	16 days	56	1,707	-300
7	Evans, Nutr Metab (1974)	8	6 wk	80	1,490	-97.5
8	Golay et al, Int J Obes relat Metab Disord (1996)	22	6 wk	37.5	1,000	-212
9	Young, Am J Clin Nutr, (1971)	3	6 wk	30	1,800	-385
10	Golay et al, Am J Clin Nutr (1996)	31	12 wk	75	1,200	-121
11	Cedarquist, J Am Diet Assoc (1952)	7	16 wk	85	1,500	-114
12	Worthington & Taylor, J Am Diet Assoc (1974)	20	21 days	17	1,182	-571
13	Rabast et al, Int J Obes relat Metab Disord (1979)	13	25 days	48	1,871	-350
14	Rabast et al, Nutr Metab (1978)	25	30 days	25	1,000	-392
15	Wing et al, Int J Obes relat Metab Disord (1995)	11	4 wk	10	800	-270
16	Alford et al, J Am Diet Assoc (1990)	11	10 wk	75	1,200	-91
17	Baron et al, Am J Public Health (1986)	66	3 mths	50	1,000	-55

Notes:

* 21 studies were included in tables 5a and 5b in the paper. Three had no results for weight change, so could not be included (Kekwick 1957, Bortz 1968 and Krehl 1967).

* I excluded Larosa et al (1980), as the table said that the study was for 12 weeks when, in fact, the article and the original journal revealed that the subjects followed their normal diet for two weeks at the start and two weeks at the end of the 12 week period. We cannot determine what the weight loss per day was in relation to a measured carbohydrate and calorie intake period.

* The 17 remaining studies are above. There was a material error in the article. This has been corrected in the table above, as follows: Study 8 (Golay et al) – the weight loss in table 5a is given as -8.0 kilograms over 6 weeks, which was commuted to -111 grams per day in table 5a. This is wrong and -8.0 kilograms over 6 weeks equates to -190 grams per day. However, the table appears to be wrong in more way than one and the original journal (and the text in the article) state that the weight change for the group on 37.5 grams CHO was -8.9 kilograms +/- 0.6 kilograms. I have taken the mid point of -8.9 kilograms and this equates to -212 grams per day. This is the number in the table for this appendix and the number I have used for the correlation.

* A number of ranges were taken at mid point level, as follows:

- Study 7 (Evans) – the range of weight loss was given as -76 to -119 grams per day, so I took the mid point of -97.5 grams per day;

- Study 11 (Cedarquist) – the range of weight loss was given as -78 to -150 grams per day, so I took the mid point of -114 grams per day.

* Five of the studies were directly comparable isocaloric studies i.e. the studies had parallel groups on a different carbohydrate level and the same calories per day (these are studies 6, 8, 10, 12 and 14). In every such isocaloric study in the article, the weight loss was substantially higher in the low carbohydrate group than in the higher carbohydrate group. At the highest calorie intake (Kasper et al, study 6, 1707 calories per day), the group consuming 56 grams of carbohydrate per day lost 300 grams per day vs. the 156 grams of carbohydrate per day group, which only lost 50 grams per day. This supports Kekwick and Pawan's findings that large numbers of calories can be consumed and weight still be lost with a low carbohydrate diet composition.

Correlation between (low) calories & (high) weight loss

	Authors	Cals (x)	Loss (y)	x*y	x*x	y*y
1	Rickman	1,325	-442	-585,650	1,755,625	195,364
2	Benoit et al	1,000	-660	-660,000	1,000,000	435,600
3	Yudkin & Carey	1,383	-200	-276,600	1,912,689	40,000
4	Fletcher	800	-223	-178,400	640,000	49,729
5	Lewis et al	1,115	-371	-413,665	1,243,225	137,641
6	Kasper et al	1,707	-300	-512,100	2,913,849	90,000
7	Evans	1,490	-98	-145,275	2,220,100	9,506
8	Golay et al	1,000	-212	-212,000	1,000,000	44,944
9	Young	1,800	-385	-693,000	3,240,000	148,225
10	Golay et al	1,200	-121	-145,200	1,440,000	14,641
11	Cedarquist	1,500	-114	-171,000	2,250,000	12,996
12	Worthington & Taylor	1,182	-571	-674,922	1,397,124	326,041
13	Rabast et al	1,871	-350	-654,850	3,500,641	122,500
14	Rabast et al	1,000	-392	-392,000	1,000,000	153,664
15	Wing et al	800	-270	-216,000	640,000	72,900
16	Alford et al	1,200	-91	-109,200	1,440,000	8,281
17	Baron et al	1,000	-55	-55,000	1,000,000	3,025
	Sum	21,373	-4,854.5	-6,094,862	28,593,253	1,865,057

$$r = \frac{n\sum xy - (\sum x)(\sum y)}{\sqrt{n(\sum x^2)-(\sum x)^2}\ \sqrt{n(\sum y^2)-(\sum y)^2}}$$

Where:

N = the number of pairs of scores (17)

$\sum xy$ = sum of the products of paired scores (-6,094,862)

$\sum x$ = sum of x scores (21,373)

$\sum y$ = sum of y scores (-4,854.5)

$\sum x2$ = sum of x scores squared (28,593,253)

$\sum y2$ = sum of y scores squared (1,865,057)

r = 0.009

Correlation between (low) carbs & (high) weight loss

	Authors	Carbs (x)	Loss (y)	x*y	x*x	y*y
1	Rickman	7	-442	-3,094	49	195,364
2	Benoit et al	10	-660	-6,600	100	435,600
3	Yudkin & Carey	43	-200	-8,600	1,849	40,000
4	Fletcher	36	-223	-8,028	1,296	49,729
5	Lewis et al	27	-371	-10,017	729	137,641
6	Kasper et al	56	-300	-16,800	3,136	90,000
7	Evans	80	-98	-7,800	6,400	9,506
8	Golay et al	38	-212	-7,950	1,406	44,944
9	Young	30	-385	-11,550	900	148,225
10	Golay et al	75	-121	-9,075	5,625	14,641
11	Cedarquist	85	-114	-9,690	7,225	12,996
12	Worthington & Taylor	17	-571	-9,707	289	326,041
13	Rabast et al	48	-350	-16,800	2,304	122,500
14	Rabast et al	25	-392	-9,800	625	153,664
15	Wing et al	10	-270	-2,700	100	72,900
16	Alford et al	75	-91	-6,825	5,625	8,281
17	Baron et al	50	-55	-2,750	2,500	3,025
	Sum	711.5	-4,854.5	-147,786	40,158	1,865,057

$$ r = \frac{n\sum xy - (\sum x)(\sum y)}{\sqrt{n(\sum x^2)-(\sum x)^2} \; \sqrt{n(\sum y^2)-(\sum y)^2}} $$

Where:

N = the number of pairs of scores (17)

$\sum xy$ = sum of the products of paired scores (-147,786)

$\sum x$ = sum of x scores (711.5)

$\sum y$ = sum of y scores (-4,854.5)

$\sum x2$ = sum of x scores squared (40,158.25)

$\sum y2$ = sum of y scores squared (1,865,057.25)

r = 0.79

Appendix 2

Study	People	Days	Deficit	Predicted (kg)	Actual (kg)	Diff/yr (kg)	In lbs
2	12	365	600	28.4	4.6	23.8	52.4
3a	2	365	400	18.9	5.7	13.2	29.1
3b	2	365	1,500	71.0	5.7	65.3	143.9
5a	1	365	600	28.4	2.5	25.9	57.2
5b	1	365	600	28.4	3.2	25.2	55.5
6	1	730	600	56.8	2.0	27.4	60.4
9	3	365	600	28.4	3.1	25.3	55.7
10	4	365	1,600	75.7	14.2	61.5	135.6
11	4	547.5	1,000	71.0	4.9	44.0	97.1
13	1	365	250	11.8	**-1.2**	13.0	28.7

Notes:

* Given that this is the evidence part of the NICE obesity paper, the lack of evidence is remarkable. From 15 studies in this table 15.14, there was no useable data for studies 4, 7, 8, 12 and 14 (i.e. no deficit and weight loss information).

* The largest study involved 12 people and the rest between 1 and 4 people.

* The studies were all for a significant period of time – at least a year.

* The predicted column is quite simply "The Calorie Formula" applied to the deficit and the time period. E.g. for Study 2, as an example, we take 365 days * 600 calories / 3,500 calories = 62.6 pounds or 28.4 kilograms. I used the same spreadsheet cell to change from pounds to kilograms and back to ensure that no accuracy was lost in conversion.

* Actual was the actual weight loss for the duration of the study – this was given by NICE in kilograms, hence my use of kilograms in the table.

* The difference is simply predicted minus actual i.e. what should have been lost minus what was actually lost. (Please note the weight *gain* in study 13).

* The final column is where the conclusion in Chapter Seven comes from: The smallest difference between the fat (alone) that should have been lost and the weight that was lost was 28.7 pounds – and this was with the study with only an approximate 250 calories deficit. The biggest difference between the fat (alone) that should have been lost and the weight that was lost was 143.9 pounds. Even if my assumptions for Study 3 were wrong, and there was no incidence of a 1,500 calorie deficit, Study 10 still gives a 135.6 pound error, which is at a similar level of enormous difference.

My assumptions:

* In Study 2, I used the median weight loss, which was given as 4.6 kilograms.

* In Study 3, the diet was not detailed more specifically than 1,000-1,600 calories, which could imply a deficit of anything from 400 to 1,500 calories depending on the limits of these ranges and the gender of the average subjects. I did 3a to represent one extreme (400 calorie deficit) and 3b to represent the other extreme (1,500 calorie deficit). The loss was specified as 5.5 kilograms for 1 person and 5.9 kilograms for the other, so I took the mid point for both (5.7 kilograms).

* For studies 5a, 5b, 6 and 9, data was taken only for the examples involving a 600 calorie deficit, since only a deficit study enabled the calorie formula to be tested.

* Study 10 was a very low calorie diet of 400 calories, so I assumed this was for an average female needing 2,000 calories a day. If any males were involved in Study 10, the difference in what should have happened (according to the calorie formula) and what did happen would have been even greater.

* Study 11 was a low calorie diet of 1,000 calories; again I assumed the 4 participants were female, with an average calorie need of 2000 calories a day.

* Study 13 was a small deficit diet of 1,700-1,800 calories day. Again, I assumed that the 1 participant was female and that the deficit was 250 calories a day. The person *gained* weight (1.2 kilograms) instead of losing 11.8 kilograms.

Appendix 3

Nutritional comparison of real vs. processed food

Nutrient (RDA/AI)	Sugars & Flour	Healthy Basket	Main source from healthy basket (Note 1)
Calories	1,076	1,077	Eggs
Carbohydrate (g)	250	62	Oats
Protein (g)	17	95	Sardines
Fat (g)	2	57	Eggs
Vit A (900 mcg) (Note 2)	0.0	8,585	Liver & spinach
Vit B1 (1.2 mg)	0.2	1.3	Liver & seeds
Vit B2 (1.3 mg)	0.0	3.5	Liver & eggs
Vit B3 (16 mg)	2.2	18	Liver & sardines
Vit B5 (5 mg) (AI)	0.7	10	Liver & eggs
Vit B6 (1.7 mg)	0.0	1.9	Liver & seeds
Folic Acid (400 mcg)	44.1	1,040	Liver & eggs
Vit B12 (2.4 mcg)	0.0	27	Liver & sardines
Vit C (90 mg)	0.0	115	Broccoli & spinach
Vit D (10 mcg) (AI)	0.0	11.5	Sardines, eggs & milk
Vit E (15 mg)	0.2	16	Seeds & sardines
Vit K (120 mcg) (AI)	0.5	1,022	K1 Spinach, K2 sardines
Calcium (1,000 mg) (AI)	26.7	1,018	Sardines & milk
Magnesium (420 mg)	37.3	506	Cocoa & spinach
Phosphorus (700 mg)	183.3	1,921	Sardines & eggs
Copper (900 mcg)	200	2,475	Cocoa, liver & seeds
Iron (18 mg)	2.0	26	Liver & spinach
Manganese (2.3 mg) (AI)	1.2	4.8	Oats & spinach
Selenium (55 mcg)	58.3	202	Sardines & eggs
Zinc (11 mg)	1.2	12	Liver & eggs

Note 1: Healthy basket: 35 grams of porridge oats; 125 grams of whole milk; 75 grams of liver; 50 grams of broccoli; 200 grams of spinach; 25 grams of cocoa powder; 125 grams of sardines; 200 grams of eggs and 20 grams of sunflower seeds.

Note 2: Please note that half the vitamin A comes from the spinach, which would have a low bio-availability and hence the intake would be much lower than indicated.

Appendix 4

Licensing Status for American States

As of June 2010, 46 states had laws to regulate dietitians or nutritionists through licensure, statutory certification, or registration.[399] For state regulation purposes, licensing, certification and registration are defined as follows:

Licensing (35) – statutes include an explicitly defined scope of practice, and performance of the profession is illegal without first obtaining a license from the state. "Interchangeable" means that the term nutritionist shall mean dietitian and the nutritionist must be a registered dietitian. "Separate" means that the term nutritionist is recognised, but that the precise qualifications deemed acceptable have been narrowly defined by the state and many have added an additional requirement to complete 900 hours work under the supervision of a dietitian.

Alabama (1989)*[lvi] - licensing of dietitian/nutritionist (interchangeable – standard ADA bill)

Alaska (1999) - licensing of dietitian/nutritionist (separate)

Arkansas (1989) - licensing of dietitian (standard ADA bill)

Florida (1988) - licensing of dietitian, nutritionist & nutrition counsellors (separate – standard ADA bill)

Georgia (1994)* - licensing of dietitian (standard ADA bill)

Hawaii (2000)* - licensing of dietitian (standard ADA bill)

Idaho (1994) - licensing of dietitian (standard ADA bill)

Illinois (1991) - licensing of dietitian & nutrition counsellors (interchangeable – standard ADA bill)

Iowa (1985) - licensing of dietitian (standard ADA bill)

Kansas (1989)* - licensing of dietitian (standard ADA bill)

Kentucky (1994)* - licensing of dietitian & certification of nutritionist (separate – standard ADA bill)

Louisiana (1987)* - licensing of dietitian/nutritionist (interchangeable – standard ADA bill)

Maine (1994)* - licensing of dietitian (standard ADA bill)

Maryland (1994)* - licensing of dietitian & nutritionist (interchangeable – standard ADA bill)

Massachusetts (1999) - licensing of dietitian & nutritionist (interchangeable – standard ADA bill)

[lvi] * Indicates year of amendment or reauthorisation. Please note, in the few cases where the records of the Commission for Dietetic Registration and those of the Alliance for Natural Health differed, I did original research and made a judgement as to which source seemed more up to date. This has no impact on the overall numbers in each category – it may simply affect a couple of dates or terms used in this Appendix.

Michigan (2007) - licensing of dietitian (standard ADA bill)
Minnesota (1994) - licensing of dietitian & nutritionist (separate – standard ADA bill)
Mississippi (1994)* - licensing of dietitian & nutritionist title protection (interchangeable – standard ADA bill)
Missouri (1998)* - licensing of dietitian (standard ADA bill)
Montana (1987)* - licensing of nutritionist & dietitian title protection (separate)
Nebraska (1995)* - licensing of medical nutrition therapists (separate)
New Hampshire (2000) - licensing of dietitian (standard ADA bill)
New Mexico (1997) - licensing of dietitian, nutritionist & nutrition associates (separate – standard ADA bill)
North Carolina (1991) - licensing of dietitian & nutritionist (interchangeable)
North Dakota (1989)* - licensing of dietitian & certification of nutritionist (separate – standard ADA bill)
Ohio (1986) - licensing of dietitian
Oklahoma (1989)* - licensing of dietitian
Oregon (1989) - licensing of dietitian (standard ADA bill)
Pennsylvania (2002) - licensing of dietitian/nutritionist (interchangeable)
Rhode Island (2007)* - licensing of dietitian & nutritionist (interchangeable – standard ADA bill)
South Carolina (2006) - licensing of dietitian
South Dakota (1998) - licensing of dietitian & nutritionist (separate – standard ADA bill)
Tennessee (1987) - licensing of dietitian/nutritionist (interchangeable)
Texas (1993)* - licensing of dietitian (standard ADA bill)
West Virginia (2000) - licensing of dietitian

Statutory certification (10) – limits use of particular titles to persons meeting predetermined requirements, while persons not certified can still practice the occupation or profession.

Connecticut (1994) - certification of dietitian
Delaware (1994) - certification of dietitian/nutritionist
Indiana (1994) - certification of dietitian
Nevada (1995)* - certification of dietitian
New York (1991) - certification of dietitian & nutritionist
Utah (1993) - certification of dietitian
Vermont (1993) - certification of dietitian
Virginia (1995)* - certification of dietitian & nutritionist
Washington (1988) - certification of dietitian & nutritionist
Wisconsin (1994) - certification of dietitian

Registration (1) – is the least restrictive form of state regulation. As with certification, unregistered persons are permitted to practice the profession.

California (1995)* - registration of dietitian

No legislation (4) – Arizona, Colorado, New Jersey and Wyoming.

Index

Reference Notes

All internet links were working as of July 2010. This list of references can be found on www.theobesityepidemic.org with click through links for your convenience.

Please note that all quotations are written as they appear in the original and hence may include abbreviations where I normally spell things out in full.

For human weight, Australia and Europe work in kilograms, America in pounds and the UK in stones and pounds. I have taken the lead from the study being reviewed and not converted original numbers. Hence one study in kilograms may be followed by another in pounds. The conversion rate is one pound equals 0.454 kilograms and there are 14 pounds in one stone.

Introduction

[1] Colleen S.W. Rand and Alex M. C. Macgregor, "Successful weight loss following obesity surgery and the perceived liability of morbid obesity", *International Journal of Obesity*, (1991). (The study results are presented in the summary of this book).

[2] British Dietetic Association's leaflet *"Want to lose weight & keep it off...?"* (http://www.bda.uk.com/foodfacts/Want2LoseWeight.pdf).

[3] https://apps.who.int/infobase/Indicators.aspx. Wadsworth M, Kuh D, Richards M, Hardy R, The 1946 National birth cohort (MRC national Survey of Health and development).

[4] Centres for disease control and prevention, National Centre for Health Statistics, United States, (2006), Figure 13, Data from the National Health and Nutrition Examination Survey (NHANES).

[5] Thomas Hawkes Tanner, *The Practice of Medicine*, (p217), (1869).

[6] "On the Method of Theoretical Physics" The Herbert Spencer Lecture, delivered at Oxford (10 June 1933); also published in *Philosophy of Science*, Vol. 1, No. 2 (April 1934), pp. 163-169.

[7] One of the forecasts of the UK Foresight Report: "Tackling Obesities: Future Choices", (October 2007).

Part 1 – The General Principle

[8] http://www.dailymail.co.uk/health/article-1200993/Why-calorie-counting-makes-fat.html

[9] http://www.dailymail.co.uk/health/diets/article-1263801/How-shed-middle-age-spread.html

[10] Anne Diamond, *Winning the Fat War*, published by Capstone, (2009).

[11] Gary Taubes, *The Diet Delusion*, published by Vermilion, (2007).

[12] The Mayer definition polled 26% of 570 votes when given 31 different options – humanthermodynamics.com. (Accessed 23 July 2010).

[13] References to the work of Rubner and Atwater are plentiful, but there is an appreciative and useful review in the *Journal of Nutrition* by William Chambers (1952). http://jn.nutrition.org/cgi/reprint/48/1/1.pdf

[14] Francis G. Benedict, *Human Vitality and efficiency under prolonged restricted diet*, (study 1917, published 1919).

[15] Ancel Keys, *The Biology of Human Starvation*, (study 1944-45, report 1950).

[16] Albert Stunkard and Mavis McLaren-Hume, "The results of treatment for obesity: a review of the literature and report of a series", *Archives of Internal Medicine*, (1959).

[17] Marion J. Franz, Jeffrey J. VanWormer, A. Lauren Crain, Jackie L. Boucher, Trina Histon, William Caplan, Jill Bowman, Nicolas Pronk. "Weight Loss Outcomes: A Systematic Review and Meta-Analysis of Weight Loss Clinical Trials with a Minimum 1-Year Follow-Up", *Journal of the American Dietetic Association*, (2007).

Chapter 1

[18] http://www.whocollab.od.mah.se/expl/globalsugar.html

(This data is for 2002. I tried to get more recent data for UK per capita sugar consumption but DEFRA confirmed to me in writing, on 18 November 2009, that this is not available).

[19] http://www.whocollab.od.mah.se/expl/globalsugar.html

[20] Anita Chaudhuri and Jon Ungoed-Thomas, with additional reporting by Justin Stoneman, "A Dieter's Dilemma", *The Sunday Times*, (4 April 2010).

[21] Eaton MacKay and H C Bergman, "The amount of water stored with glycogen in the liver", *The Journal of Biological Chemistry*, (December 1933).

[22] Rittenberg & Schoenheimer, "Further studies on the biological uptake of Deuterium into organic substances, with special reference to fat and cholesterol formation", *Journal of Biological Chemistry*, (1937).

[23] E. Wertheimer and B. Shapiro, "The Physiology of Adipose Tissue", *Physiological Reviews*, (1948).

[24] Sir Harold Himsworth, "Diabetes mellitus: its differentiation into insulin-sensitive and insulin-insensitive types", *The Lancet*, (1936).

[25] Rosalyn Yalow, Solomon Berson, "Immunoassay of endogenous plasma insulin in man", *Journal of Clinical Investigation*, (1960).

[26] William Banting, "Letter on Corpulence addressed to the public ", (1869).

[27] Yalow R.S., Glick S.M., Roth J., Berson S.A.,"Plasma insulin and growth hormone levels in obesity and diabetes", *Annals of the New York Academy of Sciences*, (1965).

[28] Edgar Gordon, "A new concept in the treatment of obesity", *The Journal of the American Medical Association*, (1963).

Chapter 2

[29] Eric Jequier, "Pathways to Obesity", *International Journal of Obesity*, (2002).

[30] Richard Feinman and Eugene Fine, "A calorie is a calorie violates the second law of thermodynamics", *Nutritional Journal*, (2004).

[31] Alan Kekwick and Dr. Gaston Pawan, "Calorie intake in relation to body-weight changes in the obese", *The Lancet*, (1956).

[32] Richard Feinman and Eugene Fine, "Thermodynamics and metabolic advantage of weight loss diets", *Metabolic Syndrome and Related Disorders*, (2003).

[33] Marjorie R. Freedman, Janet King, and Eileen Kennedy, "Popular Diets: A Scientific Review", *Obesity Research*, (March 2001).

Chapter 3

[34] A report of the Royal College of Physicians, "Obesity", *Journal of the Royal College of Physicians of London*, (January 1983).

[35] Metcalf et al, "Fatness leads to inactivity, but inactivity does not lead to fatness: a longitudinal study in children (EarlyBird 45)", *Archives of Disease in Childhood*, (June 2010).

[36] Rotterdam Consensus Workshop Group, "Revised 2003 consensus on diagnostic criteria and long-term health risks related to polycystic ovary syndrome", *Fertility & Sterility*, (January 2004).

[37] Wilhem Falta, *Endocrine diseases including their diagnosis and treatment*, (1923).

[38] George N. Wade and Janet M. Gray, "Gonadal effects on food intake and adiposity: A metabolic hypothesis", *Physiology & Behavior*, (March 1979).

Finn Molgaard Hansen, Nibal Fahmy and Jens Hoiriis Nielsen, "The influence of sexual hormones on lipogenesis and lipolysis in rat fat cells", *European Journal of Endocrinology*, (1980).

These represent two examples. The evidence is so extensive that the term "ovariectomy-induced obesity" is widely used.

[39] W.S. Leslie, C.R. Hankey and M.E.J. Lean, "Weight gain as an adverse effect of some commonly prescribed drugs: a systematic review" *QJM*, (June 2007).

[40] DCCT Research Group, "Influence of intensive diabetes treatment on bodyweight and composition of adults with type 1 diabetes in the Diabetes Control and Complications Trial", *Diabetes Care*, (2001).

[41] UKPDS Group, "Intensive blood-glucose control with sulphonylureas or insulin compared with conventional treatment and risk of complications in patients with type 2 diabetes", *The Lancet*, (1998).

[42] Marbury T., Huang W.C., Strange P., Lebovitz H., "Repaglinide versus glyburide: a one-year comparison trial", *Diabetes Research and Clinical Practice*, (1999).

[43] Must A., Spadano J., Coakley E.H., Field A.E. et al, "The disease burden associated with overweight and obesity", *Journal of the American Medical Association* (JAMA), (1999).

[44] Colditz G.A., Willet W.C., Rotnitzky A. et al, "Weight gain as a risk factor for clinical diabetes mellitus in women", *Annals of Internal Medicine*, (1995).

[45] http://www.abpi.org.uk/statistics/section.asp?sect=4

[46] http://www.mentalhealthnurse.co.uk/images/Psychopharmacology/ Clozaril%20PIL. pdf

Chapter 4

[47] Ancel Keys, *The Biology of Human Starvation*, Minnesota University Press, (1950).

[48] Todd Tucker, *The Great Starvation Experiment*, published by Simon & Schuster, (2006).

[49] Ancel Keys, *The Biology of Human Starvation*, (p894-895).

[50] Ancel Keys, *The Biology of Human Starvation*, (p833).

[51] Ancel Keys, *The Biology of Human Starvation*, (p847).

[52] ZiMian Wang, Stanley Heshka, Kuan Zhang, Carol N. Boozer and Steven B. Heymsfield, "Resting Energy Expenditure: Systematic Organization and Critique of Prediction Methods", *Obesity Research*, (2001).

[53] Harris J.A., Benedict F.G., "A biometric study of basal metabolism in man", Carnegie Institute of Washington, Publication no 279, (1919).

[54] Gerald Russell, "Bulimia nervosa: an ominous variant of anorexia nervosa", *Psychological Medicine*, (1979).

[55] National Institute for Clinical Excellence, Clinical Guidelines 43.

[56] Melvin J. Konner, *The Tangled Wing: Biological Constraints on the Human Spirit*, (2002). 2nd edition (original 1982) New York: Times Books.

Part 2 – The Calorie Formula

[57] Helen Fielding, *Bridget Jones's Diary*, (1996). First published by Picador, an imprint of Pan Macmillan. (c) Helen Fielding, 1996. Sincere thanks to Pan Macmillan for the permission to include this quotation.

[58] http://www.bda.uk.com/foodfacts/Want2LoseWeight.pdf

[59] www.bbc.co.uk/wales/bigfatproblem

[60] Gordon Wardlaw, Anne Smith, *Contemporary Nutrition*, seventh edition, McGraw Hill (2009).

[61] BUPA, *Healthy Living*, produced by BUPA's health information team, 2nd edition edited by Alastair McQueen, published September 2007.

[62] http://www.nhs.uk/Livewell/loseweight/Pages/Weightlossmyths.aspx.

[63] http://www.dh.gov.uk/prod_consum_dh/groups/dh_digitalassets/@dh/@en/ documents/digitalasset/dh_4134419.pdf

[64] NICE Clinical Guideline 43. Clause 1.2.4.30

[65] http://www.nhlbi.nih.gov/health/public/heart/obesity/lose_wt/recommen.htm

[66] http://familydoctor.org/online/famdocen/home/healthy/food/improve/795.html

[67] http://www.annecollins.com/weight-loss/calories-per-pound.htm

[68] http://en.wikipedia.org/wiki/Harris-Benedict_equation

[69] Liz Vaccariello and Cynthia Sass, *Flat Belly Diet,* published by Rodale, Pan Macmillan (2009).

[70] *Bikini Fit: The 4-week Plan*, written and published by Hamlyn, (2003).

[71] *A-Z of Calories: Britain's No 1 Calorie Guide*, published by Octavo Publications, (2010).

[72] Lorraine Kelly with Anita Bean, *Nutrition Made Easy*, published by Virgin, (2009).

[73] Gill Paul, *The Little Book of Calorie Burning*, published by Harper Collins, (2008).

[74] Bruce Byron, *Fat Bloke Slims*, published by Penguin, (2009).

[75] ITV UK, *The World's Best Diet: A Tonight Special*, aired (23 June 2009).

[76] Terry Maguire and David Haslam. *The Obesity Epidemic and its management*, (p149), published by Pharmaceutical Press, (2010).

[77] http://cruiseforums.cruisecritic.com/showthread.php?t=832239

Chapter 5

[78] http://nationalobesityforum.org.uk/families/before-you-start-mainmenu-110/34-how-weight-loss-works.html

[79] Max Rubner, "Zeitschrift fur Biologie," *Festschrift zu Voit*, (1901).

[80] Bozenraad, *Deutsche Archives Internal Medicine*, (1911).

[81] Dr. Geoffrey Livesey, "The Calorie Delusion: Why food labels are wrong", *New Scientist*, (15 July 2009).

[82] FAO Food & Nutrition paper 77: "Food energy - methods of analysis and conversion factors", Report of a Technical Workshop, Rome, (December 2002).

[83] Max Wishnofsky, "Caloric equivalents of gained or lost weight", *The American Journal of Clinical Nutrition*, (1958).

Chapter 6

[84] Lulu Hunt Peters, *Diet and Health* (with key to the calories), published by Chicago The Reilly and Lee Company, (1918).

[85] T R Van Dellen, "How to keep well", *Chicago Daily Tribune*, (15 September 1959).

[86] Louis Harry Newburgh and Margaret Woodwell Johnston, "The Nature of Obesity", *Journal of Clinical Investigation*, (1930).

[87] Michel Montignac, *Dine out and lose weight*, (1987).

[88] Richard Feinman and Eugene Fine, "Thermodynamics and metabolic advantage of weight loss diets", *Metabolic Syndrome and Related Disorders*, (2003).

[89] Ingredients from packet purchased in 2009 with sell by date of September 2009. (http://theharcombediet.com/products/least-favourite/)

Chapter 7

[90] Francis G. Benedict, *Human Vitality and efficiency under prolonged restricted diet*, (study 1917, published 1919).

[91] James M. Strang and Frank A. Evans, "The Energy Exchange in Obesity", *Journal of Clinical Investigation*, (1928).

[92] Ancel Keys, *The Biology of Human Starvation*, (study 1944-45, report 1950).

[93] Stunkard A. and M. McLaren-Hume, "*The results of treatment for obesity: a review of the literature and report of a series*", Archives of Internal Medicine, (1959).

[94] George A. Bray, "The Myth of Diet in the Management of Obesity", *The American Journal of Clinical Nutrition*, (September 1970).

[95] Search done in June 2010.

[96] Rudolph L. Leibel, Michael Rosenbaum and Jules Hirsch, "Changes in energy expenditure resulting from altered body weight", *The New England Journal of Medicine*", (1995).

[97] Gary Taubes' interview of Jules Hirsch March 2002, reported in *The Diet Delusion*, published by Random House in the USA in 2007 as *Good Calories, Bad Calories* and by Vermillion, an imprint of Ebury Publishing, in the UK in 2008.

[98] Julie E. Flood-Obbagya, Barbara J. Rolls, "The effect of fruit in different forms on energy intake and satiety at a meal", Appetite, (April 2009). (Actually, it *does* matter if people have apple in any form before a meal – it causes insulin to be released and prepares the body to store fat).

[99] Marion J. Franz, Jeffrey J. VanWormer, A. Lauren Crain, Jackie L. Boucher, Trina Histon, William Caplan, Jill Bowman, Nicolas Pronk. "Weight Loss Outcomes: A Systematic Review and Meta-Analysis of Weight Loss Clinical Trials with a Minimum 1-Year Follow-Up", *Journal of the American Dietetic Association*, (2007).

[100] Outcome of a procedure under Article 107 of Directive 2001/83/EC; http://www.nhs.uk/news/2010/01January/Documents/Sibutramine-QA.pdf

[101] James W.P.T., Astrup A., Finer N., Hilsted J., Kopelman P., Rossner S., Saris W.H.M., Van Gaal L.F., STORM study group, "Effect of sibutramine on weight maintenance after weight loss: A randomised trial", *The Lancet*, (2000).

[102] Weis E.C., Galuska D.A., Khan L.K., Serdula M.K., "Weight-control practices among USA adults 2001-2002", *American Journal of Preventative Medicine*, (2006).

[103] Sims, E. A. H., E. Danforth, E. S. Horton, G. A. Bray, J. A. Glennon, and L. B. Salans, "Endocrine and metabolic effects of experimental obesity in man", *Recent Progress in Hormone Research*, (1973).

[104] http://www.guardian.co.uk/society/2010/jul/12/weight-watchers-works-say-scientists

[105] http://www.mrc-bsu.cam.ac.uk/BSUsite/CHTMR/AM_forweb.pdf

[106] "The Science of Appetite", *Time Magazine,* special edition, (2007).

[107] The WHO data was available for the discrete points 1972 and 1982 – so I took the date before the 1974 period being analysed.
https://apps.who.int/infobase/Indicators.aspx

[108] I calculated this mathematically year on year and analysed the average calorie intake for 1975 and then that for 1976 and used the 3,500 calorie formula to work out what the average person should have gained/lost between these two years and repeated this for each year between 1975 and 1999 to calculate the overall number of pounds that should have been lost on average. The overall number was calculated cumulatively, as some years people should have gained weight and most should have produced weight loss – all according to the calorie theory.

[109] http://www.defra.gov.uk/evidence/statistics/foodfarm/food/familyfood/index.htm

[110] http://www.eatwell.gov.uk/healthydiet/seasonsandcelebrations/howweusedtoeat/changingtastes/

[111] The USA has excellent data provided by NHANES (The National Health and Nutrition Examination Survey). This shows that the average weight gain, between 1974 and 1999, for a woman was 20.1 pounds and 17.6 pounds for a male. The World Health Organisation – Deakin University study (published May 2009) concurs that the average American has gained approximately 20 pounds during this time.

[112] This derives from the 3,500 formula as follows: 20 (pounds) x 3,500 (calories per pound) = 70,000 'extra' calories. As these have been consumed over 25 years (9,125 days, ignoring leap years), that's 7.67 calories extra per day.

[113] The FSA calories burned calculator suggested 210 calories would be burned walking for an hour, which would translate 2.3 minutes walking into eight calories. Other internet calculators are more accurate and allow you to enter an average person (160 pounds) and an average walking speed (3.5 miles per hour) and this means we would need to have walked 1.6 minutes fewer a day.

[114] http://www.who.int/diabetes/facts/world_figures/en/

[115] Anita Chaudhuri and Jon Ungoed-Thomas, with additional reporting by Justin Stoneman, "A Dieter's Dilemma", *The Sunday Times*, (4 April 2010).

[116] http://www.eatwell.gov.uk/healthydiet/eatwellplate/

[117] Bozenraad, *Deutsche Archives Internal Medicine*, (1911).

Part 3 – The Diet Advice

[118] The Oxford English Dictionary.

[119] http://www.opsi.gov.uk/SI/si1998/19980141.htm.
An excellent summary is available at:
http://www.sustainweb.org/realbread/flour_fortification/

[120] http://www.whocollab.od.mah.se/expl/globalsugar.html

[121] http://www.fabflour.co.uk/content/1/31/facts-about-bread-in-the-uk.html

[122] http://www.ers.usda.gov/Briefing/Sugar/data.htm#yearbook

[123] http://www.ers.usda.gov/briefing/wheat/consumption.htm

[124] http://iom.edu/en/Global/News%20Announcements/~/media/Files/Activity%20Files/Nutrition/DRIs/DRISummaryListing2.ashx

[125] Sally Fallon Morell's presentation at the Weston Price Foundation inauguration European conference, London, (21 March 2010).

Chapter 8

[126] Ancel Keys, J. T. Anderson, Olaf Mickelsen, Sadye F. Adelson and Flaminio Fidanza, "Diet and Serum Cholesterol in Man: Lack of Effect of Dietary Cholesterol", *The Journal of Nutrition*, (1955).

[127] Anitschkow N., "Ueber die Veranderungen der Kaninchenaorta bei experimenteller Cholesterinsteatose", *Beitr Pathol Anat,* 56:379-404. (1913).

[128] http://www.health.gov/dietaryguidelines/dga2005/document/default.htm

[129] http://www.nhs.uk/Conditions/Cholesterol/Pages/Causes.aspx

[130] http://www.eatwell.gov.uk/healthissues/healthyheart/cholesterol/

[131] Keys et al, "Volume XLI: The Study Programme and objectives", *Circulation,* (April 1970).

[132] Minnesota University Archives. Author Henry Blackburn – one of the researchers on the Seven Country Study project. (http://www.sph.umn.edu/epi/history/overview.asp)

[133] Keys et al, "Volume XLI: The Study Programme and objectives", *Circulation,* (April 1970).

[134] Morris et al. "Coronary Heart Disease and physical activity of work", *The Lancet,* (1953).

[135] Minnesota University Archives. Author Henry Blackburn. http://www.sph.umn.edu/epi/history/finland.asp

[136] A.S. Dontas, A. Menotti, C. Aravanis, P. Ioannidis, F. Seccareccia, "Comparative total mortality in 25 years in Italian and Greek middle aged rural men", *Journal of Epidemiology and Community Health*, (1998).

[137] Dr. Malcolm Kendrick, *The Great Cholesterol Con*, published by John Blake, (2007).

[138] William Castelli, *Archives of Internal Medicine*, (July 1992), 152:7:1371-1372.

[139] Gary Foster et al, "A randomised trial of a low-carbohydrate diet for obesity", *New England Journal of Medicine*, (May 2003).

[140] http://www.bbc.co.uk/science/horizon/2004/atkinstrans.shtml

[141] The Horizon programme transcript says that 120 people were involved in the study, half on Atkins, half on low fat. This was not accurate. There were 63 participants in the Foster study. The programme also mentioned and interviewed Dr. Eric Westman, who had done a study with 51 subjects placed on a <25g per day low carbohydrate diet – not dissimilar to Atkins, but not strictly Atkins and there was no low fat comparator group. This was presented in the *American Journal of Medicine*, (July 2002).

[142] Atkins RC. *Dr. Atkins' new diet revolution,* revised edition, Avon Books, (1998).

[143] Brownell KD, *The LEARN program for weight management 2000*, Dallas: American Health Publishing, (2000).

[144] http://www.youtube.com/watch?v=u7AjU1QHDf8

[145] Keys et al, "Inter-cohort differences in coronary heart disease mortality in the 25-year follow-up of the Seven Countries Study", (Tables 1 and 4), *European Journal of Epidemiology*, (1993).

[146] Dr. R. Scragg, "Seasonality of cardiovascular disease mortality and the possible protective effect of ultra-violet radiation", *International Journal of Epidemiology*, (December 1981).

[147] Robert H. Lustig, "The Fructose Epidemic", *The Bariatrician*, (June 2009).

[148] Ricciuto L., Lin K., Tarasuk V., "A comparison of the fat composition and prices of margarines between 2002 and 2006 when new Canadian labelling regulations came into effect", *Public Health Nutrition*, (2009).

[149] Jakobsen M.U., O'Reilly E.J., Heitmann B.L., Pereira M.A., Bälter K., Fraser G.E., Goldbourt U., Hallmans G., Knekt P., Liu S., Pietinen P., Spiegelman D., Stevens J,. Virtamo J., Willett W.C., Ascherio A., "Major Types of dietary fat and risk of coronary heart disease: a pooled analysis of 11 cohort studies", *American Journal of Clinical Nutrition*, (2009).

[150] http://www.sph.umn.edu/epi/history/overview.asp

[151] http://www.nhlbi.nih.gov/health/public/heart/chol/wyntk.pdf

[152] G Ghirlanda, A Oradei, A Manto, S Lippa, L Uccioli, S Caputo, AV Greco, and GP Littarru, "Evidence of plasma CoQ10-lowering effect by HMG-CoA reductase inhibitors: a double-blind, placebo-controlled study", *The Journal of Clinical Pharmacology*, (1993).

[153] M.S Brown & J. L Goldstein, "A receptor mediated pathway for cholesterol homeostatis", *Science*, (1986).

[154] Garrett & Grisham, *Biochemistry*, 2nd Edition, (1995).

[155] John William Gofman, "Diet in the prevention and treatment of myocardial infarction", *American Journal of Cardiology*, (February 1958).

[156] Cystic Fibrosis Trust, UK.

[157] http://www.nice.org.uk/media/207/AA/ImplUptakeReportStatins.pdf

[158] Jensen RG, Hagerty MM, McMahon KE, "Lipids of human milk and infant formulas: a review", *American Journal of Clinical Nutrition*, (June 1978).

[159] EH Mangiapane, AM Salter, *Diet, Lipoproteins and Coronary Heart Disease: A Biochemical Perspective*, Nottingham University Press, (1999).

Chapter 9

[160] Centres for Disease Control and Prevention, (Using age adjusted data), http://www.cdc.gov/nchs/hus.htm (data page), ftp://ftp.cdc.gov/pub/Health_Statistics/NCHS/Publications/Health_US/hus09tables/09contents_tables.pdf, (detailed list of data available).

[161] http://www.census.gov/population/censusdata/table-4.pdf

[162] James P. Carter, "Eating in America; Dietary Goals for the United States; Report of the Select Committee on Nutrition and Human Needs, U.S. Senate", MIT Press, Cambridge, Massachusetts, (January 1977).

[163] Elizabeth J. Parks, "Effect of dietary carbohydrate on triglyceride metabolism in humans", *The Journal of Nutrition*, (2001).

[164] http://www.cnpp.usda.gov/Publications/DietaryGuidelines/1980/DG1980pub.pdf

[165] E. Newbrun, "Sugar & Dental Caries: A review of Human Studies", *Science* 217, (1982).

[166] Committee on Medical Aspects of Food Policy, "Diet and Cardiovascular Disease: Report of the Panel on Diet in Relation to Cardiovascular Disease", (1984).

[167] Dariush Mozaffarian, Martijn B. Katan, Alberto Ascherio, Walter C. Willett, et al, "Trans Fatty Acids and Cardiovascular Disease", *New England Journal of Medicine*, (April 2006).

[168] Peter M. Clifton, Jennifer B. Keogh and Manny Noakes, "Trans Fatty Acids in Adipose Tissue and the Food Supply Are Associated with Myocardial Infarction", *The American Society for Nutritional Sciences Journal of Nutrition,* (April 2004).

[169] John Yudkin, *Pure, White and Deadly*, (1972).

[170] Denis Burkitt, *Don't Forget Fibre in Your Diet*, (1979).

[171] http://www.health.gov/dietaryguidelines/1980_2000_chart.pdf

Chapter 10

[172] http://www.health.gov/dietaryguidelines/

[173] http://www.health.gov/dietaryguidelines/dga2005/document/pdf/Chapter3.pdf

[174] http://www.health.gov/dietaryguidelines/dga2005/document/pdf/Chapter7.pdf

[175] http://www.health.gov/dietaryguidelines/dga2005/document/pdf/Chapter6.pdf

[176] Eugine Braunwald, *Braunwald's Heart Disease: A Textbook of Cardiovascular Medicine*, 9th edition (2009).

[177] http://www.health.gov/dietaryguidelines/dga2005/document/html/executive summary.htm

[178] http://www.whitehouse.gov/blog/2010/02/09/making-moves-a-healthier-generation and www.letsmove.gov

[179] http://www.nhmrc.gov.au/publications/synopses/dietsyn.htm

[180] http://www.health.gov.au/internet/main/publishing.nsf/Content/health-pubhlth-strateg-food-guide-index.htm

[181] http://www.readnrock.com/?p=27

[182] http://www.eatwell.gov.uk/healthydiet/eighttipssection/8tips/

[183] This is called "The Government's eight guidelines for a healthy diet." I originally found the reference on www.nutrition.org.uk – the site for the British Nutrition Foundation. In March 2010, while sourcing the references for this book, I found it at http://www.food.gov.uk/multimedia/pdfs/bghbooklet.pdf - interestingly a Food Standards Agency web site. So two different eight tips can be found on the current FSA web site.

[184] http://www.nhs.uk/change4life

[185] http://www.dh.gov.uk/en/Publichealth/Healthimprovement/Obesity/HealthyWeight/ index.htm

[186] Source = http://www.whocollab.od.mah.se/expl/globalsugar.html

[187] http://www.food.gov.uk/news/newsarchive/2007/sep/plate

[188] http://www.food.gov.uk/healthiereating/eatwellplate/howdiffers

[189] http://www.food.gov.uk/multimedia/pdfs/publication/eatwellplate0210.pdf

[190] http://www.wakeuptonutella.com/faq.html

[191] http://www.nutellausa.com/nutrition.htm

[192] http://www.defra.gov.uk/evidence/statistics/foodfarm/food/familyfood/documents/ familyfood-2008.pdf

[193] Rebecca Wilcox, UK BBC 3, *Who made me fat?*, (30 October 2009). Repeated on BBC 1 (1 March 2010).

Chapter 11

[194] A. Stewart Truswell, "Review of dietary intervention studies: effect on coronary events and on total mortality", *Australian New Zealand Journal of Medicine*, (1994).

[195] World Health Organisation European Collaborative Group, "European collaborative trial of multi-factorial prevention of coronary heart disease: final report on the 6-year results", *The Lancet* (1986).

[196] The Multiple Risk Factor Intervention Trial Research Group, "Mortality Rates after 10.5 years for participants in the Multiple Risk Factor Intervention Trial", *Journal of the American Medical Association (JAMA)*, (1990).

[197] The Multiple Risk Factor Intervention Trial Research Group, "Multiple risk factor intervention trial: Risk factor changes and mortality results," *Journal of the American Medical Association (JAMA)*, (1982).

[198] George Christakis, Seymour Rinzler, et al, "The anti-Coronary Club: A Dietary Approach to the Prevention of Coronary Heart Disease - a Seven Year Report", *American Journal of Public Health*, (February 1966).

[199] George Christakis, Seymour Rinzler, Morton Archer, Arthur Kraus, "Effect of the Anti-Coronary Club Program on Coronary Heart Disease Risk-Factor Status", *Journal of the American Medical Association* (November 1966). In the intervention group there were 18 deaths from other causes and 8 from CHD compared with 6 deaths from other causes and none from CHD in the control group.

[200] Gary Taubes, *The Diet Delusion*, (2007).

[201] Schatz, Masaki, Yano, Chen, Rodriguez and Curb, "Cholesterol and all-cause mortality in elderly people from the Honolulu heart programme", *The Lancet*, (August 2001).

[202] Anderson, Castelli and Levy, "Cholesterol and Mortality: 30 years of follow-up from the Framingham Study", *Journal of the American Medical Association (JAMA)*, (1987).

[203] Elaine Meilahn, "Low serum cholesterol: Hazardous to health?" *Circulation*, (2005).

[204] Dr. Malcolm Kendrick, *The Great Cholesterol Con*, (2007).

[205] Natasha Campbell Mc-Bride, *Put your Heart in Your Mouth*, (2008).

[206] http://www.nhs.uk/conditions/cholesterol/Pages/Introduction.aspx

[207] http://www.bbc.co.uk/health/physical_health/conditions/cholesterol1.shtml

[208] Thomas Samaras and Harold Elrick, "Height, body size and longevity – is smaller better for the human body", *Western Journal of Medicine*, (May 2002). http://www.ncbi.nlm.nih.gov/pmc/articles/PMC1071721/

[209] Eugine Braunwald, *Braunwald's Heart Disease: A Textbook of Cardiovascular Medicine*, 9th edition (2009).

[210] Barbara Howard et al, "Low-Fat Dietary Pattern and Risk of Cardiovascular Disease, The Women's Health Initiative Randomized Controlled Dietary Modification Trial", *Journal of the American Medical Association*", (February 2006).

[211] Andrew Mente, Lawrence de Koning, Harry S. Shannon, Sonia S. Anand, "A Systematic Review of the Evidence Supporting a Causal Link Between Dietary Factors and Coronary Heart Disease" *Archives of Internal Medicine, (*2009).

[212] Patty W Siri-Tarino, Qi Sun, Frank B Hu and Ronald M Krauss, "Meta-analysis of prospective cohort studies evaluating the association of saturated fat with cardiovascular disease ", *American Journal of Clinical Nutrition,* (March 2010).

Chapter 12

[213] J.A.J Gowlett, "What actually was the Stone Age Diet?", *Journal of Nutritional and Environmental Medicine*, (September 2003).

[214] C. Boesch and H. Boesch, "Hunting behaviour of wild chimpanzees in the Tai National Park", *American Journal of Physical Anthropology*, (1989).

J. Goodall, "Continuities between chimpanzees and human behaviour", *Human Origins*, (1976).

[215] Peters & O'Brien, "The early hominid plant–food niche: insights from an analysis of plant exploitation by Homo, Pan and Papio in eastern and southern Africa", *Current Anthropology*, (1981).

[216] http://www.margarine.org.uk/whatisfat-types.html#unsaturated

[217] United States Department of Agriculture nutritional database. www.nutritiondata.com

[218] Mary G. Enig, Sally Fallon, *Know your fats*, (2000).

[219] McIlwain, H. and Bachelard, H.S., *Biochemistry and the Central Nervous System*, Edinburgh: Churchill Livingstone, (1985). Estimates the composition of the brain to be (approximately) 78% water, 10-12% lipids, 8% protein, 2% soluble organic substances, 1% carbohydrate and 1% inorganic salts.

[220] Solomons, N. W. and J. Bulux. "Plant sources of provitamin A and human nutriture." *Nutrition Review*, July 1993.

[221] Sally Fallon and Mary G. Enig, "Vitamin A", (March 2002).

[222] Geleijnse JM, Vermeer C, Grobbee DE, Schurgers LJ, Knapen MH, van der Meer IM, Hofman A, Witteman JC, "Dietary intake of menaquinone is associated with a reduced risk of coronary heart disease: the Rotterdam Study", *The Journal of Nutrition*, (November 2004).

[223] Alli Starter Guide – booklet that comes with a packet of Alli pills. Produced by GlaxoSmithKline

[224] http://www.gsk.com/media/pressreleases/2009/2009_pressrelease_10011.htm

[225] http://www.eatwell.gov.uk/healthydiet/fss/fats/satfat/

[226] http://www.nhs.uk/chq/pages/1124.aspx?categoryid=51&subcategoryid=167

[227] http://www.health.gov/dietaryguidelines/dga2005/document/pdf/Chapter6.pdf

[228] http://www.measureup.gov.au/internet/abhi/publishing.nsf/Content/glossary#S

[229] http://www.nhs.uk/livewell/healthyhearts/pages/cholesterol.aspx

[230] http://www.health.gov/dietaryguidelines/dga2005/document/pdf/Chapter6.pdf

[231] Beef, Porterhouse steak, raw, trimmed to 1/8" fat (USDA reference – URMIS 2145), Nutritiondata.com

[232] Beef, Sirloin, lean only (URMIS 2244), Nutritiondata.com

[233] http://www.youtube.com/watch?v=hO0OS0kBDVs

[234] Gordon Wardlaw, Anne Smith, *Contemporary Nutrition*, seventh edition, McGraw Hill (2009).

[235] http://en.wikipedia.org/wiki/Coconut_oil

[236] Felton C.V,. Crook D., Davies M.J., Oliver M.F., "Dietary polyunsaturated fatty acids and composition of human aortic plaques", *The Lancet*, (October 1994).

[237] Ewa Stachowska, Barbara Dolstrokeogongowska, Dariusz Chlubek, Teresa Wesolstrokowska, Kazimierz Ciechanowski, Piotr Gutowski, Halina Szumilstrokowicz and Radoslstrokaw Turowski, "Dietary trans fatty acids and composition of human atheromatous plaques", *The European Journal of Nutrition*, (October 2004).

[238] http://wikitravel.org/en/Georgia_%28country%29

[239] http://www.who.int/countryfocus/cooperation_strategy/ccsbrief_geo_en.pdf

[240] International Monetary Fund, "World Economic Outlook Database, for the year 2009", (April 2010). Georgia (115), Tajikistan (149), Azerbaijan (82), Moldova (125), Croatia (43), Macedonia (84) and Ukraine (112) for the low fat/high heart disease countries. Austria (10), Finland (12), Belgium (14), Iceland (19), Netherlands (7), Switzerland (4) and France (15) for the high fat/low heart disease countries.

[241] *Daily Mail*, 14 August 2009.

[242] Andrew J. Murray, Nicholas S. Knight, Lowri E. Cochlin, Sara McAleese, Robert M. J. Deacon, J. Nicholas P. Rawlins, and Kieran Clarke, "Deterioration of physical performance and cognitive function in rats with short-term high-fat

feeding", *Federation of American Societies for Experimental Biology Journal*, (10 August 2009).

[243] JR Merrill, RG Holly, RL Anderson, N Rifai, ME King and R DeMeersman, "Hyperlipemic response of young trained and untrained men after a high fat meal", *Arteriosclerosis Thrombosis and Vascular Biology, (A* Journal of the American Heart Association), *(*1989).

[244] FSA: (http://www.eatwell.gov.uk/healthydiet/fss/fats/satfat/)

NHS: http://www.nhs.uk/chq/Pages/1124.aspx?CategoryID=51&SubCategoryID=167

[245] www.nutritiondata.com

[246] http://www.uga.edu/fruit/coconut.html

[247] Bruce Fife, *The Healing miracles of coconut Oil*, (2001).

[248] World Health Organisation figures for 2002.

[249] International Margarine Association of the Countries of Europe (IMACE), "Code of Practice on Vitamin A and D fortification of margarines and fat spreads", (May 2004).

[250] DEFRA, Family Food Survey, (Table 1.1), (2008).

[251] http://www.fabflour.co.uk/content/1/31/facts-about-bread-in-the-uk.html

[252] http://www.whocollab.od.mah.se/expl/globalsugar.html

[253] http://www.just-food.com/market-research/butter-margarine-and-table-spreads-us_id65428.aspx

[254] CBC News: 9 July 2008. http://www.cbc.ca/consumer/story/2008/07/09/f-margarine.html

[255] "I can't believe it's not butter", *Marketing Week*, (29 May 1997). http://www.marketingweek.co.uk/home/i-cant-believe-its-not-butter/2023474.article

Chapter 13

[256] Lieb et al, "The Effects of an Exclusive Long-Continued Meat Diet", *Journal of the American Medical Association*, (July 1926).

[257] Karen Fediuk, "Vitamin C in the Inuit diet: past and present", MA Thesis, School of Dietetics and Human Nutrition, McGill University, (2000).

[258] Barry Groves web site: http://www.second-opinions.co.uk/diabetes-4.html and you can see Groves' demonstration of how gorillas turn carbohydrate into saturated fat at http://vimeo.com/10533993

[259] You can get any of these numbers for yourself from a molecular mass calculator on the web – I used http://www.convertunits.com/molarmass/

The precise numbers are 342.29648 g/mol for a disaccharide, 18.01528 g/mol for water and 180.15588 g/mol for a monosaccharide and 162.1406 g/mol for a polysaccharide – but I didn't want to put people off with decimals.

[260] Tuna, bluefin, raw – 23 grams of protein per 100 grams of product, Nutritiondata.com

[261] http://www.sugar-bureau.co.uk/sugar_the_facts.html

[262] http://www.kelloggs.co.uk/company/corporateresponsibility/whichreport.aspx

[263] Michel Montignac, *Dine out and lose weight*, (1987).

[264] http://www.montignac.com/en/ig_tableau.php – Montignac GI for raw carrots.

[265] Richard J Johnson et al, "Potential role of sugar (fructose) in the epidemic of hypertension, obesity and the metabolic syndrome, diabetes, kidney disease, and cardiovascular disease", *American Journal of Clinical Nutrition*, (October 2007).

[266] John Yudkin, "Evolutionary and historical changes in dietary carbohydrates", *American Journal of Clinical Nutrition*, (1967).

[267] Richard Johnson, *The Sugar Fix*, (2008).

[268] Harold Higgins., "The rapidity with which alcohol and some sugars may serve as nutriment", *American Journal of Physiology,* (1916).

[269] Togel, Brezina and Durig, *Biochemistry Zeitschrift*, (1913).

[270] John Yudkin, *Pure, White and Deadly*, (1972).

[271] Eleazar Shafrir, "Metabolism of Disaccharides and Monosaccharides with Emphasis on Sugar and Fructose and their Lipogenic Potential", (1991).

[272] Peter A Mayes, "Intermediary metabolism of fructose", *American Journal of Clinical Nutrition*, (November 1993).

[273] http://www.youtube.com/watch?v=dBnniua6-oM. There is also a paper with much of the content of the YouTube video available at http://www.cookusinterruptus.com/files/Bariatrician%20Fructose.pdf

[274] http://www.fet-ev.eu/index.php?option=com_content&task=view&id=58&Itemid=116

[275] The UK, USA and Australian references are in Chapter Eight. The other countries are detailed at the following site: http://www.eufic.org/article/en/page/RARCHIVE/expid/food-based-dietary-guidelines-in-europe/

[276] http://www.cdphe.state.co.us/pp/copan/5-a-day/5ADAY.html

[277] Ali H. Mokdad; Mary K. Serdula; William H. Dietz; Barbara A. Bowman; James S. Marks; Jeffrey P. Koplan, "The Spread of the Obesity Epidemic in the United States, 1991-1998", *Journal of the American Medical Association*, (1999).

[278] Paolo Boffetta et al, "Fruit and vegetable intake and overall cancer risk in the European Prospective Investigation into Cancer and Nutrition (EPIC)", *Journal of the National Cancer Institute*, (April 2010).

[279] www.nutritiondata.com

[280] http://goop.com/newsletter/88/en/ – Gwyneth Paltrow's personal web site.

Chapter 14

[281] Gary Taubes, "Why we gain weight. Adiposity 101 and the alternative hypothesis of obesity", (6 May 2009). http://www.brown.edu/Research/CCMB/taubes.html

[282] www.caloriesperhour.com

[283] Anton J.M. Wagenmakers, "Type 2 Diabetes: Insulin Resistance May Be the Result of Mitochondrial Dysfunction." *Public Library of Science Medicine*, (2005).

[284] William L. Haskell, I-Min Lee, Russell R. Pate, Kenneth E. Powell, Steven N. Blair, Barry A. Franklin, Caroline A. Macera Gregory W. Heath, Paul D. Thompson and Adrian Bauman, "Physical Activity and Public Health: Updated Recommendation for Adults from the American College of Sports Medicine and the American Heart Association", (2007). And in turn, the reference from within this document is:

Saris, W. H., S. N. Blair, M. A. Van Baak, et al, "How much physical activity is enough to prevent unhealthy weight gain? Outcome of the IASO 1st Stock Conference and consensus statement", *Obesity Research*, (2003).

[285] Swinburn B., "Increased energy intake alone virtually explains all the increase in body weight in the United States from the 1970s to the 2000s", *2009 European Congress on Obesity*, (May 6-9, 2009). Abstract T1:RS3.3.

[286] http://www.theheart.org/article/970183.do

[287] http://abbottnutrition.com/Products/similac-isomil-advance

[288] "Britons watch a day of television every week", *The Daily Telegraph*, (10 February 2010).

[289] www.caloriesperhour.com is the calculator used for consistency throughout this book. This is one of the more sophisticated calculators available on the internet, as it allows for weight variation and time variation for hundreds of different activities.

[290] Centers for Disease Control and Prevention, "Adult participation in recommended levels of physical activity: United States, 2001 and 2003", MMWR 54:1208–1212, (2005).

[291] Centers for Disease Control and Prevention, "Trends in leisure time physical inactivity by age, sex and race/ethnicity - United States - 1994–2004", MMWR 54:991–994, (2005).

[292] Ross C. Brownson & Tegan K. Boehmer, "Patterns and Trends in Physical Activity, Occupation, Transportation, Land Use, and Sedentary Behaviors", (2005).

[293] John Cloud, "Why exercise won't make you thin", *Time Magazine,* (17 August 2009).

[294] http://www.ingnycmarathon.org/Results.htm

[295] Robinson, J. P., and G. Godbey, *Time for Life. The Surprising Ways Americans Use Their Time*, The Pennsylvania University Press, University Park, (1999).

[296] Flegal, K. M., M. D. Carroll, C. L. Ogden, and C. L. Johnson., "Prevalence and trends in obesity among U.S. adults, 1999-2000", *Journal of the American Medical Association,* (October 2002).

[297] Mary E. Moore, Albert Stunkard, Leo Srole, "Obesity, Social Class, and Mental Illness", *Journal of the American Medical Association*, (1962).

[298] Albert Stunkard, "Obesity and socioeconomic status – a complex relation", *The New England Journal of Medicine*, (September 1993).

[299] Sproston K, Primatesta P., *Health Survey for England 2002. The health of children and young people*. London: The Stationery Office, (2003).

[300] Rebecca Wilcox, UK BBC 3, *Who made me fat?* (30 October 2009). Repeated on BBC 1 (1 March 2010).

[301] http://www.drfosterintelligence.co.uk/newsPublications/localDocuments/WeighingUpTheBurdenOfObesityReport.pdf

[302] http://www.assemblywales.org/07-051.pdf

[303] Newburgh L.H., "Obesity", *Archives of Internal Medicine*, (1942).

[304] Presenter Nick Cohen, Channel 4, "30 Minutes", (Aired 1 May 2004).

[305] *New York Post*, (13 August 2008).

[306] http://www.earlybirddiabetes.org/index.php

[307] Katie M Mallam, Brad S Metcalf, Joanne Kirkby, Linda D Voss, Terence J Wilkin, "Contribution of timetabled physical education to total physical activity in primary school children: cross sectional study", *British Medical Journal*, (2003).

[308] Ali A. Berlin, Willem J. Kop, Patricia A. Deuster, "Depressive Mood Symptoms and Fatigue After Exercise Withdrawal: The Potential Role of Decreased Fitness", *Psychosomatic Medicine*, (2006).

[309] http://www.ergoweb.com/news/detail.cfm?id=1188

[310] http://child-abuse.suite101.com/article.cfm/statistics_on_child_abduction

[311] Department of Health, *At least five a week*, (April 2004).

Part 4 – How can we stop The Obesity Epidemic?

[312] Roald Amundsen; John Cope; Frederick Hoffman; Samuel Hutton; Weston Price and Albert Schweitzer were the key explorer physicians writing around 1900. Cancer was a key study area for many of these physicians.

Chapter 15

[313] 2010 "Fortune 500" Report and International Monetary Fund, World Economic Outlook Database, April 2010: Nominal GDP list of countries, (data for the year 2009).

[314] http://www.cdrnet.org/about/index.htm

[315] Please note that the UK uses dietician and dietitian interchangeably. The USA more consistently uses just dietitian and I have used the American spelling for uniformity throughout the book.

[316] http://www.cdrnet.org/certifications/licensure/index.htm and http://www.anh-usa.org/playing-monopoly-with-our-health/

[317] Tennessee regulations: http://www.state.tn.us/sos/rules/0470/0470-01.pdf

318

http://www.eatright.org/HealthProfessionals/content.aspx?id=7454&terms=sponsors (please note this page moved during the writing of this book, so you may need to go to the main ADA web site, eatright.org and enter "sponsors"). The 2008 Annual report was also used, as not all partners and sponsors were listed on the web site.

[319] Revenue figures were obtained from on line reports: wikinvest.com; finance.yahoo.com and bizjournals.com.

[320] http://www.kelloggs.co.uk/pressoffice/pressreleases/?i=92

[321] http://www.nationalobesityforum.org.uk/about-us/our-partners.html

[322] British Nutrition Foundation annual report 2008-09. Sustaining members noted as accurate as of 31 May 2009.

[323] British Nutrition Foundation annual report 2008-09. Members noted as accurate as of 31 May 2009.

[324] http://www.nutrition.org.uk/aboutbnf/values/annual-report

[325] http://www.powerbase.info/index.php/British_Nutrition_Foundation

[326] http://www.sugar-bureau.co.uk/pl_lwko.html

[327] http://www.independent.co.uk/life-style/food-and-drink/news/is-the-british-nutrition-foundation-having-its-cake-and-eating-it-too-1925034.html (22 March 2010).

[328] http://www.ilsi.org/Pages/AboutUs.aspx

[329] http://www.ilsi.org/documents/2010_ILSI_BOT.pdf

[330] Laura Barton, "A spoonful of propaganda", *The Guardian*, (12 April 2002).

[331] http://whqlibdoc.who.int/hq/1992/a34303.pdf

[332] http://www.nhs.uk/change4life/Pages/NationalPartnerActivity.aspx

[333] http://www.marketingweek.co.uk/in-depth-analysis/change4life-partners-raise-questions-over-who-will-reap-the-rewards/2063830.article

[334] http://www.awardscentre.org/about-asa-awards/

[335] http://209.20.80.25/vsite/vfile/page/fileurl/0,,5157-1-1-117462-0-file,00.pdf

[336] http://www.guardian.co.uk/theguardian/2010/apr/09/coco-pops-healthy-snacks-children

[337] http://www.zoeharcombe.com/2010/02/kelloggs-coco-pops-advert/

[338] http://www.opsi.gov.uk/acts/acts1999/ukpga_19990028_en_1#pb1-l1g1

[339] http://www.netmums.com/food/The_Eatwell_Plate.738/

[340] http://www.food.gov.uk/aboutus/ourboard/boardmem/boardmembiogs/ (correct at June 2010).

[341] Hannah Sutter, *Big Fat Lies*, published by Infinite Ideas Ltd, (2010).

[342] http://www.dailymail.co.uk/debate/article-1220756/A-strange-lonely-troubling-death--.html

[343] http://www.sustainweb.org/pdf/Through_the_Back_Door.pdf

[344] http://www.dailymail.co.uk/news/worldnews/article-1244987/Millions-putting-health-risk-wrongly-diagnosing-food-allergies.html.

[345] http://www.guardian.co.uk/environment/2010/jan/23/margarine-butter-health-wars

[346] http://www.diabeteshealth.com/read/2010/05/21/6690/attending-weight-watchers-meetings-helps-reduce-the-risk-for-type-2-diabetes/

[347] http://express-press-release.net/70/Glamour-Partners-With-Kelloggs-Special-K-In-Year-Long-Carat-Deal.php

[348] http://www.junkfoodnews.net/mcdonalds-olympics.htm

[349] http://www.independent.co.uk/sport/olympics/golden-girl-just-wants-a-burger-with-chips-899766.html

[350] http://www.thecoca-colacompany.com/heritage/olympicgames.html

[351] http://www.independent.co.uk/news/uk/home-news/cadbury-to-sponsor-london-2012-olympics-967688.html

[352] Rebecca Wilcox, UK BBC 3, *Who made me fat?*, (30 October 2009). Repeated on BBC 1 (1 March 2010).

Chapter 16

[353] Waterman, R. Jr., Peters, T. and Phillips, J.R, "Structure Is Not Organisation", *Business Horizons*, (3 June 1980).

[354] Whitaker et al, "Predicting obesity in young adulthood from childhood and parental obesity", *New England Journal of Medicine*, (1997).

[355] Jackson-Leach et al, "Estimated burden of paediatric obesity and co-morbidities in Europe. Part 1. The increase in the prevalence of child obesity in Europe is itself increasing. *International Journal of Paediatric Obesity*, (2006).

[356] The Foresight Report, (October 2007).

[357] Terry Maguire and David Haslam. *The Obesity Epidemic and its management*, published by Pharmaceutical Press, (2010).

[358] Fearne Cotton ITV UK, "The truth about online anorexia", aired 9 April (2009).

[359] Her Majesty's Government PSA Delivery Agreement 12, "Improving the health and wellbeing of children and young people", (October 2007).

[360] Health of the Nation Report by the Comptroller and Auditor General HC 458 1995/96 (14 August 1996).

[361] The Foresight Report (October 2007).

[362] The constitution was signed by representatives of 61 states on the 22 July 1946 and the World Health Organisation came into being on 7 April 1948. http://apps.who.int/gb/bd/PDF/bd47/EN/constitution-en.pdf

[363] http://www.accessdata.fda.gov/scripts/fcn/fcnNavigation.cfm?rpt=grasListing

[364] John Yudkin, *Pure, White and Deadly*, (1972).

[365] Dr. Otto Warburg, "The Prime Cause and Prevention of Cancer", Lecture delivered to Nobel Laureates on 30 June 1966, at Lindau, Lake Constance, Germany.

[366] http://www.heartforum.org.uk/Policy_Consultations_2093.aspx

[367] http://www.dorway.com/peerrefs.html

[368] Both definitions are from The Oxford English Dictionary.

[369] John Yudkin, *Pure, White and Deadly*, (1972).

[370] Alan Johnson, Member of Parliament and Health Secretary (at the time), Statement to the UK House of commons, 17 October 2007. http://www.dh.gov.uk/en/MediaCentre/Speeches/DH_079633

[371] Liang, Maier, Steinbach, Lalic, Pfeiffer, "The effect of artificial sweetener on insulin secretion", *Hormone and Metabolic Research*, (1987).

[372] One of the forecasts of the Foresight Report: *"Tackling Obesities: Future Choices"* (October 2007).

[373] http://www.medindia.net/news/British-Expert-Calls-for-Fat-Tax-on-Unhealthy-Foods-to-Save-Children-51144-1.htm

[374] David Kessler, *The end of overeating*, published by Rodale, (2009).

[375] Kelly D. Brownell and Thomas R. Frieden, "Ounces of Prevention – The Public Policy Case for Taxes on Sugared Beverages", *The New England Journal of Medicine*, (April 2009).

[376] Nielsen SJ, Popkin BM, "Changes in beverage intake between 1977 and 2001", *American Journal of Preventative Medicine,* (2004).

[377] Rump steak was £14 per kilo (£6.36 per pound) and McDonald's had the first five items listed for 99p and the double cheeseburger listed at £1.29 (June 2010). http://www.mcdonalds.co.uk/food/saver-menu/saver-menu.mcdj?dnPos=0

[378] http://www.sustainweb.org/pdf/Thirsty_Play.pdf. Christine Haigh and Jackie Schneider, "Thirsty Play: A survey of drinking water provision in public parks" (May 2010).

[379] Cremieux PY, Buchwald H, Shikora SA, Ghosh A, Yang HE, Buessing M, "A study on the economic impact of bariatric surgery", *The American Journal of Managed Care*, (September 2008).

[380] The Association for the Study of Obesity Annual Conference, Liverpool UK, (June 2009).

[381] http://www.bda.uk.com/ced/CurriculumDocument080826.pdf

[382] http://www.qof.ic.nhs.uk/

[383] Charles Clark and Maureen Clark, "The Diabetes Revolution: A ground breaking guide to reducing your insulin dependency", published by Vermillion, (June 2008).

[384] http://www.who.int/diabetes/facts/world_figures/en/

[385] http://famouspoetsandpoems.com/poets/alexander_pope/quotes

Summary

[386] Thomas Hawkes Tanner, *The Practice of Medicine*, (p217), (1869).

[387] Letter from the FSA to Zoë Harcombe, (25 September 2009).

[388] Committee on Medical Aspects of Food Policy, "Diet and Cardiovascular Disease: Report of the Panel on Diet in Relation to Cardiovascular Disease", (1984).

[389] A Stewart Truswell, "Review of dietary intervention studies: effect on coronary events and on total mortality", *Australian New Zealand Journal of Medicine*, (1994).

[390] Letter from the FSA to Zoë Harcombe, (25 September 2009).

[391] Robert H. Lustig, "The Fructose Epidemic", *The Bariatrician*, (June 2009).

[392] Chief Medical Officer's report for England 2009 (published April 2010).

[393] http://www.fortune500s.net/pep.php
http://en.wikipedia.org/wiki/List_of_countries_by_GDP_%28nominal%29#cite_note-0

[394] The Centre for Science in the Public Interest calls McDonald's "The stranger in the playground", http://www.cspinet.org/

[395] David Kessler, *The end of overeating*, published by Rodale, (2009).

[396] Swinburn B., "Increased energy intake alone virtually explains all the increase in body weight in the United States from the 1970s to the 2000s", *2009 European Congress on Obesity*, (May 6-9, 2009). Abstract T1:RS3.3.

[397] Barry Groves' presentation at the Weston Price Foundation inauguration European conference, London, (21 March 2010).

[398] Marjorie R. Freedman, Janet King, and Eileen Kennedy, "Popular Diets: A Scientific Review", *Obesity Research*, (March 2001).

[399] http://www.cdrnet.org/certifications/licensure/index.htm and http://www.anh-usa.org/playing-monopoly-with-our-health/

Printed in Great Britain
by Amazon

40412857R00185